Chinese Medicine Essential Oils

A MATERIA MEDICA
and Practical Guide to Their Use

INCORPORATING AROMATHERAPY INTO THE PRACTICE OF ACUPUNCTURE, CHINESE HERBAL MEDICINE, AND PERSONAL HEALTHCARE WITH ESSENTIAL OILS MADE FROM TRADITIONAL CHINESE MEDICINAL HERBS

EVELYN ROBERT, L.AC.

FOREWORD BY JEFFREY YUEN

It is not the intention of the author or this book to provide specific information on disease processes or the healing of any disease or symptom. The information and statements regarding efficacy of essential oils, blends, products, or treatment strategies mentioned within this book are for informational and educational purposes only and have not been evaluated by the Food and Drug Administration. They are not to be used as a substitute for consulting a licensed medical practitioner regarding any medical advice or treatment.

Information given on the use of acupuncture or Chinese herbal medicine is based on traditional, classical Chinese medicine from historical, public and non-proprietary sources. The acupuncture and herbal strategies presented are intended solely for use by licensed acupuncturists and students under supervision of an accredited educational institution. The author and publisher do not advocate or endorse self-diagnosis, self-medication or treatment by unlicensed individuals under any circumstances. Individuals are strongly encouraged to perform their own due diligence and seek guidance from licensed professionals.

Chinese Medicine Essential Oils
A Materia Medica and Practical Guide to Their Use

by Evelyn Robert, L.Ac.

Published by Inner Palace Press
InnerPalacePress@gmail.com

Calligraphy by Jeffrey Yuen
Illustrations by Emily Lounsbury
Editor: Cathy Borders
Proofreading: Dorian Hastings
Book design: Chris Molé, booksavvystudio.com

Library of Congress Control Number: 2022900867
Softcover ISBN: 978-0-578-35065-3
Hardcover ISBN: 978-0-578-36406-3

Printed in the United States
10 9 8 7 6 5 4 3 2 1

Translation of calligraphy by Jeffrey Yuen on page x

精 Jing - Essence
動 Dong - to move, stir
係 Xin - Heart Mind
香 Xiang - to be fragrant, aromatic

DEDICATION

THIS BOOK IS DEDICATED TO MASTER, DOCTOR, JEFFREY C. YUEN, my beloved teacher, priest, shifu, and friend. The idea of making the essential oils of Chinese medicine herbs available to practitioners, and the consequent formation of Alchemica Botanica TCM essential oils as a vehicle to do so, are his brainchild. Even the name, Alchemica Botanica, and the concept for the logo—a dragon rising from an alchemical cauldron—came from his imagination. He planted the seed and I birthed the baby. All throughout the process of bringing it to fruition and beyond he has nurtured, guided, encouraged, and promoted, asking nothing in return. The book has naturally grown out of a wish to share his teachings.

I began this project as service to Jeffrey Yuen. Not because he asked for it. I am trying to think of an instance when he actually asked for anything. I can't. He gives, that is what he does. His presence in my life is a precious gift on so many levels. This book is intended as a way to give back.

Special Thanks

To fellow students of Jeffrey Yuen and others who generously spent time donating their expertise:

To Lily Robert-Foley, Ph.D. proofreader and cheerleader extraordinaire. My brilliant, beautiful daughter who took on the task of checking the text in minute, grammatically correct detail.

To Mona Dinari, L.Ac., Dipl. OM., my precious sister, who constantly encouraged me to keep going and who tirelessly scoured her many years worth of computerized notes of Jeffrey Yuen's lectures in order to add and correct what I had missed.

To Donna Keefe, L.Ac., my dear friend and advisor, whose exceptional organizational skills and good sense enormously helped to make the book more readable, understandable, and accurate. Also, for her input as a gynecology specialist.

To Cissy Majebe, OMD, founder and president of Daoist Traditions College of Chinese Medical Arts, for her insightful suggestions, drawn from many years as an educator, regarding how to make the book reader-friendly for the layperson as well as the medical professional.

To Emmylou "Junie" Norfleet, L.Ac., president of the North Carolina Acupuncture Licensing Board and founding board member of Daoist Traditions College of Chinese Medical Arts, for her friendship, encouragement, and recommendations.

To Evelyn Wu 吴姗姗, **L.Ac.**, my brilliant assistant, for her diligence and patience with the most boring, mind-numbing, but necessary tasks like creating charts and helping to build a useable general index for this book, as well as for her perceptive input from the point of view of a senior acupuncture student.

To Amy Marie Hess 劳家碧, **L.Ac.**, for their invaluable role as content editor, applying their knowledge as a practitioner of acupuncture, Chinese and Western herbalism. Their astute consideration of the point of view of both lay and practitioner readers as well as the creation of indices went a long way to make the book user-friendly.

To Alice, Wei Fang Xiang韦芳香, my precious China assistant and guide who researches and contacts essential oil factories all over China, and organizes our travel and factory visits. She does it all with grace, warmth, and perfect English.

To Christopher Dye, MS, L.Ac., my fellow essential oil enthusiast and very long-time student of Jeffrey Yuen, for checking the Materia Medica with his many years of aromatherapy, acupuncture, and Chinese medicine experience.

To Kurt Schnaubelt, Ph.D. in chemistry, founder and scientific director of the Pacific Institute of Aromatherapy, for his mentorship and guidance into the field of aromatherapy and for his kind, constructive criticism during the writing of this book.

To Will Morris, Ph.D., DAOM, MSEd, L.Ac., author and former president of AOMA for his generous time and kind advice on writing, resourcing, and self-publishing.

To Anne Cecil Sterman, MS, L.Ac. and Andrew Sterman, for giving me their encouragement, ideas, and contacts on how to self-publish based on their personal experience as authors and publishers.

To Cathy Borders, the book's midwife. My editor who skillfully and patiently birthed this book while managing to maintain my voice and point of view despite having no previous background in Chinese medicine, aromatherapy, or Daoist philosophy.

Contents

CHARTS and LISTS

ILLUSTRATIONS:

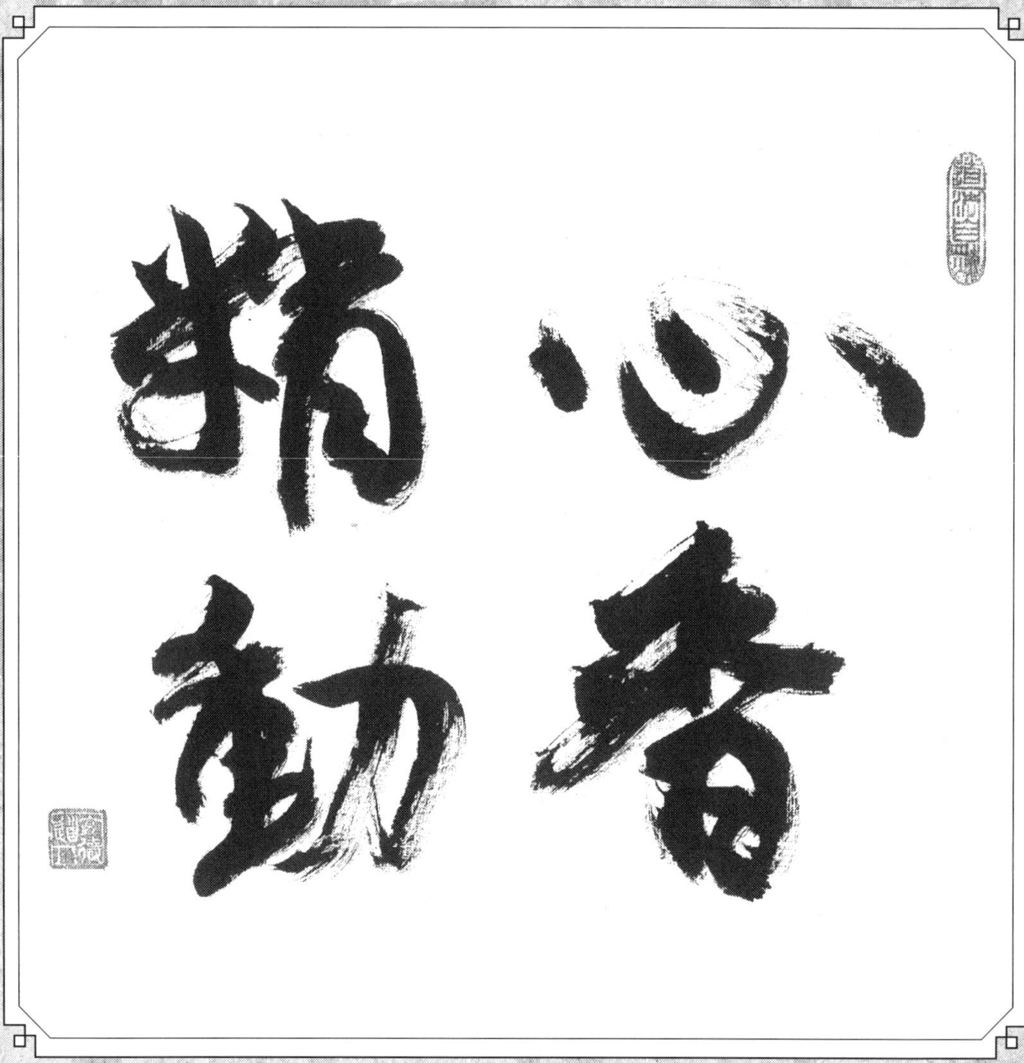

Calligraphy by Jeffrey Yuen
When the essence moves, the heart is fragrant
When the heart is fragrant, the essence moves

Foreword

Over the years, I have been fortunate to be surrounded by a circle of beloved students, friends, colleagues, and teachers—all reminding me of our interconnectedness—as we share experiences that have brought humor, wholeness, insights, and relative meanings to our lives. My gratitude to them continues to be etched upon my heart as I marvel at their efforts to broaden the scope and engage others into the richness inherent within Chinese medicine. More importantly, their endeavors are motivated by love—of their profession, patients, and humanity!

Among these individuals is Evelyn Robert, who has taken on the arduous task of sourcing, testing, and supplying high-quality essential oils of botanicals commonly used in Chinese herbal medicine. As a devout practitioner, Evelyn has meticulously introduced the merits for each of the fragrant allies discussed in this text, categorizing their attributes within the format of a Chinese materia medica (ben cao) and highlighting their potential therapeutic applications. While an enormous amount of information is presented—a reflection of decades of clinical experience and her tenacity to be comprehensive—readers should not rush to grasp the material completely. Similar to the complexity found in essential oils, the very obscurity of each botanical is its meaning, i.e., intended as an invitation for the reader to further explore, unravel, and even refine for him or herself a personalized connection to the plant. In doing so, the reader would stretch the horizons toward further understanding these essential oils and become immersed with the interdependency that lies between humanity and nature. Just as the author has nurtured an intimate bond with these oils, the reader can utilize the book as a template for his/her own cultivation.

The text serves as an important contribution to those searching for viable options in their compassionate service to healing themselves and others. Given their ready availability, essential oils offer us a reliable opportunity to take charge of our lives and witness transformations to our health. In addition, clinical discipline is provoked within the practice of Chinese medicine that often challenges reductionist and fragmented methodologies since the reader is encouraged to create a tailored blend that articulates the essence of the individual and his/her story narrated through health and medical concerns. With that in mind, may the narratives also offered by each of the essences of these botanicals serve as a salve for our pain and suffering, as their scents liberate the obstacles and torments aching within our hearts.

—Jeffrey Yuen

Preface

THE DEEP GRATITUDE AND REVERENCE THAT I FEEL toward my teachers, who generously guided and inspired me along this journey as a practitioner of Chinese medicine, is beyond words to fully express. I'll just say that I am sure it was destiny which led me to each of them and without them there is no way to explain how I got where I am today.

My very first introduction to the acupuncture meridian system came in the early 1970s by way of an encounter with a woman who was a chain-smoking Japanese macrobiotic Shiatsu practitioner ("I am Macrobiotic but not too Macrobiotic"). She gave me a Shiatsu treatment. I was fascinated and went searching for a teacher. My search led me to Ryuho Yamada, a visiting Japanese Zen priest and Shiatsu master at the San Francisco Zen Center's Tassajara retreat. Still in hippie mode, I hitchhiked from San Francisco to the beginning of the long dirt road to Tassajara, near Carmel and walked the rest of the way. Yamada Sensei agreed to teach me on the condition that I stay at the retreat and practice Zen Meditation, which I happily did. I then continued my training with Yamada Sensei after he moved to the San Francisco Zen Center. Along with Shiatsu and Zen Buddhism, he introduced me to acupuncture. I was hooked and, again, began searching for a teacher.

I began my study of acupuncture and Chinese medicine in 1982 at a California Acupuncture Board approved private tutorial program with Dr. Argon Li, an MD neurologist and traditional Chinese medicine doctor from Beijing. Dr. Li took me under his wing like a kindly father. I studied with him for two years until the third trimester of pregnancy with my second child. After my daughter was born, I continued my studies at the San Francisco College of Acupuncture and Oriental Medicine in San Francisco, where I was required to start over from the beginning of the program, graduated in 1987, received my license and began practicing out of the downstairs of my home in the Sunset District of San Francisco.

After graduation I followed Dr. Andrew Tseng, who had taught classical needling techniques and clinic at the college, to his private practice where I studied under his direct tutelage and assisted him for several years. I set up an herb pharmacy in the garage of my home in order to fill prescriptions for Dr. Tseng's patients. During this time, Dr. Tseng's weekend courses of direct translations from the classics were a treasure. Dr. Tseng's magic hands at work, alongside his Christian piety and heartfelt compassion for his patients, have had a lasting influence on me.

Specifically, in the field of herbal medicine, I was fortunate to study with Dr. Jiang Jian Fu, an oncologist and surgeon from Shanghai who had fallen in love with traditional Chinese medicine and was treating her cancer patients with herbs in the hospital. At the time of her arrival into the U.S., she had been invited here to teach, and I was lucky enough to be able to host her at my home. Her courses, drawing from herbal traditions of different periods of Chinese history were a treasure of information that went way beyond what I had been given in acupuncture school. She freely shared the treasures of her knowledge and experience in an organized, scientific way that gave clarity to creating customized formulas.

I met sinologist and scholar of Chinese philosophy Elisabeth Rochat de la Vallée in Paris in 2003. At that time, she was in need of someone to organize her classes in San Francisco. I took it on. Elisabeth's love of Daoist philosophy and her devotion to the study and translation of the classics of Chinese medicine and Daoist writings drew me into the endless wonders of these texts through exploration of the deeper meanings within the pictography of Chinese characters. As a happy result of the time we spent together, she has become a dear, treasured friend.

I first saw Daoist priest and doctor of Chinese medicine Jeffrey Yuen in 1993 just after my mom passed from colon cancer. I had gone back to Long Island, N.Y., to be with her during hospice care at her home. A friend had recommended an acupuncturist there to help. This acupuncturist happened to be a student of Jeffrey Yuen's, with whom he was consulting on behalf of my mom. This was the first time I experienced essential oils and that is how Jeffrey Yuen began teaching me before I had even met him.

After I returned to San Francisco, I received notice of a class on the treatment of cancer taught by Jeffrey Yuen. I figured I was meant to go. That was the beginning of following Jeffrey Yuen on a journey of discovery, not only of classical Chinese medicine from its Daoist roots, but of myself, of nature and human nature, of our place between Heaven and Earth, of what it means to be a healer and so much more. I hope that some of what he has imparted to me will come through in this book, with essential oils being a vehicle of discovery for the reader.

Everything I know about essential oils I learned from Jeffrey Yuen. In fact, the whole idea of Chinese medicine essential oils, their use in the context of Chinese medicine practice, and the search for them was originated, inspired, and encouraged by him. The information that I will be sharing with you is derived from his lectures, along with my clinical experience which was fundamentally informed from the time that I have spent following his teachings. Bear in mind, however, that my writing is based on my understanding of those teachings at this time. So, if you learn something from this material that you find useful, thank Jeffrey Yuen, but if you feel I have made mistakes, don't blame him.

The Quest for Chinese Medicine Essential Oils and the Founding of Alchemica Botanica TCM Essential Oils

Originally, it was Jeffrey Yuen's deep and innovative teachings on the use of essential oils as a new modality in the context of the practice of acupuncture and Chinese medicine that piqued my interest. His inspiration, together with my reverence for Chinese medicinal herbs, motivated my search for these unique essential oils and consequently, the formation of my essential oil company, Alchemica Botanica.

Jeffrey Yuen had been having great success adapting the available, standard Western essential oils into the clinical practice of Acupuncture and Chinese Medicine. He began by using essential oils as a modality to help children with congenital genetic disorders such as Down's syndrome, spina bifida, and mental retardation. Realizing essential oils' unique potential, in the mid-1990s he began teaching practitioners how to apply essential oils in their practices. At the same time, he wondered if it might be possible to access the essential oils of our own traditional Chinese medicinal herbs.

He first brought up the idea at a dinner we shared with Andy Ellis of Spring Wind Herbs; thinking that, because of Andy's involvement in supplying quality herbs to U.S. practitioners, he would be likely to have ideas about ways to produce essential oils of Chinese herbs. At that time, I owned Spring Wind Dispensary, the prescription pharmacy service offshoot of Andy's larger Chinese herb import company. Andy talked about how the oils could be produced and offered his help and contacts. As practitioners ourselves, Andy and I were excited by the idea of adding this new modality. Indeed, over the years these oils have benefited my patients enormously and getting to know these essences has been pure joy.

I began the search in 2012 by reaching out to growers of Chinese medicinal plants here in the U.S. with the idea. The problem is that roughly one hundred pounds or more of raw herb material is required to produce one kilo (about a quart) of an essential oil. Perhaps in the future we will be able to produce some "limited edition" domestic oils, but alas, at the moment, there is not enough of a consistent supply of raw material to make this work as a domestic product.

Another of Andy's suggestions was to contact some of the companies that make concentrated granules because the essential oils of the herbs are often extracted in the production process. Unfortunately, I found that supplies would likely be limited and inconsistent depending on the manufacturing needs of these companies.

That left me with the prospect of searching for ready-made essential oils directly from the source, where most of the herbs grow: China. Before I went overseas, people were constantly warning me about the pitfalls of doing businesses in China. However, diving in with an open mind, a positive attitude, and a basic trust in human nature, through trial and error, I have learned how to "weed" out the bad actors and to "sniff" out the good. I began visiting large and small extractors, distillers, and perfumers in China who are enthusiastic and dedicated to producing high-quality essential oils from authentic, medicinal herbs. I feel lucky to have been able to establish trusting business relationships and to build lasting friendships with these wonderful people.

My first successful contact and subsequent visit with such a supplier was a factory and plantation in Guangdong Province where I found several great Traditional Chinese Medicine essential oils, but also an organic Ganoderma Mushroom Ling Zhi spore oil that is extracted by Super Critical Fluid Extraction "CO2" using hi-tech equipment by a process which the company had developed themselves. This method produces essential oils with aromas that are true to the raw herbs while maintaining their water metabolites, which keeps the medicinal properties of the oils similar to traditional water decoctions of the herbs. The Ling Zhi is grown indoors using a proprietary organic food source. This is a beautiful, very impressive facility whose mission is about contributing to the health of the people and the planet.

The next good contact I made was equally impressive, although very different. This company is a small, family-run steam distillery in Jiangxi Province. Here I found two beautiful oils: Jing Jie (*Schizonepeta)* and Long Nao (natural *Borneolum*). Both of these oils are distilled from plants growing wild in the local area, giving them their especially bright, fresh aroma. In fact, the owner enthusiastically showed me the *Dryobalanops aromatica* trees growing on his property from whose sap natural borneol is distilled to produce the Long Nao oil.

Shortly after deciding to work with them, I visited a larger modern distillery in southern China whose owner proudly boasts the title of Perfumer. She specializes in floral essences and is very passionate and serious about natural, pure, and authentic aromatic essential oils. Jasmine and Chrysanthemum are two of the signature scents of this distillery and indeed, the Bai Ju Hua (White Chrysanthemum) and Ye Ju Hua (Wild Chrysanthemum) absolutes that I found there, as well as their 100% steam-distilled Damascus Rose and CO2-extracted Jasmine Sambac essential oils, are absolutely heavenly. A number of powerful Chinese medicine herb essential oils such as Qing Hao (*Artemisia annua*), Ai Ye (*Artemisia argyi*), Huang Qi (*Astragalus*) and Ren Shen (Ginseng) and others are also produced at this factory.

Since that time, I have been pleased to discover many excellent distillers and extractors who are dedicated to providing fine-quality, authentic essential oils made from Chinese medicinal herbs.

My search for earnest suppliers is ongoing. Since 2013 I have visited China twice a year in order to personally verify the authenticity of every factory and each essential oil. I am always gratified and encouraged by the enthusiastic feedback that I have gotten from healthcare practitioners and laypeople alike who are using the oils. My commitment is that I will continue to uphold the highest possible standards and do my utmost to provide safe and effective tools to augment the practice of Chinese medicine, expand the scope of aromatherapy, and to inspire people to discover the wonders of Chinese herbs and the magic of their essential oils.

—Evelyn Robert, L.Ac.

Introduction

My goal for this book is to share with you my enthusiasm for essential oils, especially those unique oils made from medicinal herbs used in Chinese medicine, and to give you a basic understanding of how to use them for personal health and wellness as well as how to apply them clinically in the context of Chinese medicine.

I am committed to the idea of making this information understandable and useful to non-practitioners and practitioners alike. In an attempt to accomplish this, for each essential oil in Part Two: the Materia Medica there is a framed section which gives an overview of the attributes and uses of that oil in layman's language flavored with Chinese medicine philosophy. This section, along with the suggested applications and blends, are intended to be an introductory guide for personal use of the oils. Practitioners will find Chinese medical language and applications bridging essential oils to acupuncture and herbs from a clinical perspective. The oils are arranged in alphabetical order by their Chinese pinyin names. At the back of the book there are pinyin/botanical/common English alternate name indexes. For those non-practitioners who wish to explore the oils in the context of Chinese medicine, I have included a chapter to explain some of the basic Chinese medicine concepts which they will encounter on the Materia Medica pages. Throughout the book, certain terms, when they are being used in their Chinese medicine context, are capitalized in order to distinguish them from strictly anatomical or common use of the words.

In my role as an acupuncture and Chinese medicine practitioner I have found that patients enjoy working with essential oils. They feel empowered by actively involving them in their healing process and encouraged by the immediately perceptible effect of aroma. Creating an essential oil blend for a particular patient is an interactive process, something we share together. It opens the door to a magical resonance that happens between the patient, the essential oil, and me.

Part One

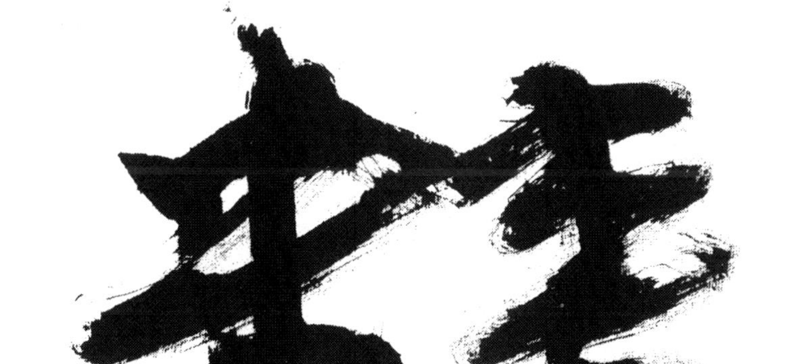

Calligraphy by Jeffrey Yuen
Jing - Essence

Magic

Essential oils and their effect on our different levels of existence, of consciousness, and of Qi are a kind of perfect blend of magic and science.

For me, there is a fuzzy line between magic and science. The myriad phenomena of the natural world look and feel like magic to me. Are the physiological and psycho-physiological workings of the human body and mind not miraculous? Are magic and miracle then not an inherent constant in everyday life?

Think about aroma. What happens when we unexpectedly encounter an aroma, or when we "stop to smell the roses"? Isn't there a shift in our mood, in our consciousness, and consequently, a change in our body chemistry, our brain's neurotransmitters? Perhaps memories are conjured up which transport us in time and space giving us an opening to relive an old experience from a new perspective. This is aromatherapy.

Sure, aromas can be broken down into their chemical components and can even be fabricated in a lab. Fragrance is a huge industry. But then again, isn't chemistry magic? Look at the structure of an atom and how it reflects the solar system, and how the nature of its parts and their interaction, their Qi, bonding with other atoms gives life and creates new molecules, each with their own distinctive character, just as our bonding with the unique molecules of a particular essential oil creates the possibility of something new in us.

When we fully experience an aroma, it changes our perception of reality, and as my teacher, Jeffrey Yuen says, "The level of consciousness that brings on disease is not the same level that can bring about healing."

If we change our consciousness, we change the course of our "dis-ease."

Essential oils, Jing You 精油, are the concentrated essence of plants.

The essence of a plant, along with the aroma that it exudes, is an expression of that plant's complete nature and innate intelligence, including its medicinal properties. In Chinese, this essence is called Jing 精. Jing Essence is the substance that contains the building blocks of life and establishes the unique blueprints of all living things. It is the genetic program that accounts for each individual's innate structure, appearance and temperament, and sets the natural patterns of growth, development, maintenance, and decline. It is the foundation of what is called the constitution in a human being, and in Chinese medicine it circulates throughout the body as what is referred to as Yuan Source Qi.

Essence resonates with essence. This means that the substance of the medicinal essential oil from a plant is able to reach and affect the constitutional, Yuan Source Qi level in a person. In other words, the essence of plants has the potential to resonate with the very essence of a person's being, helping one to be in touch with one's intrinsic nature, including one's innate ability to heal oneself.

Another medicinal aspect of Jing You includes the chlorophyll that circulates through the plant, providing nutritive substance similar to the function of blood and fluids in the human body. This means that essential oils also have the potential to reach and affect the level referred to in Chinese medicine as Ying or Nutritive Qi, the embodiment and circulation of the blood and fluids. The body fluids are called Jin Ye, which include hormonal secretions, enzymes, and the moisture that maintains the health of sensory and other organs.

AROMA IS THE EXPRESSION OF THE SPIRIT OF A PLANT.

Aroma resonates with and affects the spirit of a person. In terms of classical Chinese medicine, spirit is referred to as Shen and is embodied by the Heart Mind. Heart, mind, emotions, and spirit are inextricably linked. As the classical Chinese medicine text *Ling Shu* or *The Spiritual Pivot* (the Canon of Acupuncture, second part of *Huang Di Nei Jing* – fifth century BCE) tells us, "All diseases are rooted in the Spirit."

Disease is an opportunity to expand our awareness of our destiny and the choices that we make in life. Essential oil aromas can be an ally in the process of self-empowerment for change in our lives and ways of thinking by opening a door to the spirit and expanding consciousness. When we experience an aroma, the moment it enters the nose, the olfactory nerves transmit its spirit, affecting various functional areas of the brain, while simultaneously influencing our consciousness, changing our mood, and opening pathways to new ways of perceiving, thinking, feeling, and healing.

Aroma is also exuded by a plant to attract bees for pollination and to protect it against pests and harmful microbes. The attraction aspect is equivalent to hormonal activity triggered by aromas, such as our pheromones which stimulate sexual attraction or oxytocin which elicits feelings of love and connection. The protection aspect is acting as what is called the Wei Protective Qi in Chinese medicine. Wei Qi circulates throughout the more exterior parts of the body and is related to the Lungs. Upon inhalation, an essential oil's aromatic energy circulates to the level of the Wei Qi via breath entering the lungs, influencing all aspects of the work of Wei Qi in the body that includes autonomic and unconscious functions such as: circadian rhythm, resistance to external pathogenic factors, opening and closing of the pores, peristalsis, as well as the workings of the sinews and nerves.

With the use of essential oils in the context of Chinese medicine, there is resonance with and potential to influence all three levels of Qi: Wei Protective Qi, Ying Nutritive Qi, and Yuan Source Qi, along with the simultaneous, profound effect of aroma on the mind, emotions, and spirit. This is what makes the clinical use of essential oils aromatherapy so powerful.

Clinical Use of Chinese Medicine Essential Oils

In China, the importance of aromatic herbs as medicine has been recognized since the time of Shen Nong, the "Divine Farmer," one of the legendary gods of Chinese medicine who lived nearly five thousand years ago. Recent evidence suggests that the Chinese created distillation devices long before the Persian doctor Avicenna (980-1037 CE), previously considered the first to do so. Reference to the essential oils of Chinese medicinal plants has a long history. Most notably is Li Shi-Zhen's *Ben Cao Gang Mu* (*Compendium of Materia Medica*), first published in 1593 during the Ming Dynasty, in which twenty different essential oils and methods of extracting them are discussed. Use of the oils themselves, relative to decoctions or extracts of herbs, was limited. However, the energetic value of the aroma of plants and the aroma of the herbs while decocting—often referred to as the Qi of the herbs—as an important aspect of their medicinal properties is inherent in Chinese herbal medicine.

As a practitioner of traditional Chinese medicine today, using essential oils clinically, especially those oils produced from herbs found in the myriad Chinese herb materia medica, one can apply what is already known about the herbs to their respective essential oils by referring to their CM categories: nature, taste, and channel affinities, along with their traditional actions and indications.

As an acupuncturist, one can use essential oils on acupuncture points and channels by applying what is already known about acupuncture. Normally, these two modalities (herbs and acupuncture) are used separately. When an essential oil is placed on an acupuncture point, the two are combined simultaneously. Plus, considering the added value of essential oils' profound and rapid effect on the three levels of Qi: Wei Qi, Ying Qi, Yuan Qi, as well as on the mind, emotions, and spirit by way of their aroma and substance, there are added dimensions, providing an instant synergy beyond what acupuncture and herbal medicine can provide as separate modalities.

Another aspect to note is that essential oils work quickly. From a modern science point of view, molecules of essential oils are extremely minute and can penetrate the skin via hair follicles and sweat glands. Tests have found evidence of essential oils in the urine only one hour after application on the occipital region. The oily substance of essential oils is lipophilic, meaning fat-loving. They are attracted to fatty acids in our bodies and brain, as the substance of the brain is a fat which is called Marrow in Chinese medicine.

CO_2 Extraction and Steam Distillation

Applying one's knowledge of Chinese medicinal herbs to their use as essential oils is especially relevant when they are produced by a more modern method called Super Critical Carbon Dioxide extraction, or simply CO_2.

CO_2 is a method of extracting the essential oils of plants which retains the hydrophilic water metabolites naturally contained in medicinal herbs together with their oily lipophilic compounds, concentrated essence and aroma. This process yields a product that is closer in nature to the herbs traditionally cooked in water as a decoction than oils produced by the more traditional steam distillation where the hydrophilic compounds are separated from the oil. The relatively low temperature and stability of the CO_2 process allows compounds to be extracted by pressure rather than heat, with little denaturing or damage. Operating at a lower temperature also means that the plant waxes can be separated from the oils, yielding pure essential oil. In addition, the solubility of many extracted compounds in CO_2 varies with pressure, permitting selective extractions which eliminate the transfer of heavy metals, pesticides, and other possible contaminants into the finished product.

In other words, the CO_2 method does not use heat and steam which transform the whole essence of the plants from one state to another before yielding their essential oils, as is the case in the process of steam distillation. Whereas this transformative process of distillation may be seen as part of the magic of essential oils, my own belief is that the magic is inherent in the essence of plants either way.

APPLICATIONS OF AROMATHERAPY

There are three basic types of aromatherapy applications:

1. Aesthetic, which is focused on aroma, **inhalation**, perfumery, and personal care.
2. Holistic, which involves **topical application** and massage.
3. Medical, which involves taking essential oils by **internal ingestion.**

While essential oils may be applied topically or internally ingested, it is important to keep in mind that, at its core, the use of essential oils is about aromatherapy and the profound effect of aroma on the mind and consciousness.

INHALATION

The Physiology of the Sense of Smell

Anatomically, the sense of smell has immediate access to the cerebral cortex. The nose is like an antenna, picking up information from the outside world. Nerve endings in the nose are in direct contact with the outside, while inside of our bodies, the sense of smell has a direct connection to and immediate effect on the brain.

Receptor cells in the nose pick up messages and send them along sensory neurons, passing through a very thin, porous bone to enter the olfactory bulb, which sits just under the frontal lobe of the cerebral cortex behind the eyes. This pathway requires only two synapses to get to this specialized area of the brain which integrates and interprets information from scents, quickly influencing areas of the brain that deal with memory, emotion, metabolism, glandular stimulation, sexuality, and more. And substances influencing the nervous system can go directly from the nose to the brain, bypassing the blood.

Plus, there is a close connection between the olfactory bulb and the cerebral spinal fluid, which means a direct influence on the spine and the nervous system as well.

Inhalation is the most effective method to affect brain and nervous disorders such as Alzheimer's, Parkinson's, ADD, and mental illness.

From the Perspective of Chinese Medicine

In the brain is the union of Fire and Water. Fire represents the Heart which embodies the Shen Spirit. Water represents the Kidneys which contain Jing Essence. These opposite Yang and Yin elements of Fire and Water are harmonized and brought up to the brain by the Qi of Wood. At conception, Jing (the material Essence from the combined Yin and Yang of parents) plus Shen (the immaterial Spirit from Heaven) join together to create a complete, unique child.

Jing, Qi, and Shen are the ingredients for the Daoist cultivation practices of internal alchemy, the transformation and transmutation of one substance or one state into another, including states of physiology and states of consciousness. The Jing and Shen of essential oils, embodied in their oily substance and expressed through the Qi of their aroma, directly affect the brain and the constitution providing the potential for change on a deep level, even the possibility to influence the genetic blueprint.

Modern science has shown that experience literally changes the shape of the brain. A traumatic experience, for example, can be so profound as to influence DNA, shake one to the core, and rattle the foundation like a mental earthquake causing alteration of one's intrinsic personality. If negative experience can damage one, then positive experience can certainly reverse the damage and create new integrative neuropathways. The effect of essential oil aromas on the brain can be a powerful ally to promote the healing changes we want in our lives.

Simple, direct inhalation of an undiluted essential oil can be quite powerful. Alternatively, a few drops can be added to a steaming cup of hot water and inhaled. Using a diffuser will more widely affect the Qi of the environment and sustain the effect over a longer period of time. Adding essential oils to a bath is another way to get the benefits of inhalation. The inhalation method is useful for directly affecting the Wei Protective Qi and the respiratory system via breath entering the lungs and nasal passages. Many essential oils are strongly antibacterial, antiviral, and/or antifungal. Diffusing oils can help to clear and detoxify the air or may be used as a preventative. Diffusion may be used like incense to assist spiritual practices, and is also helpful when addressing mental emotional, and mood states such as anxiety, insomnia, or depression.

For example:

- Zi Su Ye (Perilla Leaf) diffused is effective both as a preventative during cold, flu, and allergy season, and as a decongestant for coughs and respiratory infections.
- Bai Yu Lan Ye (Magnolia Leaf) opens the nasal passages as a steam inhalation.
- Ce Bai Ye (Biota Leaf) and Bo He (Peppermint) can be diffused to clear a sick room of bacteria, such as in the case of recovery from severe burns.
- Bai Zi Ren (Biota Seed) for insomnia may be diffused in the bedroom at night.
- Jiang Xiang (*Dalbergia*) can be diffused to calm and descend the Qi and Yang as aromatherapy for hypertension and agitation.

- Mo Li Hua (Jasmine), Mei Gui Hua (Rose), or Qi Li Xiang (Orange Jessamine) are inhaled and worn as a perfume or added to the bath for recovery from a traumatic event and to lift the spirit.
- Ru Xiang (Frankincense) has been used in religious ceremonies for millennia as an incense or anointment for cleansing the body and soul, and to facilitate a connection to the divine.

Topical Application

Essential oils are highly concentrated and therefore have the potential to irritate the skin unless diluted in one of the many gentle vegetable oils which can be used as a carrier. Appropriately diluted, essential oils may be applied directly to the skin using a glass, stone, porcelain, or wooden tool. A little goes a long way in terms of effect.

Diluted single essential oils or blends of oils are helpful both therapeutically and for maintenance of health and wellness. The possibilities are endless. For example, they can be applied as massage oils or alcohol-based liniments for pain and injuries, formulated into creams or lotions for skin care, as ointments or plasters for skin conditions, rubbed over the chest or abdomen for respiratory or digestive problems, and compressed with heat for menstrual cramps.

Essential oils may be mixed with salt and added to a bath to create a therapeutic bath salt for relaxation, pain, or detoxification. A drop or two diluted into a light saline solution makes an excellent nasal wash.

Essential oils that benefit the immune system have been found to work best when topically massaged into areas of the body where the most active sweat glands are located, like the bottom of the feet or the center of the chest.

Neat Means Undiluted

Some essential oils can, cautiously, be used neat under certain circumstances. For example, a tiny drop placed directly on acupuncture points or other areas with a stone, glass, or wooden wand for medicinal use, as a perfume or anointment is safe and effective with many oils for short-term use. Therapeutically, appropriate oils may be applied neat to address an acute situation.

Spice oils such as Rou Gui (Cinnamon Bark), Gui Zhi/Gui Ye (Cinnamon Twig and Leaf), Gan Jiang (Dry Ginger), Ding Xiang (Clove), or Qing Hua Jiao (Green Sichuan Pepper) should be avoided as these can burn the skin. Allergic reactions can also happen depending on an individual's sensitivities. In case of allergic reaction, untoasted sesame oil may be applied to chelate or draw out the irritating oil.

✔ ***Information on how to dilute essential oils will be found later in the book and more application ideas are found in the Materia Medica sections on "Dosage Guidelines for Homemade Applications and Carrier Oils and Emulsifiers."***

A few examples of essential oils found to be gentle enough and helpful when applied neat are:

- Floral oils such as Mei Gui (Rose), Mo Li Hua (Jasmine), Qi Li Xiang (Orange Jessamine), or Xun Yi Cao (Lavender) can be worn as a perfume to lift the spirit or calm the mind.
- Chuan Xiong (*Ligusticum wallichii*) applied neat and even massaged directly over an area for pain has been found to be safe and effective for one-time use or according to the sensitivity of the user or the practitioner's discretion.
- Ru Xiang (Frankincense) for short-term use may be applied neat over an area for acute injuries, bruising, swelling, or burns. Apply over intact skin, not on open sores.

Topical application of essential oils, even when diluted, should always be tested first on a very small area for sensitivity. If any irritation arises, discontinue use or change the dilution percentage and test again. In the event of a skin sensitivity or allergic reaction, applying plain, untoasted sesame oil may help to chelate the irritating oil.

Applying Essential Oils with Acupuncture Theory

Essential oils may be applied topically to potentiate channels and points.

In Chinese, the word for acupuncture point, Xue Wei 穴位, means "hole or cave." Applying an essential oil into the receptive empty space of an acupuncture point infuses the very essence of the substance, intelligence, and Qi of that medicinal plant directly into the channel systems of the patient.

Essential oils may be applied directly to acupuncture points on the skin using a glass, stone, porcelain, or wooden "needle" or wand. My personal favorite is to use a needle-shaped stone or crystal with a pointed tip. In this way, I can combine the therapeutic effect of the stones with that of the oils.

A little goes a long way. A small amount of an essential oil or blend distributed over a few acupoints or along a channel as one time use, or according to the practitioner's discretion, is sufficient to achieve the desired effect. The equivalent of just one drop may be sufficient to distribute over a three-to-five-point prescription. The oils and their energetic effect will be absorbed into the points. **Do not rub in** unless you know the oils to be gentle enough for this purpose. For repeated use, dilutions are recommended.

Application can be done during treatment along with needles on the same points before or after insertion, or by applying oils alone on additional points. It is always beneficial for the patient to be able to smell the aroma of the essential oil or oils being used during treatment.

A diluted essential oil or blend of oils may also be gently spread along a channel, over an affected area of the body, used as a massage oil, applied as a compress or as an enhancement for cupping, gua sha, or moxibustion during the treatment.

Providing patients with a diluted essential oil or blend to inhale and apply on points or channels at home will extend the effect of treatment and empower them in their healing process.

The unique attribute of essential oils to reach and affect the constitutional, Yuan Source Qi level is of great benefit and absolutely revolutionizes acupuncture therapy. Essential oils are the Jing Essence of plants, and as such, they resonate with the Jing Essence of the human body. According to the Chinese medical model, Jing is stored in the Kidneys. It is the foundation of the structural material that makes up our bodies and the seed of growth, development, maturity, reproduction, and internal cyclical processes. These transitional phases are mirrored in nature in the transitional phases of the plant life cycle as directed by the essence of that plant. It is by way of this resonance that the essential oils of plants can help us through these transitional phases.

Jing contains all of the potential that we were born with. Combining essential oils with acupuncture points allows the practitioner and patient to work with this deep, constitutional level.

When using the acupuncture meridian model, the attributes of an essential oil are best able to reach the constitutional level by applying them to the points and channels that have a relationship to the Yuan Source such as those that follow:

The Eight Extraordinary Vessels (8XV)

The Eight Extraordinary Vessels are the primary conduits of Yuan Source Qi. They are the core foundation of Yin and Yang in the body, which is responsible for the materialization of human form and the source of the expression of a person's unique morphology, temperament, and destiny. Developmentally, the 8XV are the source of all the primary channels that connect with the internal organs. These are the channels which bear the names of the organs (Liver channel, Stomach channel, etc.) and are the circulating expression of the quality of the Qi of those organs.

Applying essential oils on the opening points and along the trajectories of the 8XV is a way to treat constitutional issues such as those which are congenital or familial in origin. They also address Jing Essence issues dealing with the cycles of life, growth, aging, reproduction, sexual function, menopause, and regulation of related hormonal and biological functions. Additionally, the 8XV may be used for dealing with disruptive changes to one's fundamental personality caused by traumatic events or by parental influence, especially during early childhood. Most of the opening points of the 8XV are located at the Luo Connecting points of the primary channels.

Opening-Confluent Points of the Eight Extraordinary Vessels

Extraordinary Channel	Opening-Confluent Points
Chong Mai / Thoroughfare Vessel	SP4 / Gong Sun
Ren Mai / Conception Vessel	LU7 / Lie Que
Du Mai / Governing Vessel	SI3 / Hou Xi
Dai Mai / Belt Vessel	GB41 / Zu Lin Qi
Yin Qiao Mai / Yin Motility Vessel	KI6 / Zhao Hai
Yang Qiao Mai /Yang Motility Vessel	BL62 / Shen Mai
Yin Wei Mai / Yin Linking Vessel	PC6 / Nei Guan
Yang Wei Mai / Yang Linking Vessel	TE5/ Wai Guan

Water and Fire, Essence and Spirit

Water is the source of all life. Fire provides the animating spark. In the human body, water is equated with Jing Essence. Fire is equated with Shen Spirit. The interplay of the vital fire and water relationship is essential for the creation and maintenance of life.

Certain primary channels have a greater affinity to the source, especially those belonging to the Water element and its Fire element counterparts. These are Water's Yin Yang pair of the Kidney (KI) and Bladder (BL) channels along with Fire's pair, the San Jiao (TE) and Pericardium (PC) channels.

Kidney and Bladder

Kidney and Bladder are the embodiment of the Water element in the body. In this context, Kidney, the Yin aspect of the pair, stores Jing Essence and Yuan Source Qi. Bladder, the Yang aspect of the pair, provides the pathway through which the Jing Essence and Yuan Source Qi are distributed.

San Jiao and Pericardium

San Jiao (Triple Energizer) and Pericardium (Heart Wrap) are one expression of the workings of Fire in the body. In this pairing, San Jiao is Yang and Pericardium is Yin. In a different context, that of the five element correspondences, Fire includes the Yin Yang pair of Heart and Small Intestine.

The Pericardium is the physical heart called the Xin Bao 心包 in Chinese, which translates as the "Heart Wrap," whereas the Heart, called Xin 心, is the non-physical home of the mind and spirit within the body. The San Jiao is not an organ, but rather an energetic force, a vehicle driven by the original Ming Men Life Gate fire located between the left and right Kidneys. At birth, the San Jiao mechanism distributes each individual's unique essence along the spine to the Bladder Shu Transport points of each of the internal organs. The manner by which it is distributed accounts for an individual's temperament and physical charactristics. The San Jiao then continues to be the driver of the work of metabolism: digestion, fluid regulation, temperature control, etc. Classical Chinese physiology separates the body into three burners—upper, middle and lower—in order to distinguish the particular energetic activities of these areas. San Jiao's English name, Triple Energizer, refers to its work of energizing and coordinating throughout all three burning spaces.

Essential Oils Reach the Three Levels of Qi: Wei, Ying, and Yuan

Prenatally, as the original Yuan Source Qi of the embryo begins to evolve and differentiate into Yang and Yin, it becomes Wei Protective Qi and Ying Nutritive Qi. Postnatally, Wei Protective Qi and its relationship to the lungs plays an important role in the ability to breathe and derive vitality from the air. Wei Qi also provides for the integrity of the skin, sinews, and nerves, and is the basis of the immune system.

Ying Nutritive Qi, also called Rong Flourishing Qi, is the postnatal source of the blood and all of the fluid substances that nourish and sustain life independent of those which, in utero, were automatically absorbed by the fetus from the mother through the umbilicus.

Yuan Qi, Ying Qi, and Wei Qi circulate on the deep level, moderate level, and superficial levels of the body, respectively.

Yuan Source and Luo Connecting Points

Each acupuncture channel has a Yuan Source point where essential oils can be applied to connect to the level of the constitutional Yuan Source Qi. Essential oils reach and affect the level of the Ying Nutritive Qi by applying them on the Luo Connecting points located on each channel, thereby benefiting the blood and body fluids which include secretions like hormones, enzymes, sweat, and tears.

Luo Connecting points provide a bridge connecting deeply circulating prenatal Yuan Source Qi to postnatal Ying Nutritive Qi circulating on the moderate level. This Yuan Source/Luo Connecting relationship also connects the Zang Yin organ and the Fu Yang organ pairs and their channels. Crossing the bridge can be accomplished by what is called a Source Luo treatment, where essential oils are applied on the Luo Connecting point of one channel and on the Yuan Source point of its Yin Yang pair.

Yuan-Source & Luo-Connecting Points of the Primary Meridians

Meridian	Yuan-Source Point	Luo-Connecting Point
LUNG	LU9 Tai Yuan	LU7 Lie Que
LARGE INTESTINE	LI4 He Gu	LI6 Pian Li
STOMACH	ST42 Chong Yang	ST40 Feng Long
SPLEEN	SP3 Tai Bai	SP4 Gong Sun
HEART	HT7 Shen Men	HT5 Tong Li
SMALL INTESTINE	SI4 Wan Gu	S17 Zhi Zheng
BLADDER	BL64 Jing Gu	BL58 Fei Yang
KIDNEY	K13 Tai Xi	K14 Da Zhong
PERICARDIUM	PC7 Da Ling	PC6 Nei Guan
TRIPLE ENERGIZER	TE4 Yang Chi	TE5 Wai Guan
GALLBLADDER	GB40 Qiu Xu	GB37 Guang Ming
LIVER	LR3 Tai Chong	LR5 Li Gou

The Spirit in the Blood—The Luo Vessels

In Chinese medicine, the blood—as an extension of the Heart Mind—contains the Shen Spirit including the emotions and memories of life experiences. In this regard, essential oils can be helpful by applying them topically to disperse Luo Vessels, which appear along a channel as visible superficial blood vessels or other signs of stagnation that arise as a response to unresolved emotional issues.

Shu Transport and Mu Accumulation points of the Zang-Fu Organs

Zang-Fu Organ	Shu Point	Mu Point
LUNG	BL13 Fei Shu	LU1 Zhong Fu
LARGE INTESTINE	BL25 Da Chang Shu	ST25 Tian Shu
STOMACH	BL21 Wei Shu	CV12 Zhong Wan
SPLEEN	BL20 PI Shu	LR13 Zhang Men
HEART	BL15 Xin Shu	CV14 Ju Que
SMALL INTESTINE	BL27 Xiao Chang Shu	CV4 Guan Yuan
BLADDER	BL28 Pang Guang Shu	CV3 Zhong Ji
KIDNEY	BL23 Shen Shu	GB25 Jing Men
PERICARDIUM	BL14 Jue Yin Shu	CV17 Tan Zhong
TRIPLE ENERGIZER	BL22 San Jiao Shu	CV5 Shi Men
GALL BLADDER	BL19 Dan Shu	GB24 Ri Yue
LIVER	BL18 Gan Shu	LR14 Qi Men

Mu and Shu Points

Yuan Source Qi is distributed to the Mu Accumulation and Shu Transport points. These points provide a direct connection to the internal organs. The Mu points, mainly located on the front of the body, basically accumulate the Qi of a particular organ, whereas the Shu points, mainly located alongside the spine on the Bladder channel, transport Qi to the organ.

He Sea Points

The movement of Qi through the channels can be thought of as a current of water and the channels as waterways. Beginning at the tips of the fingers and toes, and finishing at the elbows and knees, points are named for ever-widening types of waterways: Jing Well, Ying Spring, Shu Stream, Jing River, and He Sea. This grouping of points is referred to as the Antique points and each of the five is attributed to one of the five elements. They are also representative of the journey of life from the neonatal period at the Jing Well, all the way to the union of all of life's stages at the He Sea points. Mainly located near one of the large joints (elbows and knees), the He Sea points are where the fullest expression of the quality of Qi of its associated organ gathers. From this point Qi travels along its channel directly to and from the internal organ. The He Sea points are therefore a good choice for essential oil application to directly affect the functioning of an internal organ.

He Sea Points of the Primary Meridians

Meridian	He Sea Point	Lower He Sea Point
LUNG	LU5 /Chi Ze	
LARGE INTESTINE	LI11 / Qu Chi	ST37 / Shang Ju Xu
STOMACH	ST36 / Zu San Li	
SPLEEN	SP9 / Yin Ling Quan	
HEART	HT3 / Shao Hai	
SMALL INTESTINE	SI8 / Xiao Hai	ST39 / Xia Ju Xu
BLADDER	BL40 / Wei Zhong	
KIDNEY	KI10 / Yin Gu	
PERICARDIUM	PC3 / Qu Ze	
TRIPLE ENEGIZER	TE10 / Tian Jing	BL39 / Wei Yang
GALLBLADDER	GB34 / Yang Ling Quan	
LIVER	LR8 / Qu Quan	

The Extraordinary Fu

Jing Essence is distributed to the Extraordinary Fu, also referred to as the Curious Bowels. These are: Brain/Spine, Marrow, Bone, Uterus/Genitalia, Mai/Vessels, and Gallbladder. The term Fu refers to organs and structures that are hollow like the bowels and therefore have the capacity to contain and transport. These vital Extraordinary Fu contain and transport Jing Essence. For example: the cerebral spinal fluid, the spine through which it flows and its destination, the brain (which is called the "sea of marrow"), are all conduits of Jing Essence.

The Influential Hui Gathering Points

Four of the Extraordinary Fu have an influential acupuncture point called a Hui Gathering point. There are also influential points for the Qi, the Zang solid organs, and the Fu hollow organs. Applying essential oils on these special points is a way to influence their associated structures and functions on the deepest level.

All of the Influential Hui Gathering points are also included in the types of points that resonate with essential oils, since they comprise: a Yuan Source point, a He Sea point, Mu Accumulation points, points of the Bladder channel, Gallbladder channel, and two points of the Ren Mai Conception Vessel which is one of the 8XV.

It is interesting to note that the Gallbladder in its role as an Extraordinary Fu circulates throughout the Curious Bowels serving as a bridge connecting them to each other and to the ordinary Zang Fu internal organs. The Gallbladder channel traverses the uterus and brain, plus the influential point for the marrow, GB39 (Xuan Zhong), is located on the Gallbladder channel.

THE INFLUENTIAL HUI GATHERING POINTS

	INFLUENTIAL HUI-GATHERING POINTS
ZANG	LV13 / Zhang Men
FU	CV12 / Zhong Wan
QI	CV17 / Tan Zhong
BLOOD	BL17 / Ge Shu
SINEWS	GB24 / Yang Ling Quan
VESSELS	LU9 / Tai Yuan
BONES	BL 11 / Da Zhu
MARROW	GB39 / Xuan Zhong

The Superficial Wei Qi Level

Wei Protective Qi, that which circulates on the more exterior layers of the body, is regulated by the Lungs, serves as a barrier of protection from external influences, and regulates autonomic functions. This level is effectively reached by inhalation of essential oils directly entering the lungs. Wei Qi also regulates the skin, sinews, and nerves, which are well served by topical application over an affected area when dealing with skin issues or applied with massage techniques to affect the sinews and nerves.

Abbreviations and Alternate Names for Channels and Vessels

The 12 Primary Channels/Meridians:

LU – Lung
LI – Large Intestine
ST – Stomach
SP – Spleen
HT – Heart
SI – Small Intestine
BL – Bladder
KI – Kidney
PC – Pericardium
TE – San Jiao (Triple Energizer, Triple Heater, Triple Burner)
GB – Gallbladder
LR – Liver

8XV – The Eight Extraordinary Vessels:

CV-Ren Mai / Conception Vessel
GV-Du Mai / Governing Vessel
Chong Mai / Thoroughfare or Penetrating Vessel
Dai Mai/Belt or Girding Vessel
Yang Qiao Mai / Yang Heel or Yang Motility Vessel
Yin Qiao Mai / Yin Heel or Yin Motility Vessel
Yang Wei Mai / Yang Link Vessel
Yin Wei Mai / Yin Link Vessel

Internal Ingestion

Used appropriately, essential oils or blends can have great benefit when taken internally. Many essential oils are safe for internal ingestion in very small doses, but some are not for various reasons. Quality and purity are important considerations. It is advisable to know that the oils chosen for internal consumption are not adulterated or extracted with the use of solvents. Absolutes, for example, are solvent extracted to bring out more of the plant's fragrance. Essential oils are highly concentrated substances and each one should be considered carefully and diluted properly before ingesting. Beyond that, it is important to bear in mind the power of aroma on the mind and the potent effects of essential oils applied topically. Internal ingestion is most often not necessary to achieve results.

That being said, there is a practice of medical aromatherapy where essential oils are ingested. When employing this method, the oils should be diluted in an emulsifying agent like a food-grade nutritional or vegetable oil, honey, milk or soy milk, ethyl alcohol, vinegar, etc. in order to be absorbable and safe. Average for most adults is 3% to 4% essential oil to carrier for most oils. For children two to seven years old, average dilution is 0.5% to 1%, and 1% to 2% is average for children between seven and fourteen years old.

Essential oils generally work quickly and normally do not need to be taken over an extended period of time. For acute conditions, three days is normally sufficient. For more chronic issues, when it might be desirable to ingest oils over an extended period of time, it is recommended that they be taken for three consecutive days with a break for three days then continuing with this pattern. After eighteen days the blend should be re-evaluated and adjusted or rotated with an alternate blend.

For internal ingestion the patient may place 2 to 6 drops of the diluted oil or blend onto their palm to lick off or to take on a spoon. The oil can be taken as is or with a bit of honey or yogurt to further emulsify the oil. Alternatively, it can be combined as a drink with honey mixed in warm water, milk or soy milk in a cup.

Specifically, those essential oils which according to Chinese medicine tonify the Qi and blood, and those which in modern terms are considered adaptogenic, are recommended for internal ingestion. Oils in this category tend to have quite a gentle nature and are unlikely to irritate the mucous membranes. Examples of these are Huang Qi (*Astragalus*), Ren Shen (Ginseng), Gou Qi Zi (Goji Berry), and Wu Wei Zi (*Schisandra Fruit*). Also included in this category for internal ingestion are nutritional oils such as Ling Zhi (Ganoderma Mushroom).

Certain types of essential oils, due to their nature or chemical composition, need to be approached with caution or simply avoided for internal ingestion. For example, strong spice oils like Rou Gui (Cinnamon Bark), Gui Zhi/Gui Ye (Cinnamon Twig and Leaf), or Ding Xiang (Clove) can irritate the mucus membranes and need to be diluted 1% to 2% in a gentle carrier oil or as a small percentage of a diluted blend of oils. These spicy oils contain prominent percentages of phenols which exhibit many powerful beneficial properties, including antiviral and immune boosting, but should not be consumed long term. They tonify Yang and tend to be stimulating and hot-natured.

Essential oils with high ketone chemical components are potentially neurotoxic if ingested, though are safe for inhalation or topical use short-term when diluted 1% to 2%. For example, the ketone camphor in Zhang Nao (White Camphor), considered toxic if taken internally, is safe and effective as a smelling salt for loss of consciousness or applied topically to kill parasites. Another case in point is Qing Hao (*Artemisia annua*) which also contains camphor but a lesser percentage and should be diluted appropriately and considered carefully before consuming on a short-term basis. On the other hand, Qing Hao is strongly antimicrobial, and the chemical component artemisinin in Qing Hao was discovered to be a potent antimalarial drug. It has been developed as a common treatment for that disease and the Chinese doctor who developed it won a Nobel Prize for this discovery.

Phenols, when they are the dominant component of an oil, are also not recommended for internal ingestion. They can harm the liver if taken internally over an extended period of time. For example, eugenol, the phenol in Ding Xiang (Clove), although it has many beneficial properties, should only be ingested sparingly and for a short time.

Some essential oils have a psychotropic or psychedelic effect if too much is ingested, which can mean more than a few drops as a dose. Shi Chang Pu (Acorus), Rou Dou Kou (Nutmeg), and Wu Zhu Yu (Evodia) have this action. Shi Chang Pu is an interesting case in that one of its chemical components, asarone, has been shown to improve memory and mental acuity, or to treat certain mental disorders such as anxiety and depression. However, it is controversial in that at higher doses it is psychotropic and there is some evidence that asarone is neurotoxic at high concentration. These oils have strong aromas which are quite effective when inhaled or diffused and so it should be unnecessary to take them by mouth. As a matter of fact, research has shown that for mental illness or to improve memory and mental faculties, inhalation by diffusing essential oils works best.

Overall, since the Chinese herbs from which Chinese medicine essential oils are produced are traditionally intended to be taken internally—usually boiled as a decoction—they are considered safe, edible substances. Keep in mind, however, that in their essential oil form, the extraction or distillation processes brings out a unique array of highly concentrated properties, chemical components, and aromas.

✔ ***Do not be confused.** Essential oils are not the same as decocted herbs, granulated or liquid extracts, or tinctures, and cannot be dosed the same way. If unsure, it is always best to get the advice of an experienced healthcare practitioner or aromatherapist who can prescribe what is appropriate and safe.*

Choosing an Essential Oil

The choice of an essential oil may be based upon:

1. **Aroma**
2. **Note**
3. **Parts of Plants**
4. **Chemical Composition**
5. **Chinese Medicine (CM) Category, Nature, Affinities, Actions and Indications**

1. Based on Aroma

No matter what type of issue or level of imbalance is being addressed, aroma is going to be influential on account of its immediate effect on the brain, moods, emotions, and spirit. Aroma is personal and changeable. Each person has their own unique response to any essential oil, appealing or distasteful, comforting or provoking. The same aroma on a different day may strike one very differently depending on one's state of health and consciousness at that time.

Aroma Correspondences to the Five Elements:

- **Wood**: Herbaceous, woody.
- **Fire**: Floral.
- **Earth**: Sweet, musty, fruity.
- **Metal**: Sharp, spicy, pungent.
- **Water**: Musky, camphorous, balsamic.

The Five Elements Correspondences

The five element correspondences were developed in ancient China as a way to organize observations of the cosmos and the patterns of the natural world. Wu Xing 五行, what we commonly call five elements in English, translates as five phases, movements, or changes in Chinese. It is a dynamic system with each element transforming into the next just as one season turns into another.

In the Chinese medical model, the microcosm of the human body is a reflection of the macrocosm of nature and so these observations, incorporated into the basic idea of Yin and Yang, came to be integrated into the practice of Chinese medicine beginning around the time of the Warring States (475-221 BCE).

The correspondences help to identify patterns of imbalance according to the relationships among the elements and their associated internal organs in terms of how they interact with each other, and consequently affect our health, physically and emotionally. They also tell us how to live in harmony with nature, the seasons of the year, and the environmental forces at work during those times.

The qualities of the elements provide a portrait of an individual's temperament.

Whether we are living in harmony or in opposition to the temperament that we were born with, or adopted by choice, is a very important question. Has our temperament been altered against our will by social pressures or life events? The answer impacts our health, happiness, and spiritual development.

Wood

Yin Organ: Liver.

Yang Organ: Gallbladder.

Aroma: Woody, herbaceous.

Color: Blue green.

Season: Spring.

Direction: East.

Emotions: Liver: Anger, resentment, frustration;
Gallbladder: Timidity, fear of failure.

Attributes: Liver: Extroverted, directed, growth, flexibility, stability;
Gallbladder: Courage, decision making.

Sensory Portal: Eyes, vision.

Tissue: Sinews (muscles, tendons, ligaments).

Taste: Sour.

Force of Nature: Wind.

Wood is the expression of birth, growth, and new beginnings represented by springtime and reaching upward like a tree. It is responsible for the smooth flowing of the Qi and blood. When the flow is unimpeded, there is harmony among the workings of the internal organs, freedom of movement, normal cyclical processes, and an even peaceful, stable disposition. The Liver acts as a harmonizer. Emotions like anger, resentment, frustration, especially when pent-up and unexpressed, can injure the Liver and disrupt the movement of Qi and blood, causing pain, disruption of normal cycles, organ functions, and mood swings. For example, the Liver Qi, when upset by emotion, easily overacts upon the Stomach, causing indigestion and pain. Wood needs to be nourished by Water. If there is insufficient Water, Wood will become dry and brittle leading to inflexibility. When the Wood Element is flourishing, one has the ambition, courage, and stamina to accomplish one's goals in life and the ability to change the status quo.

Fire

Yin Organ: Heart.
Yang Organ: Small Intestine.
Aroma: Floral.
Color: Red.
Season: Summer.
Direction: South.
Emotions: Heart: joy, anxiety, agitation, fear of intimacy;
Small Intestine: confusion.
Attributes: Heart: excitement, passion, imagination;
Small Intestine: discernment, clarity.
Sensory Portal: Tongue, speech.
Tissue: Vessels.
Taste: Bitter.
Force of Nature: Heat.

Fire is the expression of the Shen Spirit, the mind, and emotions. It provides the warmth for love and intimacy, the excitement of childlike awe and wonder, the spark for creativity and interest in many things at once. The Heart and Mind are inextricably connected. There are two aspects of the Heart with two types of fire: the sovereign fire of the Heart and the ministerial fire of the Pericardium (also called the Heart Wrap). The Pericardium, in its role as the minister, wraps the sovereign Heart within its protective covering and takes care of its physical needs. It tempers the impulsive, fiery excitement of the Heart with reason and self-control. The Heart expresses unconditional love whereas the Pericardium's expression of love is conditional. Fire needs to be balanced by water. If fire becomes excessive, the Heart Mind will become disturbed with anxiety, agitation, hyperactivity, insomnia, even mania and delusions. The blood, as an extension of the Heart, contains the Shen, the emotions, and the memories of life experiences.

Earth

Yin Organ: Spleen.
Yang Organ: Stomach.
Aroma: Sweet, musty, earthy, fruity.
Color: Yellow.
Season: Late summer.
Direction: Center.
Emotions: Pensiveness, obsession, worry, fear of not being able to accommodate others.
Attributes: Cognition, learning, memory, focus.

Sensory portal: Mouth, taste.
Tissue: Flesh.
Taste: Sweet.
Force of Nature: Dampness.

Earth is the expression of home, family, and relationships. It is one's connection to society and deals with the influences of social demands on one's life. The Earth temperament is accommodating. The job of the Spleen and Stomach is to nourish by way of the transformation and transportation of food and fluids. Earth needs to be fed by Fire, including both the Kidneys' Ming Men fire which provides the pilot light for the metabolism of nutrients as well as the fire of the Heart and Small Intestine which completes the process of turning food into blood to be circulated throughout the body. When digestion is incomplete, dampness accumulates, slowing things down, inhibiting normal bodyfunctions. Dampness also clouds the mind, interfering with the ability to digest information and to transform thoughts which can lead to learning difficulties and obsessive thinking.

Metal

Yin Organ: Lung.
Yang Organ: Large Intestine.
Aroma: Spicy, sharp, pungent.
Color: White.
Season: Autumn.
Direction: West.
Emotions: Grief, sadness, loss, fear of vulnerability.
Attributes: Morality, judgment, logic, organization, intuition.
Sensory Portal: Nose, breathing.
Tissue: Skin.
Taste: Pungent.
Force of Nature: Dryness.

Metal is the expression of virtue and morality. It maintains the integrity of the upright Qi. It is the breath, inhalation and exhalation, holding on and letting go. It is responsible for the ability to adjust and adapt to influences from the outside world, making judgments on what to accept and what to resist. The Lung rules the skin and the Wei Protective Qi, providing the immune responses on the surface while the Large Intestine continues this process by absorbing what is useful and eliminating what is harmful. Grief and loss injure the Lung, causing the breath to be held, as if waiting to exhale. Metal needs Earth to be free of dampness, which causes phlegm to accumulate in the lungs, and obsession, which interferes with the Lung Qi's ability to let go.

Water

Yin Organ: Kidney.
Yang Organ: Bladder.
Aroma: Musky, balsamic, camphorous.
Color: Black.
Season: Winter.
Direction: North.
Emotions: Fear, fear for survival, fear of death, fear of being abandoned or alone, fear of self.
Attributes: Motivation, willpower, innate drive, comfort with self, self-love, sense of significance, of purpose.
Sensory Portal: Ears, hearing.
Tissue: Bones, joints, marrow.
Taste: Salty.
Force of Nature: Cold.

Water is the fundamental element, the source of creation. The Kidneys store the Jing Essence which is the material basis of one's constitution, growth, and development. Jing Essence and Shen Spirit, embodied by the Fire element's Heart Mind, combine together to make up a whole individual with unique physical characteristics and temperament. These combined attributes are distributed to the Shu Transport points along the Bladder channel and then to the internal organs with the help of the San Jiao's fiery Qi. Water and Fire need to be balanced and communicating in order for the body, mind, and spirit to be heathy and at peace. Fear injures the Kidneys and causes loss of belief in one's self and the will power needed to be able to fulfill one's destiny. A Water temperament enjoys solitude, is easy going, non-judgmental, and goes with the flow.

2. Based on Note

Essential oils may be classified by their note.

The note of an essential oil is determined in part by its rate of evaporation. Rate of evaporation also refers to how long the aroma of a particular oil will last. In general, oils with the fastest rates of evaporation are considered top notes; moderate rates of evaporation are middle notes; and oils that evaporate slowly and have the longest lasting aromas are called base notes. Rates of evaporation also help to determine the frequency of application. In clinical practice, the qualities of each note can be related to its activity on the level of imbalance according to the CM diagnosis from superficial to deep: top notes for Wei level, middle notes for Ying level, and base notes for Yuan level.

TOP NOTES affect the Wei Superficial level of the body and are generally for acute conditions with a floating pulse. Psychophysically, top notes address moods that have no apparent emotional cause, as when one feels "off" but doesn't know why, for example in the case of SAD (Seasonal Affective Disorder). Neurologically, it is the autonomic system. With faster rates of evaporation, they are applied more frequently, up to several times per day, for clinical use.

Top notes are called for when treating acute cases which require immediate action, and as a rule are expected to change quickly, requiring fewer applications overall. They are also used to guide something outward to the skin. Top notes are important for acclimating to the external environment, like when treating a cold or allergic reaction for example, or when the intention of the blend includes bringing something out to the surface. Inhalation using a diffuser is one method to directly affect the Wei level via breath entering the lungs. Another is application of oils on "wind" points, meaning those with the Chinese word for wind/Feng in their names, or whose actions include eliminating or expelling wind like GB20, Feng Chi ("Wind Pool").

Examples of top note oils: many mints, citruses, and peels, Bo He (Peppermint), Ding Xiang (Clove), Zhang Nao (White Camphor), An Shu Ye (Eucalyptus), and Qing Pi (Green Tangerine Peel).

MIDDLE NOTES affect the Ying, moderate level of the body and are generally for sub-acute or more chronic conditions with moderate level pulses. Their aromas evaporate more slowly than top notes. They last for several hours and are applied at a medium frequency, on average twice per day. Middle note oils are appropriate when dealing with interior imbalances; for example, those involving the blood, internal organs, body fluids, and hormonal imbalances. Psycho-emotionally, middle note oils address cognitive emotional issues. Acupuncture point application, such as on Luo Connecting points and on points of the twelve primary channels, may be used to access this level.

Examples of middle note oils: many flower, leaf, twig, needle, spice, and fruit oils such as Song Zhen (Pine Needle), Yun Shan (Spruce Needle), Xun Yi Cao (Lavender), Bai Yu Lan Ye (Magnolia Leaf), Zi Su Ye (Perilla Leaf), and Xiao Hui Xiang (Fennel Fruit).

BASE NOTES affect the Yuan Source, Jing Essence, and deep level, imbalances detected in the deepest level of the pulses. Base note oils tend to be heavy. Their aromas are long-lasting. Consequently, they may only require one application per day but overall, the course of treatment requires a longer duration. Base note oils are chosen for their resonance with the deepest levels and are important to influence a person's constitution, such as when dealing with congenital, genetic, or familial issues. Psychologically, base notes are used when there are conflicts involving one's innate temperament and fundamental personality. Acupuncture Yuan Source points are a good choice to access this level as well as the Eight Extraordinary Vessels and the Influential points of the Extraordinary Fu.

Examples of base notes are the "precious" florals (those with strong, long-lasting aromas) like pure unadulterated Rose or Jasmine essential oils, and many of the roots, woods, resins, and seeds such as Wu Wei Zi (*Schisandra Fruit*), Nan Mu (Cedarwood), Rou Gui (Cinnamon Bark), Ru Xiang (Frankincense), Mo Yao (Myrrh), and Jiang Xiang (*Dalbergia*).

BASED ON NOTE

	TOP NOTE	MIDDLE NOTE	BASE NOTE
Evaporation	Fast - less than 3 hr	Moderate - around 6 hr	Slow - up to 2 days
Affected Level	Wei / Superficial	Ying / Blood/ Moderate	Yuan / Jing / Deep
Application Frequency	Up to several times a day	Twice a day	Once a day, for longer duration
Condition	Acute	Sub-acute, or chronic w/ symptoms	Constitutional
Pulse	Floating	Moderate	Deep
Organs	Lung, Skin, Sinew	Blood, Fluids, Flesh, Fu hollow organs	Zang solid organs
Affects	Moods (psycho-physically)	Cognitive emotional states (psycho-emotionally)	Innate temperament, fundamental personality

3. Based on Parts of Plants

The Doctrine of Signatures and observations of the living metaphors found within nature's sacred designs are born out, intuitively, experientially, and often chemically, in the actions of different parts of medicinal plants and their essential oils. The Doctrine of Signatures is an ancient recognition that Mother Nature has provided a cure for all ailments, if only we allow ourselves to be in communion with her in order to see it. Even the word "signature" is made up of a combination of "sign" and "nature." Plants may express their healing properties by the similarity of their shape to parts of the human body, by the energetic purpose of their parts (root, stem, leaf, seed, fruit, flower), by the type of environment in which they thrive (damp, arid, mountainous, etc.) or by the significance of their color. These properties are often translated into the name of the plant.

As an example, She Chuang Zi 蛇床子 (Cnidium Fruit), which translates as "Snake's Bed Seed" is so named because snakes—a symbol of sexual desire—like to rest next to it and indeed it is traditionally considered a cure for impotence as well as for skin problems, represented by the shedding of snake's skin. Another example is Lian Qiao (Forsythia Fruit), which is shaped like a heart with chambers inside and is used to cool and calm Heart fire causing restlessness and irritability.

Choosing and blending essential oils for a healing transformation is like writing a poem. The evocative images, symbols, and metaphors that are conjured up help us to commune with the plants from which the oils come and to carry our intention.

Flowers & Fruits tend to affect the psyche and the exterior including the sensory orifices.

- ***Flowers*** are the most complex part of a plant and the fulfillment of its expression. They represent intelligence, metamorphosis, beauty, love, transcendence, and reaching for the divine.
- ***Fruits*** represent the maturity of one's nature, the fruits of one's labors, and what one has to offer.
- ***Peels*** represent the skin, what one presents to the world, the external appearance and attractiveness.

Leaves & Branches tend to affect the humors (blood, fluids, lymph).

- ***Leaves, Twigs, and Needles*** represent receiving nourishment from experiences. Reaching out to the outside world and the sky beyond the confines of the earthly, material plane. They serve as a bridge between the exterior and interior, heaven and earth, breaking away from old habits and ideas.

Woods, Barks, & Roots tend to affect the structure and internal organs.

- ***Woods*** represent dynamic growth, development and action, creativity and expression of individuality, decision making, and are motivational.
- ***Barks*** represent protection and hiding or numbing of pain. Many tend to be analgesic.
- ***Roots*** represent stability and belonging, connection to family, and socialization.

Resins tend to affect deep wounds and trauma.

- ***Resins*** are derived from wounds made in the wood of trees. They are a protective substance secreted by trees against disease and infestations and to heal wounds to their trunks or branches. Resins represent wound healing for both physical and emotional trauma, healing old issues around guilt and forgiveness. They are considered sacred substances used as incense or an anointment in religious ceremonies in order to summon the divine, especially when seeking healing and redemption.

Seeds tend to affect the constitution and growth patterns.

- ***Seeds*** represent potential. Most deal with altering the Jing Essence, cycles of growth, aging, and hormones. Their affinity is most often to the lower burner.

4. Based on Chemical Composition

Western aromatherapy is often based on the scientific, pharmacological effects of the major chemical constituents of essential oils. In the context of Chinese medicine, chemical composition can add to the understanding of the known properties of the herbs, specifically in their essential oil form. Thanks to Jeffrey Yuen, the actions of these major chemical constituents are translated into the language of Chinese medicine.

Essential oil chemical constituents are mainly categorized based on types of terpenes along with functional groups which are oxygenated compounds (a group of atoms responsible for the characteristic reactions of a particular compound). Listed here are many, but not all, of the chemical components commonly found in essential oils.

Terpenes: Mono, Sesqui, Di and Tri Terpenes ("ene" endings)

Monoterpenes are very common. Most essential oils contain monoterpenes. They are broad-spectrum antibacterials. Many monoterpenes are known to be anti-inflammatory and immunoregulatory. They tend to be mucolytic, break up mucus and phlegm, expectorant, and resolve fluid retention. They are antiseptic, treat exogenous conditions, expel wind-heat, tend to be cooling, and treat bacterial infections. They are analgesic, moving Qi and blood to relieve pain.

The high concentrations of monoterpenes are found in citrus oils such as the limonene in Zhi Ke (*Citrus aurantium*), Fo Shou (Buddha's Hand Fruit), and Qing Pi (Green Tangerine Peel). Other common monoterpenes are pinene in evergreens and in Du Huo (*Angelica pubescentis*), terpinene in Long Nao (*Borneolum*), and phellandrene in E Zhu (*Curcuma zedoaria*). Also, cineole, called eucalyptol in An Shu Ye (Eucalyptus), is an excellent decongestant when diffused into the air. Research on pinene has shown that it increases T cells in HIV patients.

Essential oils with a dominant percentage of monoterpenes can irritate the skin and mucus membranes if applied neat and may need to be diluted to 3%. On the other hand, it is partially due to this irritation that these oils can break up mucus and phlegm congestion. Diffusing such oils is effective to kill germs, treat sore throat and congestion.

SESQUITERPENES calm the Spirit are grounding. They regulate Qi, are analgesic, antispasmodic, nervine, hypotensive, anti-inflammatory, and antifebrile. Sesquiterpenes are antiseptic and treat exogenous viral conditions, which are more often associated with wind-cold. They tend to be gentle on the skin and can often be applied undiluted. Roots and woods have the highest concentration. Sesquiterpenes are found in most essential oils.

For example, farnesene in Chai Hu (Bupleurum), Jiang Xiang (*Dalbergia*) and Mei Gui Hua (Rose), caryophyllene in Xun Yi Cao (Lavender) and Ding Xiang (Clove), curzerene in Mo Yao (Myrrh) and E Zhu (*Cucuma zedoaria*), patchoulene in Huo Xiang (Patchouli), chamazulene in German Chamomile and Ju Hua (Chrysanthemum). Sesquiterpenes tend to be gentle on the skin, often can be applied undiluted.

DITERPENES are not as commonly found in essential oils. They are antifungal, expectorant, and antiviral for wind-damp conditions. They are also tonifying and hormone balancing, therefore useful in teenage acne, for example, as well as polycystic ovarian syndrome or menopause. Diterpenes are steroidal-like (contain phytosteroids), and moisturizing.

Diterpenes are found in Dang Gui (*Angelica sinensis*) and Ai Ye (*Artemisia argyi*), both used to regulate the menstrual cycle; and in Xiao Hui Xiang (Fennel), which can aid recovery from adrenal exhaustion.

TRITERPENES are less commonly found in essential oils. They are powerful immune-boosting agents.Triterpenes are strongly analgesic.

For example, Yi Yi Ren (Coix) as an essential oil is like aspirin due to its high triterpene content. Glycoside triterpenes such as ginsenoside in Panax ginseng and Siberian ginseng benefit the immune system. Mushroom spores as in Ling Zhi (Ganoderma) spore oil contain high concentrations of triterpenes. Generally gentle on and beneficial to the skin.

Functional Groups

ALCOHOLS ("ol" endings) are anti-infectious, antibacterial, and antiviral. They are tonifying and emotionally uplifting; they stimulate Qi. Alcohols are nontoxic, non-irritating, and are fine for long-term use. When combined with a monoterpene, which alone may be irritating, it becomes a monoterpenol that is gentle to epithelial tissue (the lining of the gut and mucus membranes) and can be taken internally.

For example: citronellol in Mei Gui Hua (Rose), linalool in Xun Yi Cao (Lavender),and Bai Yu Lan Ye (Magnolia Leaf), which calms allergic rhinitis and is safe and gentle in a light saline solution as a nasal rinse.

Examples of sesquiterpinols, which are the combination of alcohols and sesquiterpenes, are santolol in Tan Xiang (Sandalwood), and farnesol in Hu Lu Ba (Fenugreek).

PHENOLS ("ol" endings) are antidepressant; they stimulate mental faculties, tonify Qi, and powerfully boost the immune system. Studies have found that to boost the immune system, phenols work best when massaged into the skin and second best diffused into the air. Both of these methods directly affect Wei Protective Qi. They are naturally found in the amino acid tyrosine, adrenaline, and in the neurotransmitter, serotonin.

Phenols may be irritating and oils with high phenol content should always be diluted. They are not recommended for internal ingestion. Because they stimulate a lot of Qi, phenols can harm the Liver if taken internally over an extended period of time due to overstimulation. Some essential oils containing phenols are said to be toxic to cats. They are strongly antiseptic, antioxidant, antibacterial, antiviral, and break up encrustations. They may have a "hospital" smell and are often used in cleaning products. Examples are: eugenol in Rou Gui (Cinnamon Bark) and Ding Xiang (Clove), which are both considered to have restorative and anti-aging properties. Phenols are also found in Mei Gui Hua (Rose) and Xi Xin (Asarum).

KETONES ("one" endings) are anticoagulant; they break up Qi and blood stasis. They can be helpful in Luo Vessel treatments but use caution during pregnancy. Ketones are lipolytic, mucolytic and decongestant, break up fat, mucus, phlegm, goiters, and cancerous tumors. They can also be anti-inflammatory, analgesic, and vulnerary (promotes wound healing). Essential oils with high percentages of ketone constituents should always be considered cautiously. Many essential oils containing some types of ketones are safe, nontoxic, and beneficial.

Examples: Menthone in Bo He (Peppermint) and chrysanthenone in Ju Hua (Chrysanthemum), which is anti-inflammatory, clears heat and cholesterol. Jasmone in Jasmine flower is actually beneficial to the skin. Nepetalactone found in Jing Jie (*Schizonepeta*) is the same chemical in catnip that makes cats euphoric. Certain ketones, such as camphor, if they constitute a major component of an essential oil, are potentially neurotoxic and should never be ingested or used in high dosages, but are still safe for diffusing or applied topically for short-term use diluted to 2%. For example, the camphor in Zhang Nao (White Camphor) is toxic if taken internally, but safe and effectiveas a smelling salt for loss of consciousness or diluted and applied topically to kill parasites.

ALDEHYDES ("hyde" or "al" endings) calm spirit, are sedative, nervine, hypotensive, vasodilating, antiviral, antipyretic (brings down fever), and anti-inflammatory. A case in point is Chai Hu (Bupleurum), which is cooling and sedating and contains a few prominent aldehydes. Their relaxing effect on the nervous system can calm tremors, hypersensitivity, and anxiety. Aldehydes tend to have a typical lemon-scent like citral and geranial, which is a terpene aldehyde found in Bi Cheng Qie (Litsea). Another example is perillaldehyde in Zi Su Ye and Zi Su Zi (Perilla Leaf and Seed). These are all considered warming as herbal medicines in traditional Chinese medicine, although in their essential oil form, aldehydes give them a somewhat more cooling action, and Bi Cheng Qie (Litsea), which is in the Warming Interior category as an herbal medicine, brings heat out to the surface for release as an essential oil. Aldehydes can irritate the skin if not sufficiently diluted, and prolonged use may cause an allergic reaction.

ESTERS ("acetate" endings) are considered one of the most balancing and harmonizing chemical components. They regulate Qi, are antispasmodic, anti-inflammatory, and nervine. Esters tend to be antifungal. They act as harmonizers and are very safe. They are often found as major components in florals and fruits. Examples include: linalyl acetate in Xun Yi Cao (Lavender) and benzyl acetate, both of which are responsible for the pleasant, sweet, fruity aroma of many flowers and fruits such as Qi Li Xiang (Orange Jessamine), Jin Yin Hua (Honeysuckle), and Mei Gui Hua (Rose). Esters are gentle on the skin and easy to use.

OXIDES AND ETHERS are closely related, the terms are often used interchangeably. Both relax muscles including the smooth muscle that deals with digestive, respiratory and diaphragmatic constriction. Oxides increase oxygen in the body. They can be diffused to create a more aerobic atmosphere for altitude sickness, migraines, or heart conditions. The most abundant and important oxide found in many essential oils is 1-8 cineole also known as eucalyptol. Found in An Shu Ye

(Eucalyptus), Ai Ye (*Artemisea argyi*) and Bo He (Peppermint) to name a few, this oxide is expectorant and mucolytic. It promotes the elimination of excess water in the body and can be applied to reduce swelling or to reduce fluid retention in the chest as in the case of congestive heart failure.

COUMARINS are anticoagulant, antifungal, antiviral, balancing for moods. For example: osthole in She Chuang Zi (Cnidium Fruit), Gui Zhi/Gui Ye (Cinnamon Twig and Leaf), and Bai Zhi (*Angelica dahurica*). This is an important component in She Chuang Zi (Cnidium Fruit) which is very useful in formulations for fungal or vaginal yeast infections. The high osthole content in She Chuang Zi is also thought to be what accounts for its Viagra-like, pro-libido action. Caution should be used with coumarins as some are photo-sensitive, should be well diluted 2% to 3% and need to avoid sun exposure.

5. Based on Chinese Medicine (CM)

Category, Nature, Taste, Affinities, Actions and Indications

Thanks to the classics of Chinese herbal medicine, practitioners have the benefit of thousands of years of documented knowledge and experience to support an understanding of the qualities and properties of medicinal herbs, which can then be applied to their essential oils.

Modern Chinese herbal materia medica organize the herbs according to their category and each herb is given a nature (hot, cold, warm, cool, neutral) and taste (bland, sweet, spicy, pungent, acrid, bitter, salty, sour), as well as organ channel affinities, all of which help explain the actions and indications of each herb. These assigned characteristics are meant to be considered in combination. Taken together they paint a more complete picture of an herb's medicinal properties.

Nature

Nature refers to the nature of an herb in terms of the energetics of temperature and its effect on the Qi of the body.

- **Hot:** Yang, stimulating, rising.
- **Cold:** Yin, settling, descending.
- **Warm:** Comforting, antidepressant, circulating.
- **Cool:** Calming, relaxing, anti-inflammatory, moistening.

Taste

Each type of taste refers to its action in the body.

- **Acrid/Pungent:** Dispersing, moving, venting outward, releasing the exterior, promoting sweating.

- **Spicy:** Digestive, increasing secretions, transforming dampness.
- **Sweet:** Tonifying, nourishing, harmonizing.
- **Sour:** Stabilizing, binding, preventing or reducing loss of body fluids.
- **Bitter:** Detoxifying, purging, draining downward, drying dampness.
- **Salty:** Retaining Yin fluids, softening hardness (masses, hematomas, arterial hardening, plaque).
- **Bland:** Promoting urination, reducing swelling.

Category

Typical herb categories and subcategories include:

- **Releasing the Exterior:** wind-cold or wind-heat.
- **Clearing Heat:** purging fire, clearing damp heat, cooling blood, eliminating toxins.
- **Downward Draining:** purgatives, moist laxatives, harsh expellants.
- **Draining Dampness and Regulating Water.**
- **Dispelling Wind-Damp:** relieving pain, opening channels and collaterals, strengthening tendons and bones.
- **Transforming Phlegm and Stopping Cough.**
- **Aromatic Transforming Dampness.**
- **Relieving Food Stagnation and Improving Digestion.**
- **Qi Regulating.**
- **Regulating Blood and Stopping Bleeding.**
- **Invigorating Blood and Removing Blood Stasis.**
- **Warming the Interior and Expelling Cold.**
- **Tonifying:** nourishing blood, tonifying Qi, tonifying Yin, tonifying Yang.
- **Stabilizing and Binding.**
- **Calming the Spirit and Nourishing the Heart.**
- **Aromatic Opening Orifices.**
- **Extinguishing Wind and Stopping Tremors.**
- **Expelling Parasites.**
- **Topical Application.**

Please refer to the "Essential Oils and CM Categories List" in the Appendices section. This list demonstrates how the essential oils of Chinese herbs can fit into the traditional Chinese medicine categories. It shows the versatility of the oils beyond the limits of the one category normally assigned to each raw herb. Considering the unique qualities of each oil allows the practitioner to fine-tune their choices within a category. Additionally, combining oils from multiple categories is a way to address the complete picture of an individual's needs. Keep in mind that many oils fit into more than one category and therefore can fulfill multiple roles.

As an example, Jin Yin Hua (Honeysuckle) traditionally fits into the CM category of Clearing Heat and Eliminating Toxins. However, as an essential oil, you will also find it in the categories of Calming Spirit, Eliminating Wind-Heat, Improving Digestion, and Tonifying Yin. Its sweet floral nature is calming, clarifying, and uplifting for the spirit, and nourishing for the body fluids. Its chemistry, aside from being antipathogenic, also benefits the digestion as a prebiotic.

It is important to remember, however, that the categories, natures, tastes, channel affinities, and the actions and indications assigned to herbs are not written in stone and have varied depending on the historical circumstances, social needs, and philosophy of a particular clinician or era of Chinese medical history.

Beyond that, in their essential oil form, the possibilities open up even further dimensions. The affect of aroma is immediate and powerful, yet also very personal and individual. Even chemical components will affect different people differently depending on their body chemistry and temperament.

Aromatherapy is an interactive and dynamic art. Practitioners should always feel free to discover for themselves new channel affinities, natures, tastes, and actions from their own experience with the herbs and their essential oils. The oils emit life-force and intelligence. Let them become familiar friends and allies in carrying your healing intention and expanding your knowledge. Invite them to become your teachers in your personal quest for wisdom and self-realization.

The Materia Medica of essential oils contained in this book will describe each oil from the point of view of traditional Chinese medicine combined with the factors that distinguish them in their essential oil form.

CHEMOTYPES

The energetics of plants, and consequently their essential oils, will change due to the environment in which they grow. Plants dynamically respond and adapt to the ecosystem around them. They are influenced by climate, geography, altitude, types of soil, moisture, dryness, temperature, pests, and the other plants and animals in their surroundings. For example, a plant growing on the top of a sunny, windy mountain will yield an essential oil with different energetic, aromatic, and medicinal qualities as well as percentages of chemical components than that same species will when found near a shady stream at the base of the mountain. Another important factor is the season and climatic conditions at the time of harvesting.

Throughout the long history of Chinese herbal medicine, there has been a tradition of regarding certain herbs grown in a particular geographical location as superior. Often that location was added to the name of the herb such as Guang Huo Xiang (Patchouli) to indicate that it was grown in the Guangzhou area. Or in the case of Xing Ren (*Prunus armeniaca*) for which there are two types with different medicinal attributes: Bei Xing Ren from the north is Bitter Almond, Nan Xing Ren from the south is Sweet Almond.

Recently the Chinese government has been encouraging the cultivation of products involving traditional medicine, including essential oils. This has led to increased interest by essential oil factories to learn more about Chinese herbs and how to choose those which yield oils that contain the best medicinal, aromatic components. In other words, they are paying attention to chemotypes.

Li Ting 李婷, is the manager of a wonderful essential oil factory in southern China which supplies Alchemica Botanica with beautiful products. I am so grateful for the time she has spent teaching me, as well as, and especially, for her friendship and hospitality each time I visit. Fostered by her background in Chinese medicine and chemistry, Li Ting is a treasure of expertise in the innovative production of the highest quality essential oils and their medicinal attributes. She explains chemotypes this way:

Li Ting

"In China, we have a saying about your question, "淮南生橘，淮北生枳," that means even the same plant will change because of planting in different places. Genuine medicinal material is the most important thing in our producing process. When we chose the raw material for producing, first thing we will consider is the place where the material is growing. Like you said, different growing places will change the content of chemical components. Another thing we will consider is the species. For example, Osmanthus has four main varieties (golden, silver, red, and seasons) but we only use the golden one (var. *thunbergii*) for producing because it has the most beautiful scent of all kinds. And for all the places that are planting golden Osmanthus, the ones growing in Guilin are the best. And the weather will affect the chemical components too. For example, when the rain is more than average annual level, you will find that the scent of the flower may not be as strong as usual. So, the harvest timing is crucial too.

"To summarize, this is how we chose raw material: 1. Look for the varieties (species) we want. 2. Look for the best place of growing. 3. Choose the best time to harvest. 4. Use the most suitable producing process."

SOME CHINESE MEDICINE CONCEPTS EXPLAINED

FOR READERS WHO DO NOT PRACTICE CHINESE MEDICINE, here is a brief explanation of some of the basic precepts of Chinese medicine and some of the concepts and terms you will see in the actions and indications section of each oil in Part Two, The Materia Medica.

Over the long history of Chinese medicine, during different periods, beginning with *The Yellow Emperor's Classic of Internal Medicine* (second century BCE), methods of categorizing and differentiating states of wellness and illness developed.

THE MICROCOSM REFLECTS THE MACROCOSM

The design, internal environment, and functioning of the human body mirror the cosmos and are influenced by the forces of nature. This also applies to the fundamental relationship of one's intrinsic temperament, morphology, and destiny to cosmic forces at the time of conception and birth. Another significant factor is the effect of the social environment on one's thoughts, emotions, actions, and on the course of one's life. Living in harmony with nature and adapting to challenges are the keys to maintaining balance and consequently, health of body and mind.

THE EIGHT PRINCIPLES

The Eight Principles are described by four sets of Yin Yang opposites. These help the doctor to identify the location and nature of an illness or pattern of disharmony, and then to assess the body's ability to respond to a pathogenic process as it attempts to restore balance.

Yin and Yang are what make the world go round. They are constant and, simultaneously, the mutually unifying and mutually opposing forces behind all phenomena and all manifestation. In the cosmos, the sun is Yang and the moon is Yin. Daytime, brightness, and warmth are Yang. Nighttime, darkness, and coolness are Yin. Yin and Yang arise from the same source which has many names: Tai Ji, The Grand Ultimate, The Void, The Mystery, The One.

The *Dao De Jing* tells us, "The one gives birth to the two, the two gives birth to the three, the three gives birth to the myriad of all things." Heaven and Earth are the Yang and Yin from which we human beings are created and between which we stand. In our bodies, Yin essences are the material, structural building blocks and nutritive substances like blood. Yang on the other hand, is the spark of life, energy, Qi, the metabolic fire that makes everything move and work.

YIN / YANG are the root principles from which the others arise. In this context, exterior, excess, and heat are considered Yang, while interior, deficiency, and cold are Yin.

EXTERIOR / INTERIOR identify the location and origin of the illness. In general, exterior conditions originate from outside the body, like an airborne pathogen such as a cold virus or allergen. They express with symptoms on the outer body such as the skin, pores, or muscles. Interior conditions may be the result of the progression of an illness that began on the outside of the body, or from an illness that originated in the interior affecting the functioning of an organ, or problem with the blood circulation, for example. Interior conditions are often due to issues relating to the emotions, diet, or lifestyle.

EXCESS / DEFICIENCY identify the response to the illness and body condition of the patient. In general, excess conditions occur when the body's resistance to a pathogen is strong, causing an active struggle between the pathogen and the disease-fighting forces such as high fever, production of a lot of phlegm, or constipation. Deficiency patterns result when the body condition and resistance is weak, allowing the pathogen to go deeper into the body and the disease process to be prolonged. Common deficiency signs are fatigue, sweating, low-grade fever, and loose stools.

HEAT / COLD describe the nature of the illness as well as the nature of the person. Heat and cold do not only literally refer to temperature. They also describe the balance of Yin and Yang forces in the body. An insufficiency of one will cause the other to become overly dominant. Conversely, an overabundance of either will interfere with the expression of its opposite. Heat and cold can describe the nature of an exogenous pathogen. Heat expresses with responses such as over-excitation, irritability, hyperactivity, redness of the skin and face, thirst for cold drinks and aversion to heat. Cold manifests as hypoactivity, fatigue, pale skin and complexion, preference for warmth, cold limbs.

The Six Excesses / Six Pathogenic Factors

The six excesses are related to types of climatic or environmental factors that can affect the body from the outside. Each factor commonly causes a particular set of symptoms. Determining which combination of factors are at play, such as wind-cold, wind-heat, or wind-damp helps the practitioner to predict the course of an illness and decide on a treatment strategy, which may include essential oils, herbal medicine, and/or acupuncture techniques. The general idea is that wind, the overriding causative factor, which carries the others into the body, needs to be expelled. At the same time, cold needs to be warmed, heat needs to be cooled, dryness moistened, and dampness transformed.

The six excesses are each related to a certain season and one of the five elements:

Wind – Wood – Spring
Cold – Water – Winter
Heat – Fire – Summer
Dryness – Metal – Autumn
Dampness – Earth – Late Summer
Summer Heat – Fire – Summer

Common Syndromes and Symptoms of the Six Excesses

WIND is the overriding, initial manifestation of an exterior syndrome. It may include symptoms such as aversion to drafts, mild fever, sweating, dizziness, headache, nasal congestion, itchy throat, cough, and a floating pulse. Wind is further differentiated according to other climatic factors.

WIND-COLD basically describes the common cold with symptoms like strong aversion to wind and chill with mild fever, headaches, generalized body aches, a runny nose, and a cough with clear thin mucus.

WIND-HEAT is accompanied by fever, sweating, headaches, red eyes, sore throat, photosensitivity, thirst, nasal congestion, and cough with yellow and dense or even bloody phlegm, respiratory problems, and constipation.

WIND-COLD-DAMP has effects similar to those of the common cold but the addition of dampness causing a feeling of heaviness in the body with sore limbs, listlessness, and digestive upset like nausea, no appetite, and diarrhea.

WIND-COLD-DAMP BI PAINFUL OBSTRUCTION SYNDROME happens when cold and damp get into the channels, muscles, tendons, and joints causing pain and other symptoms such as heavy sensation of the limbs, numbness, spasms, joint and deep bone pain with difficult movement. Symptoms are worse with cold damp weather. This is a common cause of arthritis and rheumatism. Bi syndromes can also include pain such as headaches and toothaches.

HOT BI PAINFUL OBSTRUCTION SYNDROME can result from long term, unresolved wind-cold-damp, Bi or other factors. The joints and sinews become inflamed, very painful with redness and swelling, numbness, atrophy, and poor mobility.

WIND-HEAT-DAMP has symptoms of intermittent fever, sweating with no resolution of the fever, epigastric fullness, poor appetite, loose stools, fatigue of the limbs and body.

SUMMER HEAT results in fever, profuse sweating, strong thirst, dark urine.

SUMMER HEAT-DAMP symptoms include lack of appetite, nausea, vomiting, loose stool, abdominal and epigastric stuffiness, fever (low-grade), sticky/difficult sweat.

DRYNESS AND COOL (Late Autumn) results in light headache, aversion to cold, no sweating, cough, dry throat and lips, stuffy nose.

DRYNESS AND WARMTH (Early Autumn) symptoms include fever, sweating, thirst, dry throat, dry nose, dry cough possibly with blood in sputum, chest tightness.

✔ *In Chinese medicine, fever often refers to a subjective sensation of heat and not necessarily an elevated thermometer reading.*

Causative Factors of Some Common Skin Conditions Using the Six Excesses Model

- **Urticaria:** Wind interferes with the circulation of Qi and blood under the skin.
- **Psoriasis:** Dryness, or dryness with heat, interferes with the circulation of blood and moistening fluids to the skin.
- **Eczema:** Damp accumulation under the skin.
- **Ulcers, Abscesses:** Damp-heat accumulation under the skin.
- **Skin Cancer:** Chronic unresolved heat and stagnation or exposure to toxic substances turn into fire toxin expressing on the skin.

The Seven Injuries / The Seven Emotions

The seven injuries categorize states of mind and emotions that can cause illness. Unlike the six excesses which are external factors, the seven injuries are generated internally. They are a way to explain the mind/body connection. Each of these seven emotions is associated with one of the internal organs. A certain emotion is said to injure its related organ, causing symptoms of disharmony and distress which interfere with the normal flow of the Qi and blood and impair the organ's function. These associations help the doctor to identify the origins of the patient's physical complaints.

JOY – Heart. A state of overexcitement and agitation that scatters the Qi. The spirit feels ungrounded. May cause insomnia, palpitations.

ANGER – Liver. Includes resentment, frustration, irritability. Interferes with the smooth flow of the Liver's Qi and often causes heat to rise upward. May result in headaches, dizziness, hypertension, or menstrual irregularities.

ANXIETY – Heart. Extreme worry over things that have an unknown outcome. A feeling of restless nervousness that, over time, puts a strain on the heart, mind, and nervous system.

PENSIVENESS – Spleen. Excessive thinking, obsessive worry over something with a known outcome. Tends to interfere with normal digestion and absorption.

GRIEF – Lung. Sadness over a loss and difficulty letting go. Affects the chest, respiration, and elimination.

FEAR – Kidney. Fear of the unknown, of being alone, of death. Loss of self-worth, self-empowerment. Affects the lower back, joints, urination.

FRIGHT – Heart and Kidney. Shock caused by sudden, unexpected events. Initially may cause tachycardia, sweating, incontinence, and even loss of consciousness. Lingering effects cause post-traumatic stress disorder (PTSD).

The Internal Organs From the Chinese Point of View

Along with the Western physiological functions of the organs, Chinese medicine ascribes certain additional functions. For one thing, the organs are not simply thought of as a physical conglomeration of cells and tissue but as entire systems encompassing the special qualities and movements of their Qi and the relationships among the organs as integral parts of the whole. Harmony among the workings of organs is essential for maintenance of health. Each organ system is a very complex story which readers are encouraged to explore in texts devoted to the subject.

The organ systems are organized into Yin Yang pairs called the Zang Fu: one Yin Zang solid organ and one Yang Fu hollow organ. They are: Lung/Large Intestine, Spleen/Stomach, Heart/Small Intestine, Pericardium/San Jiao, Kidney/Bladder, and Liver/Gallbladder. Basically, the solid organs gather and store, whereas the hollow organs receive and move. Each Yin Yang pair is associated with one of the five elements which describe the many natural correspondences for each of the organs including associated emotions and mental states. You will find the five element correspondences on page 20, "Choosing an Essential Oil Based on Aroma."

The organs are discussed in the *Su Wen* or Simple Questions, a part of *The Yellow Emperor's Classic of Internal Medicine*. As you will see in the quotations below, each from Chapter 8 of the text, translated by Elisabeth Rochat de la Vallée, likens the organs to government officials, each playing their role in the governing of the body.

For the sake of a clearer understanding of some of the information presented in the Materia Medica, here is a basic list of those organ qualities which are unique to the Chinese point of view:

Lung

"The Lung has the charge of minister and chancellor. Thus, the regulation of the relays for animation is brought about."

- Rules the Qi.
- Governs reception of Qi/air/breath.
- Controls respiration, inhalation and exhalation.
- Disseminates the Qi.
- Administers Wei Protective Qi.
- Descends the Qi to the Kidneys which anchors inhalation of breath.
- Regulates water passages.
- Houses the Po (corporeal soul).
- Opens to the nose.
- Controls the skin, the pores, and body hair.

Large Intestine

"The Large Intestine is responsible for transit. The residue from transformation stems from it."

- Completes the process of transformation and transportation of foods and fluids, the absorption of fluids and nutrients.
- Receives turbid fluids and products of digestion from the small intestine and excretes waste.
- Regulates absorption and excretion, holding on and letting go, judgment.

Spleen

"The Spleen and Stomach are responsible for the storehouses and granaries. The five tastes stem from them."

- Governs transportation and transformation of foods and fluids.
- Responsible for transformation of dampness.
- Rules the muscles and flesh and strength of the four limbs.
- Produces the blood from food and fluids and sends the blood to the heart and lungs to provide oxygenation and circulation.
- Banks the blood, keeps the blood within the vessels, controls bleeding.
- Ascends the Qi.
- Source of postnatal, acquired Jing Essence.
- Houses the Yi (thought, intellect, and intent).
- Opens to the mouth, saliva, sense of taste.
- Manifests on the lips.

STOMACH

- Governs reception, rotting and ripening (fermentation) of foods and fluids.
- Directs the digestive Qi downward to the intestines.
- Initiates production of nutritional substance.
- First step in the production and separation of Jin Ye pure and turbid fluids.

HEART AND PERICARDIUM

"The Heart holds the office of Sovereign Emperor. The Radiance of the Spirit stems from it."

- The Heart is the home of the Shen Spirit, mind, consciousness, and emotion.
- The Pericardium is the Heart Wrap (Xin Bao) and Heart Protector which manifests symptoms of the physical heart.
- Rules the blood, the blood vessels, and circulation.
- Finalizes the production of the "red substance" (complete oxygenated blood).
- Maintains the nervous system.
- Controls sweat.
- Opens to the tongue and regulates speech.
- Manifests in the face.

SMALL INTESTINE

"The Small Intestine is responsible for receiving and making things thrive. Transformed substances stem from it."

- Further separates the pure and turbid in the process of digestion, absorption, and assimilation of vital fluids and nutrients.
- Descends unabsorbed fluids to the bladder.

TRIPLE ENERGIZER (*Triple Heater, San Jiao, Triple Burner*)

"The Triple Burner (San Jiao) is responsible for the opening up of passages and irrigation. The waterways stem from it."

The San Jiao is not literally an organ *per se* but rather an energetic mechanism which basically controls metabolic processes throughout the upper, middle, and lower burners, as well as the distribution of fluids and Jing Essence:

UPPER – Chest, heart, and lungs

MIDDLE – Diaphragm and upper abdomen, liver, gallbladder, stomach, spleen

LOWER – Lower abdomen, intestines, kidneys, bladder

- Controls passage of the waterways.
- Promotes the movement of Qi and fluids throughout the body.
- Distributes Yuan Qi, the manifestation of the constitution, from the Kidneys to the internal organs by way of the Back Shu points of the Bladder channel. The manner of this distribution accounts for the expression of one's temperament according to the five element model.

Kidney

"The Kidneys are charged with arousing the power. From them come skill and ability."

- Foundation of Yin and Yang in the body.
- Stores Jing Essence also referred to as Kidney Yin.
- Provides the basis for growth, development, and reproduction.
- Foundation of Ming Men Life Gate fire, also referred to as Kidney Yang. It is the metabolic spark which warms the body, provides the pilot light for digestion, and promotes the functioning of the internal organs.
- Origin of Yuan Source Qi also referred to as the constitution.
- Provides the basis for growth, development, and reproduction.
- Source of marrow which is the product of Jing Essence plus Shen Spirit. It includes the brain, also referred to as the "sea of marrow," and the bone marrow, the source of blood cells.
- Rules water metabolism.
- Grasps the Lung Qi, anchors the inhalation of breath.
- Rules the bones and joints.
- Houses the Zhi (will, motivation).
- Opens to the ear.
- Manifests in the head hair.

Bladder

"The Bladder is responsible for regions and cities. It stores the body fluids. The transformations of the Qi then give out their power."

- Responsible for storage and expulsion of water as directed by the Kidney Qi.
- Bladder's Yang Qi brings Kidney Essence along the spine to support the back, brain, and senses.

LIVER

"The Liver holds the office of the general of the armed forces. Assessment of circumstances and conception of plans stem from it."

- Controls the smooth flow of the Qi and blood.
- Stores the blood.
- Regulates the emotions.
- Liver blood nourishes Heart Qi.
- Houses the Hun (ethereal soul).
- Initiates creating and planning.
- Harmonizes the relationship among the Zang solid and Fu hollow organs.
- Nourishes and rules the sinews, flexibility, and movement of the limbs.
- Rules the nerves.
- Manifests in the nails.
- Opens to the eyes.

GALLBLADDER

"The Gallbladder is responsible for what is just and exact. Determination and decision stem from it."

- Called the pivot, coordinates side to side movement.
- Directs the manifestation of the Liver's creative plans.
- Source of courage and decision making.
- Assists clarity of vision, and the senses.
- Has a direct relationship with the head and brain.
- Stores and excretes bile produced in the liver into the small intestine to aid digestion.
- One of the Extraordinary Fu, also called the Curious Bowels. Connects and harmonizes them all.

Qi

Qi is everywhere. Without Qi there is no life. All things have Qi, even those things that are normally not thought of as living, such as stones. We are able to discern Qi by its effects. In nature, for example, the Qi of wind is constantly moving and creating change. In the human body, qualities of Qi are differentiated. The Qi of an organ, such as the Liver, has its own particular quality which then flows through the Liver channel, meeting up with channels of other organs, creating relationships between the organs, structures, and humors of the body. In another example of these dynamic relationships, we say that the Qi moves the blood, and in turn, the blood nourishes the Qi.

Qi is also differentiated in the body according to the level or depth at which it moves. Each level of Qi has its special qualities and functionality.

The Levels of Qi

Wei Qi

Wei Protective Qi circulates throughout the more exterior parts of the body referred to as the superficial level, including the skin, nerves, muscles tendons, and ligaments. It is regulated by the Lungs and is responsible for protecting the body from outside influences and resistance to external pathogenic factors. In this way, it is an important aspect of the immune system. Included in the Wei Qi are the workings of the autonomic nervous system, the unconscious functions such as: respiration, circadian rhythm, opening and closing of the pores, and movement of the smooth muscles like those that account for peristalsis.

Ying Qi

Ying Nutritive Qi circulates throughout the interior aspects of the body referred to as the moderate level. It includes the blood, body fluids, hormonal and enzymatic secretions that provide nourishment and functionality to the internal landscape, including the internal organs. It is especially influenced by the spleen, heart, and liver whose jobs are, respectively, to produce, circulate, and store the blood.

Yuan Qi

Yuan Source Qi supports the deepest level. It is the basis of the constitution. It is stored in the Kidneys as Jing Essence and circulated by the San Jiao mechanism. It provides the foundation of the bone structure, joints, marrow, the brain, and the potential for reproduction.

Diluting Essential Oils

Dilution of essential oils depends on the nature of the particular oil and its chemical components, skin sensitivity, age, and usage. It can range anywhere from 0.5% to 50% or higher essential oil to carrier oil.

Direct application of essential oils on the skin may be done after testing for sensitivity. For application on acupuncture points, test on a single point first. The equivalent of just one drop may be sufficient to distribute over a three-to-five-point prescription using a thin glass, stone, porcelain, or wooden tool. Rubbing essential oils into points or channels is often not necessary and not recommended with most oils unless sufficiently diluted.

Jeffrey Yuen's Dilution Method

- **1% dilution** means 10 to 12 drops of essential oil diluted in 1 oz (30ml) of carrier oil.

Therefore:

- **2% dilution** means 20 to 24 drops of essential oil diluted in 1 oz of carrier oil.
- **4% dilution** means 40 to 48 drops of essential oil diluted in 1 oz of carrier oil.
- **6% dilution** means 60 to 72 drops of essential oil diluted in 1 oz of carrier oil.
- **10% dilution** means 100 to 120 drops of essential oil diluted in 1 oz of carrier oil.

Average Therapeutic Dilution Guidelines

- **Adults:** Average dosing dilutions for adults are from 4 to 6% of essential oil to carrier oil.
- **Children:** Pediatric dosing is 0.5% to 2%. 0.5% to 1% from two years of age up to seven or eight. 2% for children over seven or eight years old.
- **Animals:** Animal dosing is like that for children. 0.5% to 2%, depending on age and weight. ***Note: Special caution with cats—they metabolize differently and there is possibility of liver toxicity with harsher oils.***

Clinical Strategy Dosing for Adults

- Prevention: 2%
- Restoration: 2 to 4%
- Treatment: 4 to 6%

Dilutions vary depending on the type of oils used and skin sensitivity. More gentle oils may be used in higher percentage dilutions. Children and elders or those with more sensitive skin may require lower percentage dilutions.

✔ **Always test for skin sensitivity on a small area before applying essential oils topically. Unexpected sensitivity or allergic reactions are possible.**

Creating Essential Oil Blends

THE ART OF CREATING AN AROMATHERAPY BLEND in the context of Chinese medicine is the art of combining oils, similar to the way a Chinese herbal prescription would be formulated using a combination of herbs, taking into consideration the nature, taste, channel affinities, and therapeutic actions of the herbs. Likewise, in an essential oil blend, each oil plays its role.

Traditionally, herbal formula-making strategy would assign each herb a job modeled after historical, Confucian court hierarchy:

Principal / Sovereign and Minister

Herbs that address the main issue as determined by the main signs and symptoms; diagnosis and treatment principal based on the CM pattern or five element imbalance.

Assistant / Deputy

Herbs that assist the principal to keep focused on the main issue, or deal with secondary symptoms. They can be added in order to harmonize and/or regulate.

Envoy

Provides directionality toward areas of the body, channels, and organs, and to correct the movement of the Qi, blood, and fluids. For example, ascending for a headache or descending for hypertension, bringing outward to the surface for a skin problem or consolidating inward for a weak constitution.

We apply these same principals of prescription formulation to essential oils by creating blends. An essential oil blend is a combination of essential oils and a carrier oil suitably chosen for a particular purpose which satisfies the treatment principle derived from a diagnosis. The percentage of each ingredient in the blend reflects the degree of emphasis intended for each oil in the formula.

The choice of essential oils for a blend may take into consideration various factors, including their combined aromas, the parts of plants, the therapeutic properties of the individual oils, their chemical constituents, and the relationship of the note of each oil to the area of the body or level of imbalance being addressed.

THE ROLE OF NOTES IN AN ESSENTIAL OIL BLEND

TOP NOTE OILS provide the first impression, tend to be awakening and uplifting, affect unconscious moods, and the Wei Protective level. Added last but first to hit the nose. Usually 20% to 30% of the blend, but the percentage will depend on the intention of the blend. For issues involving exterior conditions like a cold, for example, or when dealing with the skin, nerves, and sinews, or when addressing acute illnesses or pain, then the percentage could be higher.

MIDDLE NOTE OILS give body to the blend. They provide a harmonizing effect, are the bridge between deep and superficial, and they affect the conscious emotions, expression, and the Ying nourishing blood level. Added second, middle notes are usually the biggest percentage of the ingredients: 50% to 60%.

BASE NOTE OILS provide depth to the blend and act as a fixative. They are grounding and centering, affect the temperament, one's intrinsic nature, and the constitution. Added first, usually 10% to 20% of the blend, but dependent on the level of the issue being addressed. For deep level, constitutional, or congenital issues affecting the Yuan Source Qi, the percentage might be greater. It is also important to consider the strength of the aroma. Base oils are often quite strong and can overpower other oils in the blend.

✔ ***Percentages are always flexible depending on the intention of the blend and the desired balance of aromas.***

	TOP NOTE	MIDDLE NOTE	BASE NOTE
Affects	Unconscious Moods	Conscious Emotions	Temperment Constitution
Provides	First Impression	Body, Harmonizing	Depth, Fixative
Role	Awakening, Uplifting	Bridge between Deep & Superficial	Grounding, Centering
Added	Last, but first to hit the nose	Second	First

Frequency of Application Guidelines for Blends

Jeffrey Yuen prefers to formulate a blend with a top, a middle, and a base note in order to address the whole individual within the context of their life. His suggested average application frequency for blends which contain all three notes is twice per day for three days, then take three days off and repeat for a total of eighteen days, at which point the blend is adjusted if continued treatment is needed.

For acute conditions which require immediate attention and are expected to resolve quickly, more frequent applications per day but overall a shorter course of treatment—on average three days—is expected to be sufficient.

For chronic conditions requiring long term use, application is one or two times per day, three days on, and three off. Blend formulas should be rotated every eighteen days. Re-evaluate after three months.

The Math: Determining Percentages and Numbers of Drops

First decide what total quantity is needed—1 oz for example. Next, determine what total dilution percentage is appropriate for the particular case, and then, within the total, what percentage of each oil in the blend satisfies your goal. Finally, calculate how many drops of each oil to mix into the chosen carrier oil.

For example:

To create a 4% dilution (40 to 48 total drops in 1 oz of carrier oil), do the math to determine how many drops of each oil to combine. Math can be done simply by moving the decimal point in your percentage number, in which case 50% of a 4% dilution becomes 5 x 4 which equals 20 drops. In this example we are formulating a blend of three oils: one top, one middle, and one base note.

Middle note oil 70%:	7 x 4 = 28 drops
Top note oil 20%:	2 x 4 = 8 drops
Base note oil 10%:	1 x 4 = 4 drops
	Total = 40 drops in 1 oz of carrier oil

To create a 6% dilution (60 to 72 total drops in 1 oz of carrier oil), multiply by 6. In this case, we are formulating a blend of four oils: two middle, one base, and one top note.

Middle note oil 50%:	5 x 6 = 30 drops
Middle note oil 30%:	3 x 6 = 18 drops
Base note oil 5%:	0.5 x 6 = 3 drops
Top note oil 15%:	1.5 x 6 = 9 drops
	Total = 60 drops in 1 oz of carrier oil

Case Study Example

One case example is that of a thirty-three-year-old woman with depression three months after the death of her father. She doesn't want to get out of bed, has a poor appetite (loss of appetite for life), along with obsessive thoughts of guilt and remorse. In short, she is having difficulty letting go and moving on.

This is primarily a Ying level imbalance dealing with the emotions. It is a 6% dilution (60 drops in 1 oz of carrier oil).

Base Note: Mei Gui Hua (Rose) 10% – 1 x 6 = 6 drops
Heart, Liver, and Kidney affinities.
Assists recovery from emotional trauma. Thorns address wind, ability to change.
Flowers inspire feelings of nourishment, beauty, love, reaching for the divine and transcendence.

Middle Note: Hou Po (Magnolia Bark) 45% –4.5 x 6 = 27 drops
Lung, Large Intestine, Stomach, and Spleen affinities.
Neuroprotective, addresses mood swings, fright palpitations, depression, pain. Barks represent protection. Spleen affinity deals with pensiveness and obsession. Lung affinity deals with grief, loss, and guilt. Descends the Lung Qi to the Kidneys to help regain vitality and motivation.

Middle Note: Song Zhen (White Pine) 25% – 2.5 x 6 = 15 drops
Lung and Kidney affinities.
Aids and eases the dying process, for the one moving on and for those left behind, release of the Po (corporeal soul), letting go and ascension of the Hun (ethereal soul).

Top Note: Fo Shou (Buddha's Hand Fruit) 20% – 2 x 6 = 12 drops
Liver, Lung, Stomach, Spleen affinities.
Relieves emotional indigestion, poor appetite.
Fruits and peels allow for release of what is pent up inside to the exterior, and the full expression of one's nature, unencumbered by the past.

Carrier Oil: Jojoba oil – Nourishes blood, a good carrier for perfumes to allow the rose aroma to come out.

Dosage Guidelines for Homemade Applications

Here are some ideas for essential oil applications using safe and commonly accepted dosages and dilutions. Dosages may vary dependent on skin sensitivity, age, constitution, severity of condition, and treatment goal (prevention, maintenance, or therapeutic). Care should always be taken to avoid irritation especially with spicy oils and oils with ketones. The following are average dosages. You are encouraged to experiment for yourself and to discover the oils and dosages that work best for you or your patients.

- **Aroma lamp:** 3-10 drops.
- **Body/facial oils:** 15-20 drops per 2 oz of carrier (1%).
- **Bath oils:** 40-50 drops per 2 oz of carrier (2%). 1 tsp per bath. Mix with an emulsifier to evenly blend oil and water. For example, with 1/2 to 1 cup of full fat dairy milk, cream, or soy milk.
- **Bath salts:** 10-20 drops per 1/2 cup of Tibetan sea salt, Epsom salt, etc. (0.5-1%).
- **Candles:** 30-50 drops to 4 oz of wax.
- **Cleansing mask**: 4-8 drops added to clay or clay powder and water.
- **Compresses**: A compress is applied warm and may be allowed to cool if less heat is required or kept warm with a hot water bottle over the compress. Retain the compress for approximately 20 minutes each time. Dosage and application method are dependent on the condition being treated and the sensitivity of the patient's skin. In order of increasing strength:
    1. 10-20 drops of the oil or blend of oils, neat, in 1 pint of warm water, soak flannel cloth and apply over the area.
    2. Soak flannel cloth in a diluted oil or blend, seal in a plastic bag, immerse in hot water, remove the warm cloth and apply over the area.
    3. Gently spread 3 drops of the diluted oil or blend directly on the skin over the area, place a warm, soft cloth over it with or without a hot water bottle.
- **Dermatological oils:** 60 drops per 2 oz of carrier (3%) for skin conditions.
- **Diffuser:** 5-10 drops for most diffusers. Dosage depends on size of receptacle.

- **Douche:** 3-5 drops per quart of water and vinegar (1-2 tbsp white vinegar to 1 quart water).
- **Exfoliant:** 1-2% essential oils in papaya or pineapple juice which contain enzymes that aid exfoliation.
- **Foot bath:** 6-8 drops with emulsifier such as Epsom salt, alcohol, vinegar per quart of water.
- **Gargle/mouthwash:** 1-2 drops in 1/4 cup warm honey water or light saline solution.
- **Hair oil:** 50 drops to 2 oz jojoba carrier oil (2.5%).
- **Inhalation:** 5 drops in 1-2 pints of steaming hot water.
- **Hand sanitizer:** 2/3 alcohol (ethanol 70% or higher) and 1/3 aloe vera gel as the base with 2-4% essential oils.
- **Liniments:** 30 drops in 1 oz (3%) in ethyl alcohol (vitalizes blood), vinegar (decalcifies, relieves pain), witch hazel (astringent, anti-inflammatory).
- **Lymphatic massage oil:** 40 drops per 1 oz carrier (4%).
- **Massage oils:** 25 drops per 2oz of carrier (1%). May vary depending on the chosen oils for specific therapies.
- **Nasal wash:** 1-2 drops in light saline solution for use in a Neti Pot or Navage. Mix oil and salt before adding water.
- **Salves:** 3% dilution (60-68 drops essential oils per 1/4 cup of salve base). Base: 2 tbsp melted beeswax, 2 tbsp coconut oil, 2 tbsp shea butter, 1/4 cup jojoba or sweet almond oil.
- **Shampoo:** 50 drops to 4oz shampoo.
- **Sitz bath:** 15-30 drops of diluted oil or blend in basin of water. Emulsifier depending on the use.
- **Spray:** 10-12 drops in one cup of distilled water or 50% water and 50% ethyl alcohol. Shake before spraying.
- **Suppositories/boluses:** 10-20 drops in 1/4 cup coconut oil or cocoa butter (1-2% dilution). Keep refrigerated to solidify. Cut into small cubes. For rectal suppositories, bolus must reach the rectal/colon area.
- **Toothaches:** 1% dilution of essential oil in sesame oil on a small wad of cotton or cotton swab soaked with the blend. Apply directly on the affected tooth.
- **Washes:** 6-15 drops per quart of water. Heat water then add oil emulsified with 1 tbsp of vinegar, ethyl alcohol, or other emulsifier depending on the use. Gently apply or spray on the skin.

Carrier Oils and Emulsifiers

CARRIER OILS ARE MILD, USUALLY COLD EXPELLER-PRESSED vegetable oils, and are used as the medium in which one or more essential oils are diluted. They serve the purpose of keeping essential oils from irritating the skin while enhancing the function of the blend.

Saturated oils are more shelf-stable, with jojoba being the most stable of all. Most vegetable oils can become rancid over time (6-12 months) and should be stored tightly closed in a cool, dark, and dry place. Some may need to be refrigerated. More stable oils such as jojoba, vitamin E, or wheat germ oils may be added to extend shelf life. A rancid carrier will ruin the effects of an essential oil blend.

Emulsifiers allow oils to mix evenly in water or other liquids. They are useful when making sprays or lotions, for example.

Tips for Mixing Essential Oils and Carrier Oils

To make an essential oil dilution or diluted blend, first combine the number of drops of essential oil needed to achieve the percentage of dilution, then add the desired quantity of carrier oil and mix with intention.

Using Jeffrey Yuen's dilution method as the guide:

- A 1% dilution is 10 to 12 total drops of essential oil in 1 oz of carrier oil.
- By extension then, for example, to make a 4% dilution, combine 40 to 48 drops of essential oils in a 1 oz glass bottle then add the appropriate carrier oil and mix well.
- With floral essential oils, the carrier should be light, like jojoba or rapeseed for example.
- To make a gao/paste/ointment, use something with a thick consistency, such as coconut oil, cocoa butter, shea butter or honey. Add beeswax to thicken.
- To make a bolus for suppositories, use beeswax or coconut oil as a carrier (they melt with body heat, but are solid at cool temperatures or refrigerated). For example, a bolus can be made with 1% She Chuang Zi (Cnidium Fruit) essential oil for vaginal yeast infections.
- To draw out, one method is to make a paste by mixing essential oils with the powdered, raw herb of Ge Gen (Kudzu Root), or Yi Yi Ren (Coix seed), or with green clay powder. For example: to draw out and dry up pustular swellings or insect bites, Jeffrey Yuen suggests Bai Zhi (*Angelica dahurica*) essential oil as a 2% dilution in sesame oil (20 to 24 drops of Bai Zhi to 1 oz of sesame oil) mixed with green clay powder and applied directly over the affected area.

Carrier Oils

Bai Zi Ren – Biota Seed

Cold expeller-pressed Platycladus orientalis

Yuan level

Biota seed is used in essential oil dilutions and blends where nourishing the Heart and calming the Spirit is the focus. As such, it is helpful in cases of insomnia, anxiety, or irritability including when there is deficient Yin, or menopausal night sweating. Bai Zi Ren oil is a good carrier choice for a formulation benefiting the Qi and blood. Also, consider for blends when descending the Lung Qi is the goal, as in coughing, wheezing, or asthma, for example. Bai Zi Ren also moistens the intestines for constipation. This oil has a very slight evergreen aroma.

Shi Liu Zi – Pomegranate Seed Oil

CO2-extracted

Ying level

Balancing and nourishing for the skin. Contains omega 5 fatty acids. Supplements the Yin and the Ye/Thick body fluids including hormonal secretions. Internal ingestion for blood sugar regulation and to nourish Yin. Beneficial to heart health and helps to remove cholesterol. Reduces oxidative stress and aids chelation of heavy metals. Apply topically with mucolytic essential oils (those containing ketones or phenols) to break up fatty deposits, break down adipose tissue, and to promote fluid metabolism. For example: combine with Hu Lu Ba (Fenugreek) essential oil to break down adipose, fatty tissue, and cellulite.

Zi Su Zi – Perilla Seed

Cold expeller-pressed Perillae fructescens Fructus

Ying level

An excellent carrier oil for essential oils and blends when the lungs, large intestine, and respiratory system are the focus. As a Chinese medicinal herb, its function is to stop coughing and wheezing by dissolving phlegm and directing the Lung Qi downward. It is widely used in traditional herbal formulas for asthmatic and cough conditions of various types, for example with essential oils of Song Zhen (Pine), Yun Shan (Spruce), or An Shu Ye (Eucalyptus). Perilla seed is moistening and lubricates the intestines and so would be useful in blends for dryness and constipation. The aroma of Zi Su Zi cold-pressed oil is subtle and slightly nutty.

Black Cumin Seed – Black Seed

Cold expeller-pressed Nigella sativa

Ying level

Cumin seed is antispasmodic and relaxing. It clears heat in the blood and lowers blood pressure. A useful carrier for blends addressing menopausal symptoms. Aids digestion. Recently, human studies have shown benefits for relief of indigestion and heartburn. Breaks up mucus and stagnation. Thymoquinone, a major chemical component of *Nigella sativa*, has been extensively studied for its pharmacological benefits. Numerous research studies have shown anti-inflammatory, antioxidant, antimicrobial, antiviral, anticancer, and immune-enhancing properties.

Calophyllum – Tamanu

Cold expeller-pressed

Ying level

Balances the skin. Breaks up stagnation. This oil has strong antiviral, antibacterial, anti-inflammatory, and antineuralgic properties. It is healing and regenerating for the skin. For example, calophyllum may be considered in blends when clearing pathogenic factors and regenerating healthy skin is the goal, as in cases of herpes or shingles. Calophyllum is antifibrotic and mucolytic, which means it helps to break up mucus and phlegm accumulation, fibrotic tissue, clusters, and decongest the lymphatic system. It has some similar properties to castor oil but is gentler.

Sweet Almond Oil – Nan Xing Ren

Wei level

Balanced and gentle for the skin. A good all-purpose oil. Absorbs quickly. Useful for Wei level imbalances with top note oils. An appropriate carrier oil for blends to address the lungs and exterior wind syndromes.

Castor Oil – Ba Ma Zi

Ying level

Mucolytic, breaks up mucus and phlegm, clears the lymphatic system, breaks up fibrotic tissue and stagnation. For example, it provides a good base for a compress with essential oils to break up uterine fibroids, or for congestion or stones in the Gallbladder with essential oils of Yin Chen Hao (*Artemisia scoparia*), Zhi Zi (Gardenia Fruit), and Qing Pi (Green Tangerine Peel). Nan Mu (Cedarwood) is one option with castor oil to clear lymph congestion.

Calendula-Infused Oil or Ointment – Jin Zhan Hua

Wei level

Healing, cooling, antiviral. Good in blends to apply on burns, irritations, herpes sores, etc. Use as an ointment with Yin Chen Hao (*Artemisia scoparia*) and Xun Yi Cao (Lavender) for burns or with Qing Hao (*Artemisia annua*) for herpes.

Argan Oil

Wei level

Regulates pH balance in the skin. Works well as both a cleanser and a moisturizer. A good carrier for blends addressing skin repair and protection.

Coconut Oil – Ye Zi

Ying level

Contains saturated fatty acids, therefore is quite stable at room temperature. A balanced, gentle, multipurpose oil. Nourishing, provides a good base for blends to tonify the Yin, for example with Mei Gui Hua (Rose) or Mo Li Hua (Jasmine), and Wu Wei Zi (*Schisandra Fruit*) or Bai Zi Ren (Biota Seed).

Cod Liver Oil – Xue Yu Gan

Ying level

Aids processing by the liver. Breaks down fats. Use Hu Lu Ba (Fenugreek) essential oil with cod liver oil to break up belly fat and cellulite, combine these with Wu Wei Zi (*Schisandra Fruit*) and vigorously apply over the waistline area, then compress with a hot washcloth to insulate the heat. To increase libido, use cod liver oil as the carrier with She Chuang Zi (Cnidium Fruit) essential oil.

Grapeseed Oil – Pu Tao Zi

Wei level

Drying effect on the skin, absorbs quickly, astringent. For Wei level imbalances. Use as a carrier with top note oils and blends where top notes are prominent as in acute illnesses or formulations for rash, itching, or damp skin conditions. A good alternative to almond oil for those with nut allergies.

Hazelnut Oil – Zhen Zi

Ying level

Moistening for the skin and nourishing for the eyes. A great carrier for blends addressing eye conditions. Moistens and draws out.

Jojoba Oil – He He Ba

Ying level

Has a very stable shelf life. Nourishes blood. One of the best carrier oils for perfume. Balancing for the skin. Nourishing for the Jin/Thin body fluids which moisten the skin and sense organs like the eyes and nasal passages. Good for oily skin, clears sebaceous glands by encouraging full release.

Hemp Oil – Ma You

Yuan level

Enters the blood brain barrier. Breaks up plaque in the brain. A good carrier for brain disorders related to aging such as Alzheimer's or to guide blends to the brain.

Olive Oil – Lan

Ying level

Nourishes blood, moistens skin. A good carrier for blends addressing blood deficiency with essential oils such as Gou Qi Zi (Goji Berry), Dang Gui (*Angelica sinensis*), Bai Zi Ren (Biota Seed), or to benefit the skin for dryness and rashes due to blood deficient wind. It also nourishes the Liver blood and calms Liver wind. Contains mostly monounsaturated fatty acids and therefore is fairly stable at room temperature.

Palm Oil – Zong Lu

Wei level

Contains saturated fatty acids (like coconut oil) and is therefore quite stable at room temperature. It is called resilient, hardy, and tolerant. Helps to carry intention for therapeutic massage treatment.

Papaya and Pineapple Juices

Wei Level

Contain enzymes that are helpful to exfoliate the skin along with citrus peel essential oils such as Qing Pi (Green Tangerine Peel).

Rapeseed Oil – Yun Tai Zi

Ying level

Very stable shelf life. Good carrier for perfume. Non-greasy, light and smooth as a massage oil carrier. High in omega 3, 6, and 9. Rich in Vitamin K, E, and antioxidants.

RICE BRAN OIL – MI KANG

Wei and Ying level

Benefits the skin and the eyes. Its vitamin E content helps to prevent rancidity when storing oils. Vitamin E is an antioxidant, important in cell maintenance, repair, and anti-aging. A good, gentle, all-purpose oil.

SAFFLOWER OIL – HONG HUA

Ying level

Moves blood. It is derived from the same plant as the Chinese medicine herb Hong Hua (*Carthami Flos*). Good for blends where relieving pain and invigorating the blood is the goal, such as for menstrual pain with Chuan Xiong (*Ligusticum wallichii*) and Dang Gui (*Angelica sinensis*), and for injuries or cardiovascular issues.

SESAME OIL – ZHI MA

Yuan level

Moistening for the skin. Nourishing for the Kidneys and Jing Essence. Use as a carrier oil for blends addressing constitutional issues: Kidney deficiency, sexual dysfunction, infertility, supporting the aged, etc. Swish 1-2 tablespoons sesame oil in mouth with 1 drop of Ding Xiang (Clove), Mo Yao (Myrrh), or Ju Hua (Chrysanthemum) for "oil pulling" to draw out toxins, protect teeth, or oral cavity pain. Rub on the gums with 1 drop of Ju Hua (Chrysanthemum) for pain, toothache, periodontal disease, or inflammation.

WALNUT OIL – HE TAO

Ying level

Moistening for the skin. Nourishes blood. Based on the Doctrine of Signatures, the walnut is used in Chinese medicine to benefit the kidneys and brain. The shape of the walnut, with its two hemispheres, is a reflection of the hemispheres of the brain and of the two kidneys. Consequently, walnut oil is a good choice for blends addressing the Yuan level, the constitution and the marrow.

Emulsifiers

Alcohol

Use an edible ethyl alcohol, such as grain alcohol or other neutral spirits. Isopropyl/rubbing alcohol is not recommended due to its strong odor. Alcohol vitalizes the blood. Use in blends to increase circulation and ease pain as a liniment or to emulsify essential oils for a spray with distilled water (50% alcohol, 50% water).

Egg White

Albumin has a similar crystal structure to that found in the central nervous system, such as in cerebrospinal fluid. Use as a carrier to gravitate an essential oil blend to the Central Nervous System. Dries on the skin and may be applied as a paste to hold an essential oil or blend on the skin. Used this way it has a drawing out effect.

Honey

Nourishing. A good emulsifier for internal ingestion. Soothing for the mucus membranes. Directs essential oils and dietary therapy to the uterus.
Dark honey nourishes Yuan Source Qi—**Red honey** nourishes blood.

Lecithin (Soy, Sunflower, etc.)

A useful emulsifying and lubricating agent for blends containing oil and water or other liquids. As an example, it provides a smooth consistency for lotions. Source of essential fatty acids and phosphatidylcholine. On average, add 0.5% to 1% of liquid lecithin by weight. Combine the oils with lecithin first before adding water.

Vinegar

Use as a carrier with essential oils to make a liniment for pain, tendonitis, bursitis, etc. Decalcifies, use for blends addressing calcification of joints, bunions, etc. A good carrier for antifungal preparations or yeast infections. Mildly acidic and astringent. Cleansing and toning. White or apple cider vinegar.

Yogurt, Milk

Use with appropriate essential oils to promote clear complexion and eliminate dark spots such as: Bai Zhi (*Angelica dahurica*), Bai Yu Lan Ye (Magnolia Leaf), Jin Yin Hua (Honeysuckle), Mei Gui Hua (Rose), or Mo Li Hua (Jasmine). Keep refrigerated. Milk is soothing and nourishing as an emulsifier for bath oils. Full fat milk or cream works best. Soy milk can also be used to emulsify oils.

Salt

Combine essential oils with salt to:

- Create a bath salt.
- Dissolve masses. For example, a saline solution with essential oils to reduce polyps.
- Promote a drawing out effect. Make a saltwater blend by adding essential oils, shake well, and rub on skin.
- Awaken the senses as a smelling salt for inhalation with essential oils that open the sensory orifices such as: Long Nao (*Borneolum*), Zhang Nao (White Camphor), Su He Xiang (Styrax), Xi Xin (Asarum).
- Warm, invigorate, and stimulate Yang Qi. Add a diluted essential oil or blend to coarse salt, wrap in a cloth, and rub onto the skin along a channel or area.

Types of salt:

- **Land salts:** invigorating, more Yang, absorbs the sun's energy.
- **Sea salts:** nourishing, calming, more Yin, Water Element.
- **Mineral salts:** detoxifying, drawing out, cooling, moving. Epsom salt (magnesium sulfate) or Mang Xiao (Mirabilitum).

Witch Hazel

An astringent with anti-inflammatory, antibacterial, and antiviral properties. It may be used in blends for leakages, such as bleeding and discharges. It can also be used for swellings or varicose veins. It dries dampness and energetically anchors downward. It is often used topically for acne, insect bites, poison ivy, or to tighten the skin. Useful as a carrier for blends to treat swollen joints with Yi Yi Ren (Coix) and Yun Shan (Black Spruce) essential oils for example.

DMSO

Helps to drive essential oils into an area. Especially good for arthritic pain. Considered to be anti-inflammatory and analgesic for nerve pain such as shingles or nerve blockage. Also, a muscle relaxant. May be used topically for amyloidosis, keloid scars, as well as scleroderma, bunions, calluses, and foot fungus.

✔ **Caution may cause rash. Test for sensitivity.**

Part Two

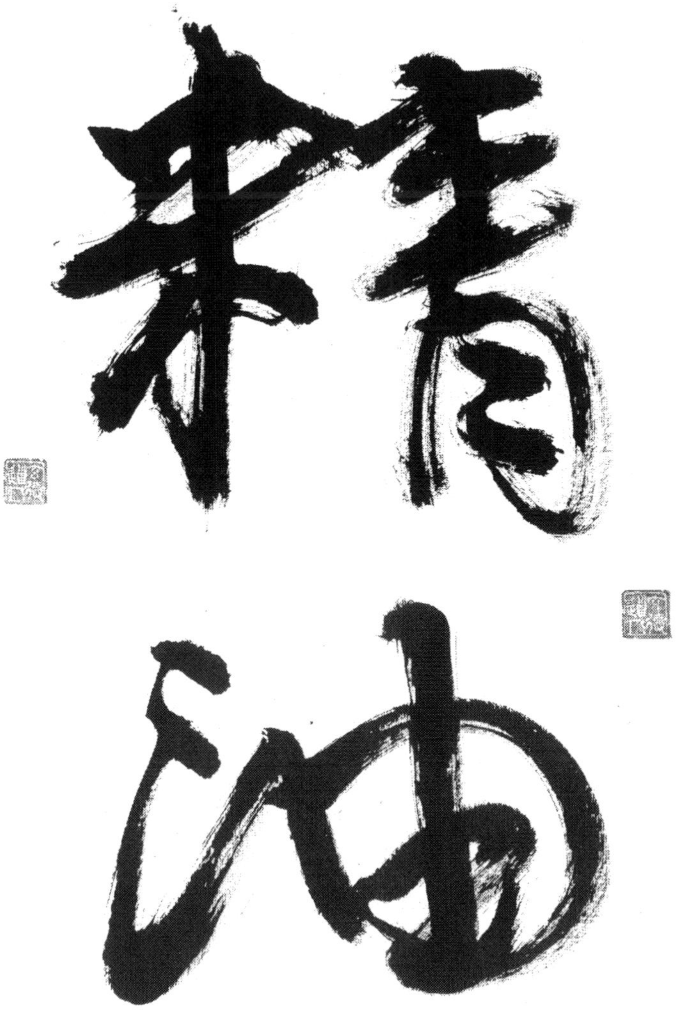

Calligraphy by Jeffrey Yuen

Jing You - Essential Oil

Materia Medica

Chinese Medicine Essential Oils
Materia Medica and Reference Guide

The following monographs of essential oils are a synthesis of notes compiled from Jeffrey Yuen's lectures along with my own and other practitioners' clinical experience, as well as information taken from traditional Chinese medicine materia medica, acupuncture, and aromatherapy sources, including the producers of the oils. Resources for chemical component analysis are compiled from testing done by independent labs, analysis reports from extractors and distillers, and research articles.

The framed section in each oil's entry presents its basic characteristics, in a manner accessible to the lay and professional audience alike. In the 'Actions and Indications' sections, I have attempted to blend user-friendly, commonly understood terms with Chinese medicine concepts, many of which are explained in the 'Chinese Medicine Concepts Explained' chapter of this book. The oils are arranged in alphabetical order by their Chinese pinyin names for ease of searching. At the back of the book there are pinyin/botanical/common English alternate name indexes for those who are unfamiliar with the Chinese names.

Many of the treatment strategies presented are from Jeffrey Yuen's teachings and from my understanding of those teachings. Strategies are also drawn from my own and other practioners' experience with the clinical application of essential oils. Dilution percentages suggested are, by and large, fairly conservative for safety. Whether you are a practitioner or an individual essential oil lover, you are encouraged to test the oils yourself, work interactively with your patients, play with the blends presented, and create your own blends as you gain experience with the oils. In other words, create your own materia medica. Where space allows, lines are provided for your notes.

The acupuncture points mentioned are not fixed-point prescriptions but rather intended as ideas using the types of points that resonate with essential oils because of their connection to the Yuan Source Qi. Practitioners are urged to come up with their own ideas based on the relationships that they have developed with the points and what works for them. It is my hope that non-practitioners will explore using essential oils on the points and channel systems. There are many excellent resources available that describe their indications and locations.

Where the major chemical components are listed, a bracketed number refers to an endnote at the back of the book, providing points of interest from research.

When you see the phrase, "create an aromatic blend," this means to encourage the aromatherapist, or practitioner and patient, to experiment with the oils and to collaborate on blending oils to produce an aroma that has the desired psycho-physical, emotional, mental, or spiritual impact when inhaled.

In this materia medica, you will notice I quote from *The Shen Nong Ben Cao Jing/The Divine Farmer's Materia Medica Classic.* I am aware that the original "Divine Farmer," the Daoist alchemist naturalist, Shen Nong, and later, Tao Hong Jing—a Daoist shaman and herbal physician of the Shang Qing School who compiled and organized Shen Nong's work—were not writing about essential oils. However, their understanding of the herbs came from a highly cultivated, deeply personal and experiential connection to nature and to the essence and spirit of the plants. For that reason, their impressions seem to resonate with the essential oils, and their descriptions enhance the information presented here with a connection to the Daoist roots of Chinese medicine.

Ai Ye 艾葉 / Qi Ai 蕲艾

MUGWORT LEAF

Artemisiae argyi Folium

Ai Ye is called "Yang within blood," Blood is a Yin substance like all of the fluids of the body including secretions such as hormones, which are a product of the Ye aspect of the Jin Ye (thin and thick fluids). Production and regulation of the blood and fluids is the job of the Yang Qi. Yang is warming and vitalizing while Yin is cooling and nourishing. Yang and Yin need to be balanced in order for the systems of the body to function normally and for metabolic and cyclical processes like the menstrual cycle to be regulated. Ai Ye essential oil with its strong pungent aroma provides Yang energy to warm and regulate the blood and stimulate the production and release of hormones. This Yang energy is also needed to support the Spleen's functions of producing blood and keeping the blood within its banks, preventing it from overflowing. For these reasons, it is widely used in gynecology. Ai Ye essential oil also warms and opens the lungs to free the breath and resolve congestion. When the Lung Qi is dispersing freely, the body fluids will circulate, and the blood will be oxygenated.

Aroma: Herbaceous, pungent, earthy.

Note: Middle.

Part of Plant: Leaf.*

Extraction Method: Distillation.

Color: Light yellow-green.

Growing region: Hubei Province, China. The variety called Qi Ai from Hubei has a stronger aroma and contains more oil than other varieties and its use can be traced back to the Ming Dynasty. Harvested in early June to mid July when the oil is at its peak.

Major Chemical Components: Monoterpene ether oxide: 1-8 cineole (eucalyptol). Monoterpenes: pinene, cymene, phellandrene, camphene. Monoterpene Ketones: camphor. Ketone: artemisia ketone. Sesquiterpenes: selinene, caryophyllene. Monoterpene alcohols: borneol, terpineol. Triterpenoids. Diterpenes.

CM Category: Regulating Blood.

Nature and Taste: Pungent, bitter, warm.

Affinities: Spleen, Liver, Kidney. As an essential oil, also Lung.

Average Dilution: 2-4%.

Cautions and Contraindications: Ketone components, dilute well. Caution for children, cats, and pregnancy.

---

* Artemisia argyi, *in its dried leaf form, is the main ingredient of moxibustion, as is the closely related species of* Artemisia vulgaris.

Pharmacological Actions: Hemostatic, analgesic, antibiotic, antibacterial, antitussive, anti-asthmatic, expectorant, hormonal stimulant, gastrointestinal stimulant, insect repellent.

ACTIONS AND INDICATIONS:

- Warms and regulates the blood and stops irregular or excessive bleeding especially when there is cold and when deficient Spleen Qi is not banking the blood.
- Regulates menstrual bleeding, relieves cramping and pain, treats infertility, when cold is the cause.
- Benefits respiration for cough, phlegm, wheezing, asthma. Soothes skin inflammation, irritation and itching, clears up damp skin conditions such as eczema.
- Effective as insect repellant.
- Benefits the endocrine system, regulates secretion of adrenal, thyroid, and gonadal hormones (TSH, FSH, LH, ACTH) and helps the Kidney Yang to ascend to the pituitary gland to support hypoactive pituitary with symptoms such as poor appetite, low libido, dull headaches, low stamina, and endurance.

CM CONCEPTS, CHANNEL SYSTEMS, AND PATTERNS:

- Open the Du Mai/Governing Vessel.
- Tonify Kidney Yang.
- Regulate blood.
- Warm the channels.

APPLICATION AND BLENDS:

- To make an insect repellant spray, blend Ai Ye with other essential oils that repel insects such as Bi Cheng Qie (Litsea) whose strong lemony scent keeps the bugs away. Make a 4% to 10% dilution, depending on skin sensitivity, using 1/2 ethyl alcohol and 1/2 water as the carrier. Avoid contact with the eyes. Shake well before use.
- Diffuse Ai Ye with Song Zhen (Pine) to treat cough and asthma.
- To treat infertility due to cold in the uterus, deficiency of Kidney Yang, obstruction in the Chong and Ren Mai (Thoroughfare and Conception Vessels), blend Ai Ye 40%, Dang Gui (*Angelica sinensis*) 40%, and Rou Gui (Cinnamon Bark) 20%. Dilute 3% in olive oil and apply a few drops spread over the lower abdomen area of the uterus and ovaries. To increase sperm and egg counts, include Mei Gui Hua (Rose). Apply three days on and three days off.
- Ai Ye treats a variety of bleeding disorders including:
  - Profuse menstrual bleeding due to deficiency and cold, combine Ai Ye 45% with Gan Jiang (Dry Ginger) 10% and Wu Wei Zi (*Schisandra Fruit*) 45%. 10% dilution in Bai Zi Ren (Biota Seed) cold-pressed carrier oil. Apply on acupoints that stop uterine bleeding, warm the uterus and strengthen the Yuan Source Qi such as on SP1, LR1, LR6, CV4, CV3, ST29, BL20, BL32.
  - For nosebleed, coughing with blood, combine Ai Ye with Ce Bai Ye (Biota Leaf) equal parts, 20% dilution in grapeseed oil. Apply on LU6, LI2, ST44.

An Shu Ye 桉樹葉

EUCALYPTUS LEAF

Eucalyptus globulus and *Eucalyptus radiata Folium*

Eucalyptus essential oil, with its strong, pungent aroma and anti-infective, decongestant properties make it an excellent addition to diffusions and chest rubs for colds, sinus congestion, coughs, and respiratory infections. It effectively breaks up mucus and phlegm including swollen lymph glands. Diffusing Eucalyptus in the sick room can quickly resolve seemingly serious deep coughs, wheezing and difficult breathing. For adults and cold conditions use *Eucalyptus globulus*. For children, or conditions with more heat and fever, use *Eucalyptus radiata*, which tends to be more gentle and cool-natured.

Aroma: Strong, pungent, camphorous.

Note: Top/Middle.

Part of Plant: Leaf.

Extraction Method: Distillation.

Color: Clear.

Growing Region: Guangdong, Hainan, Yunnan, and Fujian Provinces, China.

Major Chemical Components: Monoterpene ether oxide: 1-8 cineole (eucalyptol) [1]. Monoterpenes: pinene, phellandrene, limonene. Aldehyde (benzaldehyde): cuminaldehyde.

CM Category: Releasing the Exterior.

Nature and Taste: Spicy, warm.

Affinities: Lung, Stomach.

Average Dilution: 4-6%.

Cautions and Contraindications: Contraindicated for cats. Caution for adults with a history of seizure disorders. For acute care, not for long term use.

Pharmacological Actions: Antiviral, antimicrobial, antibacterial, antifungal, mucolytic, antitussive decongestant, antipyretic, anti-inflammatory, diuretic.

Actions and Indications:

- Releases exterior wind-cold to resolve colds with chill and fever, headache, body ache, thin mucus, and nasal congestion.
- Treats respiratory infections, cough, dyspnea, copious mucus, and thick-colored phlegm congestion.
- Breaks up congestion in the lymphatic system.

Application and Blends:

- Diffuse alone or with other essential oils 15-20 drops total of essential oils in the diffuser.
- As a chest rub, dilute 4-6% in almond oil and apply over the lung area. Blend with other essential oils depending on the nature of the condition. For example: wind-cold use Eucalyptus (*Eucalyptus globulus)* with Jing Jie (*Schizonepeta*), and Gui Zhi/Gui Ye (Cinnamon Twig and Leaf) 4% dilution; wind-heat use Eucalyptus (*Eucalyptus radiata)* with Bo He (Peppermint) and Xun Yi Cao (Lavender) 4-6% dilution; cough and phlegm congestion with Zi Su Ye (Perilla Leaf) and Song Zhen (Pine) 6% dilution.
- For nasal congestion blend Eucalyptus with Xi Xin (Asarum), and Bai Zhi (*Angelica dahurica*) 10% dilution in grapeseed or almond oil applied on LI4, LI20, BL3.

NOTES:

Bai Dou Kou 白豆蔻

ROUND CARDAMOM

Amomi rotundus Fructus, Amomum krervanh

THIS SHARP AROMATIC SPICE CUTS THROUGH DAMPNESS that weighs down the body and clouds the mind. Just a whiff of its strong aroma is enough to clear fuzzy thinking or settle an upset stomach. It helps clear obsessive thoughts and emotions that often accompany sluggish digestion and metabolism, poor concentration, and fatigue. It does this by energizing the Earth and Metal elements, restoring proper transformation and transportation of foods and fluids, and increasing respiratory capacity. The small round fruit of *Amomum rotundus* doesn't look like much from the outside but break open its shell and the crushed seeds inside explode with strength.

Aroma: Strong menthol-like with sharp spice.

Note: Middle.

Part of Plant: Fruit.

Extraction Method: CO2 extraction.

Color: Yellow-orange.

Growing Region: India, Sri Lanka.

Major Chemical Components: Monoterpene ether oxide: 1-8 cineole. Monoterpene: pinene, terpinene. Monoterpene alcohol: terpineol. Sesquiterpenes: humulene, caryophyllene.

CM category: Aromatic Transforming Dampness.

Nature and Taste: Acrid, warm, aromatic.

Affinities: Lung, Spleen, Stomach.

Average Dilution: 4-6%.

Pharmacological Actions: Digestive, stomachic, anti-reflux, antiemetic, decongestant, antiviral, antibacterial, antispasmodic, deodorant

Actions and Indications:

- Moves the Qi and dissolves dampness for interior and exterior syndromes.
- Regulates the digestive Qi and strengthens the spleen and stomach function to improve poor appetite, relieve nausea, vomiting, reflux, fullness, distention, and pain.
- Relieves morning sickness.
- Descends the Qi of Stomach and Lung and resolves chest congestion.
- Treats flu-like conditions with digestive and respiratory symptoms.
- Transforms dampness to resolve summer heat conditions.

APPLICATION AND BLENDS:

- To transform accumulation of dampness in the middle burner due to dysfunction of Spleen and Stomach Qi, with epigastric and abdominal fullness, distention, and poor appetite, combine equal parts Bai Dou Kou with Cang Zhu (Atractylodes), Hou Po (Magnolia Bark) and Chen Pi (Aged Tangerine Peel) as a 4-6% dilution in black cumin seed oil to gently rub on the abdomen.

- For exterior wind-damp flu-like conditions with both digestive and respiratory symptoms, chest congestion, feeling of heaviness in the body, mild feverishness, poor appetite, nausea, vomiting, or diarrhea, combine Bai Dou Kou 35%, Zi Su Ye (Perilla Leaf) 40%, and Zhi Ke (*Citrus aurantium*) 25%. Dilute 4-6% in black cumin seed carrier oil. Apply on chest and stomach areas as well as on points such as LU7, LI4, ST40. For children, dilute 0.5 to 1% for under seven years old, 2% for seven to fourteen years.

- To make a children's "tummy rub" to warm and strengthen digestive function and treat indigestion, Bai Dou Kou can be applied as a single oil, diluted in black cumin seed oil to 0.5% to 1% for under seven years old, 2% for seven to fourteen years. Apply a few drops, occasionally, as needed, or three days on and three days off for more persistent issues.

- When obsessive thoughts and emotions affect the digestion, metabolism, and mental clarity, the acrid, transforming aroma of Bai Du Kou can be inhaled neat and applied to acupoints that strengthen the Earth Element to improve the Spleen and Stomach's transformative function. Points may include: SP3, ST40, and the Spleen's Shu Transport point on the outer Bladder channel named Abode of Thought, Yi She, at BL49.

- Bai Dou Kou is an option to relieve morning sickness, either as a single oil or together with Huo Xiang (Patchouli). Use as needed by direct inhalation, neat or diluted according to the expectant mother's preference.

BAI JU HUA 白菊花 / JU HUA 菊花

WHITE CHRYSANTHEMUM

Chrysanthemi morifolium Flos

IN CHINA, BAI JU HUA, THE WHITE CHRYSANTHEMUM FLOWER, represents nobility, elegance, and endurance. Chrysanthemum is hardy and grows abundantly all year round. In essays and poems, writers used the terms "Jade Bone," "Icy Body," and "Pearl Petal" to praise the Chrysanthemum flower. On cold autumn days, when all other flowers fade away, only the chrysanthemum is able to flourish in the harsh winds.

The combination of dainty elegance with strong character describe Ju Hua essential oil's attributes. As a flower oil, it represents the full outward and free expression of one's temperament and beauty. Its strength is in its ability to clear away heat, pressure, inflammation, and infections.

The heady aroma of Ju Hua essential oil is a sweet floral with a clean, sharp edge. Upon inhalation it cools and clears the head and eyes while leaving a fresh taste in the mouth. It benefits the skin, eyes, throat, head, and blood pressure. It is soothing for pent up emotion by providing pathways for release.

The Shen Nong Ben Cao Jing/Divine Farmer's Materia Medica Classic classifies Ju Hua as a superior grade herb and says, "Ju Hua is sweet and balanced. It mainly treats head wind, head dizziness and painful eyes as if they were fit to burst from their sockets, tearing, dead skin and muscles, aversion to wind and damp impediment. Protracted taking may disinhibit the blood and Qi, make the body light, slow aging and prolong life."

Aroma: Light, heady, sweet, with a clean, camphorous, and sharp edge.

Note: Middle.

Part of Plant: Flower.

Extraction Method: CO2 extraction.

Color: Olive-amber.

Growing Region: Tongxiang, Zhejiang Province, and Guilin, Guangxi Province, China. Harvested in November on a sunny day when the aroma is strongest.

Major Chemical Components: Monoterpene alcohols <30%: endo-borneol, isoborneol, alpha-terpineol. Monoterpene ketone: camphor. Ketone: chrysanthenone. Monoterpenes: alpha and beta pinene, camphene. Esters: bornyl acetate, isobornyl acetate. Phenol: thymol.

CM Category: Releasing the Exterior.

Nature and Taste: Sweet, bitter, cool.

Affinities: Lung, Liver.

Average Dilution: 2-4%. Contains ketones which may irritate certain skin types. Dilute and test.

Pharmacological Actions: Antipyretic, anti-inflammatory, antibacterial, antiseptic, antihypertensive, vasodilator, nervine.

ACTIONS AND INDICATIONS:

- Dispels wind-heat for colds or flus with fever, headache, eye redness and pain, sore throat, thirst, respiratory infection.
- Benefits the eyes to relieve pressure, swelling, inflammation.
- Supplements Liver Yin and clears Liver fire and Liver wind with blurry vision, dizziness, headache, high blood pressure, tremors, restlessness, insomnia.
- Heals cuts, wounds, and insect bites.
- Use in dermatology includes psoriasis, eczema, abscesses, ulcerations, sores, inflammation, and regenerative for damaged skin.

CM CONCEPTS, CHANNEL SYSTEMS, AND PATTERNS:

- Expel exogenous wind-heat.
- Nourish Liver Yin.
- Pacify Liver wind.
- Ascend and release outward for Divergent meridian SDS treatment (superficial-deep-superficial needling technique).
- Facilitate Yang Qiao Mai/Yang Heel Vessel treatment.
- Benefit the Abundance Palace of the Nine Palaces.

APPLICATION AND BLENDS:

To dispel wind and heat for colds and flus, combine Ju Hua with equal parts Bo He (Peppermint), Jin Yin Hua (Honeysuckle) and Lian Qiao (Forsythia) as a 4-6% dilution in grapeseed or almond oil, or with ethyl alcohol as a carrier. Diffuse the blend neat into the air and apply diluted to the upper back area around GV12, 13, 14 on the forehead and occipital region. Gua sha may be applied prior to application. 3-6 drops may be added neat to a pint of steaming hot water for steam inhalation with eyes closed.

For dermatological use, to treat psoriasis, eczema, abcesses, ulcerations, sores, or inflammation, combine Ju Hua 40% with Lian Qiao (Forsythia) 40%, and Jing Jie (*Schizonepeta*) 20% as a 3% dilution in grapeseed or calophyllum (tamanu) oil. Apply to the affected areas. If the condition is more damp, with swelling or pustules, replace Jing Jie (*Schizonepeta*) with Yi Yi Ren (Coix Seed) and increase its percentage to equal parts. In order to draw out, combine the carrier oil with green clay powder to make a paste for application on the lesions.

To benefit the eyes, depending on the condition:

- If there is deficiency or the patient is over fifty years old, combine Ju Hua with Hu Luo Bo Zi (Carrot Seed), Man Jing Zi (Vitex), Wu Wei Zi (*Schisandra Fruit*), Du Huo (*Angelica pubescentis*), Gou Qi Zi (Goji Berry), and Xi Xin (Asarum) or Gui Zhi / Gui Ye (Cinnamon Leaf and Twig).
- If younger and there is stagnation, or phlegm accumulation (eye screens), combine Ju Hua with Chai Hu (Bupleurum), Jing Jie (*Schizonepeta*), Su He Xiang (Styrax), Bai Yu Lan Ye (Magnolia Leaf), Chuan Xiong (*Ligusticum wallichii*), and Bai Zhi (*Angelica dahurica*).
- If there is redness, swelling, heat and inflammation, Ju Hua with Jin Yin Hua (Honeysuckle) and Man Jing Zi (Vitex).

Any of the above eye blends may be diluted to 2-3% in a gentle carrier oil such as almond and prepared as a compress over the eye area. Be sure to wring the cloth completely and do not let the oil drip into the eyes. Or steam the eyes with 3-5 drops of the blend in 1 pint of hot water. May also be applied on distal acupoints that affect the eyes such as GB37, LR3, ST36, SI6. Add gentle moxibustion on BL18 for deficiency conditions and for those over fifty years old.

To supplement Liver Yin when there are signs of Liver fire and wind rising up such as blurry vision, dizziness, headache, high blood pressure, tremors, restlessness, and insomnia, create an aromatic blend of Ju Hua 30% with Wu Wei Zi (Schisandra Fruit) 20%, Jiang Xiang (*Dalbergia*) 20%, Mei Gui Hua (Rose) 20%, and Bo He (Peppermint) 10%. Spread a drop of the blend on the temples and on the bottom of the feet. Apply on Liver's Shu Transport point BL18, Liver's Yuan Source point LR3, Pericardium's Luo Connecting point PC6, and on GB20. Deeply inhale the aroma. May be applied neat for occasional acute symptoms. For longer term use, dilute to 4-6% in Bai Zi Ren (Biota Seed) cold-pressed carrier oil.

BAI JU HUA ABSOLUTE 白菊花
HANG BAI JU 杭白菊
WHITE CHRYSANTHEMUM
Chrysanthemi morifolium Flos

BAI JU HUA ABSOLUTE, with its lovely sweet fragrance and smooth, thick consistency makes it an excellent choice for a soothing skin cream. Its cooling, anti-inflammatory, and antiseptic properties help to clear up problem skin such as acne, psoriasis, eczema, allergic reactions, or infections. It is a good choice wherever there is redness and irritation. Additionally, Bai Ju Hua can be applied to calm the nerves, relax the vessels, and bring down high blood pressure.

Aroma: Strong, heady, sweet, floral.

Note: Base.

Part of Plant: Flower.

Extraction Method: Solvent extraction using edible hexane.*

Color: Opaque, dark green.

Growing Region: Tongxiang, Zhejiang province and Guilin, Guangxi province, China. Harvested in November on a sunny day when the aroma is strongest.

Major Chemical Components: Monoterpene alcohol: borneol, isoborneol, a-terpineol. Monoterpene ketone: camphor >3%. Ketone: chrysanthenone. Sesquiterpene: zingiberene, beta-elemene. Ester: Bornyl acetate. Essential fatty acids: palmitic acid, linoleic acid, decanoic acid.

CM Category: Releasing the Exterior.

Nature and Taste: Sweet, bitter, cool.

Affinities: Lung, Liver

Average Dilution: 2-4%. Contains ketones which may irritate certain skin types if not sufficiently diluted.

Pharmacological Actions: Antipyretic, anti-inflammatory, antibacterial, antiseptic, antihypertensive, vasodilator, nervine.

---

* *Although the hexane solvent used is considered edible, absolutes are not recommended for internal consumption.*

Actions and Indications:

Generally, the same for both CO2-extracted Bai Ju Hua (White Chrysanthemum) and Bai Ju Hua Absolute, except that the absolute is solvent-extracted to bring out its perfume fragrance and has a much thicker consistency. Absolutes are usually considered to have more of a base note quality. It's aroma benefits the Home Palace of the Nine Palaces.

Application and Blends:

- For skin conditions, dilute 2-4% in the appropriate carrier. If there is dryness, use shea butter. For wet, weeping, or swollen skin, use green clay powder and grapeseed oil.
- For symptoms of hypertension such as headache, red irritated eyes, and irritability, apply a 4% dilution of Bai Ju Hua in coconut oil on the temples.

NOTES:

Bai Yu Lan Ye 玉蘭葉

MAGNOLIA LEAF

Magnoliae denudata Folium

Bai Yu Lan Ye essential oil is aromatically unique in that it is a leaf with the soft, sweet, comforting aroma of a flower. Its complex spice and citrus tones cut through damp turbidity. Since ancient times in China, the Magnolia has been considered a symbol of purity and planted in temple gardens.

Its Chinese name, White Jade 玉蘭, represents its affinity with the Metal element and, like Jade, it helps to bring about completion of a transformative process. It works with the Lungs to free up the passage of breath and the process of letting go. It assists the Earth element, the Spleen, to clarify thought.

Linalool, a prominent chemical component of Magnolia Leaf essential oil, produces antinociceptive effects. In psychology, this is a factor that increases tolerance for or reduces sensitivity to perceived dangerous or harmful stimuli. Hyper-reactivity to outside stimuli, on the physical level, can result in allergic or pain responses. Psychologically this is a description of the type of nervous reactions seen in Post Traumatic Stress Disorder. Bai Yu Lan Ye calms both types of reactions.

Aroma: Light sweet floral, citrusy, mild spice.

Note: Middle.

Part of Plant: Leaf.

Extraction Method: Distillation.

Color: Clear.

Growing Region: Hunan province, China.

Major Chemical Components: Monoterpene alcohol: linalool [2]. Sesquiterpene: germacrene. Sesquiterpene alcohol: eudesmol. Monoterpene: pinene. Ester: bornyl acetate (an ester of borneol).

CM Category: Transforming Damp, Releasing Exterior Wind.

Nature and Taste: Acrid, bitter, warm, aromatic.

Affinities: Lung, Spleen.

Average Dilution: 4-6%.

Pharmacological Actions: Decongestant, mucolytic, anti-inflammatory, nervine, analgesic, antinociceptive, antifungal, anti-allergic.

Actions and Indications:

- Aromatically transforms dampness.
- Benefits respiration, eliminates wind, cough, phlegm, and congestion.
- Opens sinuses, relieves sinus pressure and headaches.
- Transforms damp terrain to kill parasites and yeast overgrowth.
- Regenerates tissue.
- Eliminates pain, inflammation, hypersensitivity, allergies, and fibromyalgia.
- Treats post-traumatic stress disorder (PTSD).
- Benefits mental clarity, obsessive-compulsive disorder (OCD), and mood disorders.
- Benefits the Global Palace of the Nine Palaces.

Application and Blends:

- Add 1-2 drops to a light saline solution for a nasal rinse to reduce allergic reactivity, nasal and sinus congestion, inflammation, and swelling. May use a neti pot or Navage, for example. To emulsify the oil, mix with salt before adding water.

- As a preventative during allergy season, diffuse Bai Yu Lan Ye and Zi Su Ye (Perilla Leaf) into the air with 10-15 drops of combined essential oils in the diffuser.

- To calm PTSD, create an aromatic blend with Bai Yu Lan Ye, Qi Li Xiang (Orange Jessamine), Jiang Xiang (*Dalbergia*), Mei Gui Hua (Rose), and Xiang Fu (*Cyperus*) for inhalation with deep breaths, to wear as perfume and in the bath. Apply to points of Yin Wei Mai/Yin Link Vessel such as PC6, KI9, LR14.

- Include Bai Yu Lan Ye in blends for fibromyalgia, to reduce hyper-reactivity, cool inflammation, relax the sinews, calm the nerves and the mind, with other essential oils such as Chuan Xiong (*Ligusticum wallichii*), Xun Yi Cao (Lavender), Hu Po (Amber), and Bo He (Peppermint). Create an aromatic 4-6% dilution liniment in ethyl alcohol for topical application.

BAI ZHI 白芷

ANGELICA DAHURICA ROOT

Angelicae dahuricae Radix

THE CHINESE NAME, BAI ZHI 白芷, means "White Analgesic," which refers to the potency of this general pain-relieving essential oil. More specifically, it is famous for relieving pain and pressure on the head and sinuses. The color white in its name means that it especially addresses pain related to the Metal element and the Lungs, which, on an emotional level, have to do with the pain of holding on to grief and loss or guilt and shame. The Lungs open to the skin and the nose. Applied topically, this essential oil promotes clear complexion, lightens dark spots, and treats a variety of skin conditions and irritations. Upon inhalation, its warming, leathery pungent aroma rises upward permeating the frontal sinuses, freeing the breath.

Aroma: Rich, leathery, pungent.

Note: Middle/Base.

Part of Plant: Root.

Extraction Method: CO2 extraction.

Color: Orange-amber.

Growing Region: Eastern Siberia and Northern China

Major Chemical Components: Monoterpenes: pinene, myrcene, sabinene, cymene, limonene, cryptone. Monoterpene alcohol: terpinen-4-ol. Triterpenes. Furanocoumarins.* Alcohol: 1-dodecanol.

CM Category: Releasing Exterior Wind-Cold.

Nature and Taste: Pungent, warm.

Affinities: Lung, Stomach, Spleen.

Average Dilution: 4-6%.

Cautions and Contraindications: Photosensitive, may cause skin irritation in high concentrations when exposed to direct sunlight.

Pharmacological Actions: Analgesic, antispasmodic, anodyne, antidote, antifungal, antibiotic, antiseptic, antimicrobial, anti-inflammatory, carminative, diaphoretic, antipyretic, diuretic, stimulant.

ACTIONS AND INDICATIONS:

- Relieves headaches, especially in the forehead and sinus regions.
- Clears sinus and nasal congestion, relieves swelling, pressure, headache, toothache.

**Furanocoumarins are the chemical component in* Bai Zhi *that causes it to be photosensitive.*

- Expels head wind affecting vision or hearing or causing dizziness.
- Promotes blood circulation.
- Relaxes muscular tension, spasms, and cramps.
- Dermatology: eliminates blemishes, pustular swellings, sores, abscesses, rashes, itching, and insect bites.
- Alleviates breast abscess, lymph congestion, and vaginal discharge.
- Promotes healthy tissue growth.

CM Concepts, Channel Systems, and Patterns:

- Relieves Yang Ming channel headache.
- Expels wind and eliminates dampness.

Application and Blends:

- For headaches especially affecting the Yang Ming (Stomach and Large Intestine channels), whether chronic or acute, blend Bai Zhi 45% with Chuan Xiong (*Ligusticum wallichii*) 45% and Bo He (Peppermint) 10%. Dilute 4-6% in safflower oil for topical application on the affected area of the head and on LI4.
- For nasal congestion and pressure, mix Bai Zhi and Xi Xin neat as a steam inhalation with 5 drops in 1-2 pints of hot, steaming water. May also be applied to LI20, LI4, BL3.
- To promote clear complexion, eliminate blemishes and dark spots, make a paste with essential oils of Bai Zhi 40%, Jin Yin Hua (Honeysuckle) 40%, and Qing Pi (Green Tangerine Peel) 20%. Dilute to 3% in 1 oz coconut oil and milk. Keep in the refrigerator. Apply to skin overnight. To lighten single dark spots, apply directly. Do not expose to sunlight.
- For damp dermatological disorders such as abscesses or pustular swellings, make a paste with grapeseed oil (to dry up) and green clay powder (to draw out). Use Bai Zhi alone or with other essential oils such as Lian Qiao (Forsythia) and Jin Yin Hua (Honeysuckle) to further clear heat toxin, plus a citrus peel top note oil such as Qing Pi (Green Tangerine Peel) to exfoliate. Dilute to 4%. Apply the paste directly on the lesions, cover and keep in place overnight, three days on, three days off.
- To reduce breast abscess and lymph congestion, combine Bai Zhi 30% with E Zhu (*Curcuma zedoaria*) 25%, Lian Qiao (Forsythia Fruit) 15%, Jing Jie (*Schizonepeta*) 15%, and Zhi Ke (*Citrus aurantium*) 15%. Dilute 4-6% in calophyllum. Apply over the local area and associated distal points, two to three times per day, three days on, three days off. A warm compress may be applied.
- To aid the release of painful grief and loss or guilt and shame, create an aromatic blend of Bai Zhi with other essential oils such as: Song Zhen (White Pine), Hou Po (Magnolia Bark), Bai Yu Lan Ye (Magnolia Leaf), Mo Li Hua (Jasmine), and Fo Shou (Buddha's Hand). For deep inhalation and diffusion, to wear as perfume, or use as bath salt.

BAI ZI REN 柏子仁

BIOTA SEED, CHINESE ARBORVITAE, THUJA

Biotae orientalis Semen, Platycladus orientalis

BAI ZI REN ESSENTIAL OIL IS BEST KNOWN FOR ITS ABILITY TO TREAT INSOMNIA. The sweet evergreen aspect of its aroma elicits a sense of quietude, while its bitter base note is grounding. Deep inhalation stimulates the pineal gland, to calm the mind, secrete melatonin, and regulate circadian rhythm. It also has tonifying qualities. It nourishes the Heart blood and boosts the Qi which give one the strength to deal with emotional difficulties and traumatic experiences.

The Shen Nong Ben Cao Jing/Divine Farmer's Materia Medica Classic gave Bai Zi Ren the distinction of an upper grade herb and says it can "treat fright palpitations, quiet the five viscera, boost the Qi, make the body light, and never senile, reduce hunger, sharpen the eyes and ears, render the facial complexion shiny and attractive."

Aroma: Sweet evergreen spice with bitter base notes.

Note: Base.

Part of Plant: Seed.

Extraction Method: Distillation.

Color: Gold.

Growing Region: Shanxi and Shandong provinces.

Major Chemical Components: Sesquiterpene alcohols: cedrol [3], platydiol. Monoterpenes: pinene, carene. Sesquiterpenes: cuparene [4], δ-cadinene. Monoterpene alcohol: linalool.

CM Category: Nourishing the Heart, Calming the Spirit.

Nature and Taste: Sweet, neutral.

Affinities: Heart, Liver, Large Intestine, Lung.

Average Dilution: 6-10%.

Pharmacological Actions: Sedative, nervine, anxiolytic, antioxidant, adaptogenic, antitussive, hemotonic, hemostatic, insulin regulating, vulnerary.

ACTIONS AND INDICATIONS:

- Stabilizes and pacifies to treat insomnia, forgetfulness, fright palpitations, dizziness, disorientation, blood pressure.
- Treats restless organ syndrome, also referred to as Zang Zao or visceral dryness. A state of agitation with frequent crying, depression, anxiety, mood swings, poor sleep, generalized physical discomfort, shakiness, rapid heartbeat, and fatigue.

- Benefits Qi and nourishes blood.
- Strengthens the Will and the Qi to keep moving.
- Opens the Heart, strengthens the Will, treats PTSD.
- Protects and strengthens red blood cells.
- Aids adaptation to internal or environmental stressors.
- Regulates blood sugar to manage diabetes.
- Anchors the Lung Qi to alleviate coughing, wheezing, and asthma.
- Moistens the intestines.
- Regenerative for the skin.

CM Concepts, Channel Systems, and Patterns:

- Open Yin Wei Mai/Yin Link Vessel.
- Treat Zang Zao Visceral Dryness.

Application and Blends:

- For insomnia, Bai Zi Ren may be ingested using 2 drops as a dose with an emulsifier such as Bai Zi Ren cold-pressed carrier oil or honey, as well as diffused in the sleeping room or added to the bath before bed.

- To ease post-trauma, strengthen the Will, conquer fear, and open the Heart, create an aromatic blend of Bai Zi Ren with any combination of: Qi Li Xiang (Orange Jessamine), Bai Yu Lan Ye (Magnolia Leaf), Jiang Xiang (*Dalbergia*), Mei Gui (Rose), and Wu Wei Zi (*Schisandra Fruit*). For inhalation with deep breaths, to wear as perfume, or use in the bath. Apply to points of Yin Wei Mai/ Yin Link Vessel such as PC6 and KI9.

- To regulate blood sugar, combine equal parts Bai Zi Ren with Wu Wei Zi (*Schisandra Fruit*) and Hu Lu Ba (Fenugreek), diluted 4% in pomegranate seed oil, and ingest 1/3 tsp twice per day along with appropriate diet and exercise. Take three days on and three days off. Keep refrigerated.

- As an aid to anchor the Lung Qi to the Kidneys for chronic coughing, wheezing, asthma, and dyspnea with deficiency, blend Bai Zi Ren 25% with Yun Shan (Black Spruce) 40%, Wu Wei Zi (*Schisandra Fruit*) 25%, and Chen Pi (Aged Tangerine Peel) 10%. Diffuse neat, and dilute 10% in cold-pressed Zi Su Zi (Perilla Seed) or sesame seed oil for application on acupoints such as Shu points and Yuan Source points of Lung and Kidney, BL23, BL13, LU9, KI3. Gently spread over the area of the Front Shu points of the Kidney Channel on the chest that affect the Lung, represented by KI24 through KI27.

Bi Cheng Qie 蓽澄茄 / Shan Ji Jiao 山雞椒

LITSEA FRUIT

Litseae cubeba Fructus

Litsea essential oil has a restorative, strengthening effect on the Qi and Yang functions of the body mainly by improving digestion and absorption of vital nutrients. At the same time, its strongly lemon-scented prominent aldehyde component kills germs and insects including ticks and has been used to treat Lyme disease. In Chinese medicine, Bi Cheng Qie is categorized as an herb that warms the interior, while as an essential oil it has the added attribute of being able to draw heat and toxins from deep within the body outward to be released. Litsea essential oil has beneficial effects on the brain and nervous system as well. As an example, it has been shown to help restore post-stroke loss of sensory motor function by topical application on the skull over the affected area of the brain.

Aroma: Bright, strong, sharp, lemon pepper.

Note: Middle.

Part of Plant: Fruit.*

Extraction Method: Distillation.

Color: Gold.

Growing Region: Guangxi and Hunan provinces, China. Harvested in July and August when the fruit turns dark purple to black in color and the oil is abundant.

Major Chemical Components: Monoterpene aldehydes (< 60%): citral, neral, geranial. Sesquiterpene alcohol: cubebol. Monoterpene alcohol: citronellol. Monoterpenes: limonene, pinene, myrcene, camphene. Monoterpene ketone: camphor (> 0.03%).

CM Category: Warming the Interior.

Nature and Taste: Pungent, warm. As essential oil: anti-inflammatory and releases heat to the exterior.

Affinities: CM: Spleen, Stomach, Kidney, Bladder. As essential oil, also Lung, and Liver.

Average Dilution: 4-6%.

Pharmacological Actions: Stimulant, antioxidant, anti-inflammatory, analgesic, antispasmodic, osteopromotive, antimicrobial, antibacterial, antiseptic, antiparasitic, insecticidal, insect repellant, antifungal, carminative, stomachic, antidysenteric, diuretic, expectorant, anti-asthmatic, anticancer [5].

* *Dou Chi Jiang refers to the root and stem of* Litsea cubeba. *It is in the same CM category as the fruit and shares many of the same properties.*

Actions and Indications:

- Strengthens Spleen and Kidney Yang for chronic poor digestion and absorption, "cock's crow" early morning diarrhea, poor appetite, low back weakness and aching. Increases digestive enzyme activity, treats malabsorption syndrome. Inhibits intestinal yeast and bacteria.
- Treats dysentery.
- Relieves pain and spasms of musculoskeletal or smooth muscle tissue, including of the digestive tract and uterus.
- Promotes blood circulation.
- Invigorates Qi and blood in the lower abdomen to relieve dysmenorrhea.
- Expels wind-damp Bi Obstruction with painful swollen joints, and especially when manifesting as pain in the lower back.
- Heals bone fractures, traumatic injury.
- Releases exterior wind-cold with underlying deficiency to resolve lingering colds with strong chills, fever, profuse sweating, muscle aches, and fatigue or asthmatic conditions.
- Goes to the pituitary gland to stimulate Yang Qi.
- Restores loss of function due to brain injury or stroke.

CM Concepts, Channel Systems, and Patterns:

- Clear heat as part of Divergent Meridian SDS (superficial-deep-duperficial needling strategy of drawing heat from the deep, Yuan level out to the surface).

Application and Blends:

- To benefit Spleen and Kidney Yang and general health, apply as a single oil or combine Bi Cheng Qie 50% with Ding Xiang (Clove) 25%, and Chen Pi (Aged Tangerine Peel) 25%. Dilute 4% in black cumin seed oil and apply on Source points and Shu points of Spleen and Kidney channels as well as on the area around the navel. Three days on and three days off.

- To mend broken bones and relieve pain, make a compress of equal parts Bi Cheng Qie with She Chuang Zi (Cnidium Fruit), Hu Lu Ba (Fenugreek), Ce Bai Ye (Biota Leaf), Ru Xiang (Frankincense), and Mo Yao (Myrrh) 4-6% dilution in safflower oil. Apply over the break. Wrap and leave in place overnight, three days on, and three days off.

- To relieve abdominal or muscular spasm and pain, apply a compress of Bi Cheng Qie with Chuan Xiong (*Ligusticum wallichii*), and Xun Yi Cao (Lavender) diluted 10% in safflower or black cumin seed oil for application over the painful area. Or make a liniment using ethyl alcohol as the carrier.

- Bi Cheng Qie with Ai Ye (*Artemisia argyi*) is an effective insect repellant. Equal parts, 4-10% dilution, depending on skin sensitivity, in 1/2 ethyl alcohol and 1/2 distilled water as a spray.
- To restore the loss of sensory motor function, Bi Cheng Qie may be applied as a single oil, diluted 4-6% in sesame oil or other carrier oil and applied on the head over the affected, functional part of the brain such as the speech, vision, or particular motor function centers, three days on and three days off.
- To stimulate the pituitary and Yang Qi, apply as a single oil or with Ai Ye (*Artemisia argyi*). Dilute 4-6% in walnut or sesame oil and apply on points of Du Mai/Governing Vessel including GV20. Moxibustion is applicable.

NOTES:

Bo He 薄荷

PEPPERMINT

Menthae haplocalyx Herba

PEPPERMINT ESSENTIAL OIL'S BRIGHT PUNGENCY IS A TRUE TOP NOTE. It works on the Wei Qi level, venting out what needs to be released, whether it be a cold, a rash, pain, or constrained emotions. Either inhaled or applied on the skin it produces an immediate, refreshing, dispersing, and cooling effect. Its aroma quickly lightens a dark mood and clears the mind.

Aroma: Strong, bright, pungent, minty.

Note: Top.

Part of Plant: Leaf.

Extraction Method: Distillation.

Color: Light golden yellow.

Growing Region: Xinjiang province, China.

Major Chemical Components: Monoterpene alcohol: menthol. Monoterpene ketones: menthone, pulegone. Ester: menthyl acetate. Monoterpene ether oxide: 1-8 cineole (eucalyptol).

CM Category: Releasing Exterior Wind-Heat.

Nature and Taste: Pungent, cool.

Affinities: Lung, Liver.

Average Dilution: 2-8%. Higher dilutions tend to be stimulating. External use only. Not recommended for young children. May cause irritation.

Pharmacological Actions: Antipyretic, antiseptic, anti-inflammatory, antipruritic, diaphoretic, analgesic, antispasmodic, sedative, carminative, hepatoregenerative.

Actions and Indications:

- Dispels wind-heat, resolves fever, headache, sore throat, and congestion.
- Opens the nasal passages. Brightens vision and clears heat from the eyes: eye pain, redness, allergies, inflammation, conjunctivitis, blepharitis.
- Benefits the liver, regenerates liver cells, decongests and smoothes Liver Qi.
- Releases pent up emotions, eases symptoms of PMS.
- Vents rashes, stops itching due to wind-heat, inflammation, eczema, dermatological conditions, measles or bug bites.

CM Concepts, Channel Systems, and Patterns:

- Ascend and release outward for Divergent SDS (superficial-deep-superficial) needling strategy.
- Free constrained Liver Qi

Application and Blends:

- Apply alone, or with other essential oils, diluted in almond oil to dispel wind heat illnesses, and relieve symptoms of common cold such as headache, fever, sore throat and stuffy nose. Bo He may be combined with Jin Yin Hua (Honeysuckle), Lian Qiao (Forsythia), Ju Hua (Chrysanthemum), and Chen Pi (Aged Tangerine Peel) for more feverish flu-like conditions as a 4-6% dilution. Gua sha may be applied on the upper back and occipital area prior to application and apply on points such as LI4 and LU7. For nasal congestion, add LI20. For higher fever or painful sore throat apply on LI1.
- To open the nasal passages and break up congestion, place 3-5 drops of Bo He in 1-2 pints of hot, steaming water and inhale the steam with eyes closed.
- For headache, especially of the Shao Yang channel (temple) or Yang Ming channel (forehead) areas. Apply Bo He diluted 6-10% as a single oil or together with Chai Hu (Bupleurum) for Shao Yang, or Bai Zhi (*Angelica dahurica*) for Yang Ming, equal parts. If there is heat, dilute in ethyl alcohol, otherwise may be diluted in almond oil. Apply to the painful areas of the head.
- For red, irritated eyes, blend Bo He with Bai Ju Hua (Chrysanthemum) in equal parts diluted to 2% using Gou Qi Zi (Goji Berry) essential oil as the carrier and apply as a cool compress over closed eyes. Wring out the compress cloth well. Do not allow the oil to drip into the eyes.
- To stop itching, apply Bo He as a single oil or together with Jing Jie (*Schizonepeta*). If there is a great deal of inflammation such as with eczema or hives, use Bo He with Ye Ju Hua (Wild Chrysanthemum Absolute). Prepare a salve to apply topically, 2-6% dilution depending on skin sensitivity, with coconut oil or shea butter as the emulsifiers. May be kept refrigerated for a cooling, soothing sensation.
- For PMS with symptoms such as moodiness, bloating, breast distention, cramping, and headache, create an aromatic blend of Bo He, Chai Hu (Bupleurum), Dang Gui (*Angelica sinensis*), and Xun Yi Cao (Lavender). Neat for inhalation and as a bath salt or a 4-6% dilution in safflower oil for application as a compress on areas of discomfort.

Cang Zhu 蒼術

ATRACTYLODES

Atractylodis lancea Rhizoma

The Chinese character for zhu/shu 術 in Cang Zhu, refers to artistry and skill. It can hold and conduct the intention of the practitioner. Cang Zhu's aroma and essence embody the magic of transformation. In the body it transforms accumulation of dampness and directs the movement of water. Too much dampness slows things down and interferes with proper bodily functions internally; and in the limbs, it causes swelling, aching, and difficulty with movement. By clearing up the dampness, Cang Zhu brings that which was inhibited back to life.

Dampness is also a state of mind. It is a kind of depressive heaviness, and a foggy lack of clarity. If damp accumulates over time, it becomes thick and sticky phlegm which eventually can block the senses causing mental confusion. Cang Zhu's magic helps to break through the fog to transform thoughts, settle the mind, build up low self-esteem and self-worth to do away with hopelessness, and more extreme suicidal tendencies.

In *The Shen Nong Ben Cao Jing/Divine Farmer's Materia Medica Classic,* Cang Zhu is considered an upper grade herb. It says, "It mainly treats damp impediment, dead muscles, tetany, and jaundice. It stops sweating, eliminates heat, and disperses food. It can be used as a conductor in decoctions."

Aroma: Fresh, sharp, earthy.

Note: Middle/Base.

Part of Plant: Rhizome.

Extraction Method: CO2 extraction.

Color: Dark red-brown

Growing Region: Mao Shan area of Jiangsu province, China.

Major Chemical Components: Sesquiterpenoids: atractylodin, atractylone [6], hinesol, eudesmol, atractylenolide, caryophyllene, elemene, selinene.

CM Category: Aromatic Transforming Dampness.

Nature and Taste: Pungent, bitter, cool.

Affinities: Spleen, Stomach, Lung, Liver. As essential oil, also Kidney.

Average Dilution: 8-10%.

Pharmacological Actions: gastrointestinal relaxant, anti-inflammatory, anti-allergic, antispasmodic, anti-ulcer, vulnerary, nervine, diuretic, antiviral, antibiotic, antiparasitic, antidiabetic.

Actions and Indications:

- Aids digestion, strengthens the Spleen, and transforms Spleen damp which can lead to epigastric and abdominal fullness, distention, nausea, vomiting, loose stools, diarrhea, as well as a feeling of heaviness in the body and extremities.
- Tonifies postnatal Qi by strengthening Spleen and Lung thereby supporting digestion and respiration.
- Transforms damp accumulation, damp-cold or damp-heat in the lower burner, with signs such as leucorrhea (white or yellow discharge), cystitis, prostatitis, genital itch, and low backache.
- Circulates fluids throughout the extremities.
- Regulates sweating.
- Treats damp Bi painful obstruction syndrome with painful, stiff, swollen joints and decreased mobility.
- Repairs necrotic flesh.
- Transforms phlegm to unblock the senses.
- Benefits the eyes, diminished vision, cataracts, glaucoma, night blindness.
- Eliminates parasites.

CM Concepts, Channel Systems, and Patterns:

- Yin Qiao Mai/Yin Heel, Motility Vessel treatment.
- Treat Tai Yin Stage headache.

Treatment Strategies:

To transform damp accumulation in the Spleen, combine Cang Zhu with Hou Po (Magnolia Bark), Bai Dou Kou (Cardamom), and Chen Pi (Aged Tangerine Peel). If there is more cold, add Gan Jiang (Dry Ginger). Dilute 10% in grapeseed oil and apply on SP3, ST40, LR13 (Mu Accumulation point of Spleen), and compress over the abdomen. Make necessary dietary changes.

For damp accumulation in the lower burner, blend equal parts Cang Zhu with Nan Mu (Cedarwood) and Ai Ye (*Artemisia argyi*). Apply on Dai Mai/Belt Vessel points, GB26, CV3, BL32, BL40. For genital area symptoms, blend with She Chuang Zi (Cnidium Fruit) dilute 3% in coconut oil. Apply on the affected area and on LR5.

To treat damp Bi syndrome with painful, swollen joints, make a liniment with Cang Zhu 30%, Yi Yi Ren (Coix) 25%, Song Zhen (Pine Needle) 30%, and Fo Shou (Buddha's Hand) 15%, as a 10% dilution in ethyl alcohol. Massage into affected areas.

- To tonify postnatal Qi, combine Cang Zhu with Huang Qi (*Astragalus*) and Chen Pi (Aged Tangerine Peel). Dilute 10% in black cumin seed oil. Apply to acupoints such as SP3, LU9, BL20, BL13, CV12, CV17.
- To build self esteem, wear Cang Zhu as an amulet and inhale the aroma. Place Cang Zhu neat on KI6 and points of the Yin Qiao Mai/Yin Heel Vessel.
- To transform phlegm blocking the senses, causing mental confusion, add 27 drops of Cang Zhu to 2.7 oz spray bottle of Yuan Zhi (*Polygala tenuifolia*) hydrosol, shake well before spraying on the face and head, and apply Cang Zhu, neat, on ST40 and Jing Well points.

NOTES:

CE BAI YE 側柏葉

BIOTA LEAF, CHINESE ARBORVITAE, THUJA

Biotae orientalis Cacumen, Platycladus orientalis

THREE KEY WORDS DESCRIBE THE ACTIONS OF CE BAI YE ESSENTIAL OIL: regulate, repair, restore. It regulates the blood to stop bleeding and eliminate blood stasis. It repairs damage to flesh, bone, and blood vessels. It restores blood cells, hair loss, and bone loss. Ce Bai Ye oil is distilled from the leafy twigs of the Chinese Arborvitae, which means Tree of Life. Its unique tart evergreen aroma and consolidating essence embody its many benefits, conveying a sense of hope and renewal.

Aroma: Tart evergreen with sharp, acrid edge.

Note: Middle/Base.

Part of Plant: Leaf and Twig.

Extraction Method: Distillation.

Color: Pale yellow.

Growing Region: Shanxi and Shandong provinces, China.

Major Chemical Components: Monoterpenes: carene, pinene, sabinene, limonene. Sesquiterpene: thujopsene. Sesquiterpene alcohol: cedrol [3]. Diterpene: pinusolide.

CM Category: Regulating Blood.

Nature and Taste: Astringent and cool.

Affinities: Lung, Liver, Large Intestine. As essential oil, also Kidney.

Average dilution: 10%.

Pharmacological Actions: Hemostatic, platelet agonist, astringent, vulnerary, hemotonic, osteopromotive, antioxidant, anti-inflammatory, antibacterial, antifungal, antitumor, antipyretic, stomachic, insulin regulating.

ACTIONS AND INDICATIONS:

- Cools blood and stops bleeding in various bleeding disorders, bruising, pernicious anemia, ruptured vessels, hemorrhage.
- Eliminates blood stasis and heals damaged tissue to treat traumatic injuries, broken bones, or scarring, and promotes healing of burns and gastric ulcers.
- Enhances calcium absorption to bones.
- Nourishes blood.
- Protects and strengthens red blood cells.

- Regulates blood sugar and insulin according to recent research.
- Promotes hair growth.
- Eliminates phlegm and stops cough, bronchitis.
- Exerts strong antioxidant and antitumor activity.

CM Concepts, Channel Systems, and Patterns:

- Facilitate Luo Vessel treatment.

Application and Blends:

- To promote hair growth, blend Ce Bai Ye 60%, Mu Xiang (Saussurea) 30%, and Gan Jiang (Dry Ginger) 10%. Add 50 drops of the blend to 4oz of shampoo or conditioner.

- To stop bleeding combine equal parts Ce Bai Ye and Wu Wei Zi (*Schisandra Fruit*). Apply neat for acute conditions on acupoints that regulate blood, cool blood, and stop bleeding: SP1, LR1, LR2, HT5. May be ingested, short term, for hemorrhage or internal bleeding disorders, diluted 20% in grapeseed oil or Bai Zi Ren (Biota Seed cold-pressed) carrier oil. Take 3-6 drops per dose, three times per day.

- Dilute Ce Bai Ye 10% in witch hazel as a liniment for topical application on bruising, ruptured vessels, and varicose veins.

- For respiratory infections with profuse hot (yellow/green) phlegm, diffuse Ce Bai Ye 40% with An Shu Ye (*Eucalyptus radiata*) 40%, and Zhi Ke (*Citrus aurantium*) 20% or breathe the steam of 5 drops in a pint of hot water. Dilute 10% in Zi Su Zi (Perilla Seed) or almond carrier oil for topical application on the chest.

- Apply topically on areas of injury, damaged tissue, broken bones, scaring, burns with equal parts Ce Bai Ye, Ru Xiang (Frankincense), and Mo Yao (Myrrh). Dilute 10% in safflower oil to vitalize blood, in calophyllum (tamanu oil) to break up scar tissue. To mend broken bones and promote bone density, add She Chuang Zi (Cnidium Fruit) essential oil.

CHAI HU 柴胡

BUPLEURUM ROOT

Bupleuri chinensis Radix

THE AROMA OF CHAI HU ESSENTIAL OIL IS STRONG. Just a few drops activate a blend. It is provoking when change needs to be facilitated and pent-up emotions need to be released. Yet its ultimate effect is soothing, even sedating, because it smoothes the flow of the Liver's Qi. In short, it's a "chill out" oil. Its energetic intention is to harmonize. It brings opposing forces back into balance. It gets rid of the old and welcomes the new.

One of Chai Hu's common uses is for treatment of PMS. This is because the Liver rules that phase of the menstrual cycle. When the Liver Qi is constrained during the premenstrual time, emotional mood swings and physical discomfort will occur. Aromatic essential oil blends including Chai Hu are helpful to ease these symptoms.

The Shen Nong Ben Cao Jing/Divine Farmer's Materia Medica Classic classifies Chai Hu as a superior grade herb. It says, "It mainly treats bound Qi in the heart, abdomen, intestines and stomach, drink and food accumulation and gathering, cold and heat and evil Qi. It weeds out the stale to bring forth the new."

Aroma: Strong, woody, acrid.

Note: Middle.

Part of Plant: Root.

Extraction Method: Distillation or CO2 extraction.

Color: Distilled - transparent pale green. CO2 - opaque pale green.

Growing Region: Shanxi province, China. Harvested in October.

Major Chemical Components: Triterpene saponine: saikosaponin [7]. Aldehydes: hexanal, furfural carbaldehyde, heptanal. Sesquiterpenes: cedrene, cuparene, thujopsene, cadinene, beta elemene. Sesquiterpene alcohol: cedrol. Monoterpenes: fenchene, pinene, sabinene.

CM category: Releasing the Exterior.

Nature and Taste: Bitter, pungent, slightly cold.

Affinities: Liver, Gallbladder, Pericardium, San Jiao.

Average Dilution: 4-6%.

Pharmacological Actions: Sedative, analgesic, antipyretic, anti-inflammatory, antibiotic, antiviral, immune modulatory, hepatoprotective, cholagogue, antibiotic.

Actions and Indications:

- Regulates Qi and blood.
- Clears heat.
- Releases Qi Bind in head, throat, chest, heart, diaphragm, abdomen.
- Relieves headaches, migraines. Clears heat and inflammation from the eyes.
- Harmonizes Wood and Earth (Spleen, Stomach, Liver, Gallbladder), digestive upset with epigastric and flank pain, stifling sensation in the chest, abdominal bloating, nausea, and indigestion.
- Resolves interior/exterior disharmony in lingering illness with alternating fever and chill, bitter taste in the mouth, dry throat, poor appetite, nausea, vertigo, irritability, chest and ribs area distention.
- Smoothes the flow of Liver Qi and blood, regulates menses, hormonal balance, PMS.
- Releases Liver Qi constraint, pent up emotion, anger, frustration.
- Benefits, protects, and repairs the liver.
- Controls cravings, addictions, and OCD.

CM Concepts, Channel Systems, and Patterns:

- Ascend and release outward for Divergent meridian (SDS superficial-deep-superficial) strategy.
- Regulate the Hun.
- Harmonize Shao Yang Stage patterns.

Application and Blends:

- For premenstrual syndrome (PMS), to regulate the menstrual cycle, and smooth the movement of Liver Qi and blood, blend Chai Hu 25% with Xiang Fu (*Cyperus*) 30% Dang Gui (*Angelica sinensis*) 20%, Ho Luo Bo Zi (Carrot Seed) 20%, and Mei Gui Hua (Rose) 5%. Inhale directly or diffuse and apply, neat, on acupoints such as LR3, LR14, SP6, CV3.
- For headaches and migraines blend Chai Hu 15% with Chuan Xiong (*Ligusticum wallichii*) 35%, Bai Yu Lan Ye (Magnolia Leaf) 30%, and Bo He (Peppermint) 20% as 4-6% dilution in ethyl alcohol or safflower oil. May be applied neat for acute, short-term use. Dilute for repeated applications or sensitive skin. Apply directly over the painful area and consider points of the Shao Yang channels that address head wind such as GB41, GB20, GB14, GB8, TE5.
- For Shao Yang Stage lingering illness, combine Chai Hu with Gui Zhi/Gui Ye (Cinnamon Twig and Leaf) if there is more cold; if more heat, with Zhi Zi (Gardenia Fruit). Dilute 4-6% in almond oil. Apply to TE5 and other acupoints depending on the symptoms.

- To harmonize Spleen, Stomach, Liver, Gallbladder when there is digestive upset due to constraint of the Liver Qi, create an aromatic blend of Chai Hu with Fo Shou (Buddha's Hand), Mu Xiang (Saussurea) and Xiang Fu (*Cyperus*). Dilute 4-6% in black cumin seed oil and gently apply over the upper abdomen and lower ribs area. To release pent up emotion, add a floral oil like Qi Li Xiang (Orange Jessamine), Mo Li Hua (Jasmine), or Mei Gui Hua (Rose). Deeply inhale the aroma and wear as perfume. Consider application on acupoints such as BL18, BL21, LR13, GB24, ST23, PC6, PC7, LR3, LR5.
- As a support for difficulty with control of cravings, addictions, obsessive-compulsive behaviors, create an aromatic blend with Chai Hu, Huo Xiang (Patchouli), Jiang Xiang (*Dalbergia*), and Fo Shou (Buddha's Hand) for deep inhalation to find stable ground, clear the obstacles, and start anew.

NOTES:

Chen Pi 陳皮

AGED TANGERINE PEEL

Citri reticulatae Pericarpium

Chen Pi essential oil is extracted from the aged peel of mature tangerine fruit. Its tart yet earthy aroma reflects its character, which is like that of a wise and doting grandmother who wants to feed and nurture, lovingly, while at the same time making sure that her loved ones do not become lazy but rather keep moving in the right direction. The rich crimson color of the essential oil, due to the aging of the peel prior to distillation, indicates an affinity to the Fire element, Heart, and Pericardium. It warms the Heart and Spirit and directs the Earth element's digestive Qi to produce nourishing blood. Chen Pi is a useful top note addition to blends addressing weakness of digestive, respiratory, or cardiac functions.

Aroma: Citrusy, fruity, tart, subtly earthy.

Note: Top.

Part of Plant: Peel.

Extraction Method: Distillation.

Color: Crimson.

Growing Region: Guangdong province, China.

Major Chemical Components: Monoterpenes: limonene, terpinene, pinene, myrcene, cymene, sabinene, thugene. Monoterpene alcohols: linalool, terpineol, citronellol. Monoterpene aldehyde: perillaldehyde. Methyl esters. Phenol: thymol.

CM Category: Regulating Qi.

Nature and Taste: Acrid, bitter, warm, aromatic.

Affinities: Lung, Spleen, Stomach. As essential oil, also Heart and Pericardium.

Average Dilution: 4-8%.

Pharmacological Actions: Smooth muscle relaxant, mucolytic, antitussive, anti-asthmatic, antimicrobial, antiviral, antibacterial, antioxidant, antihistamine.

Actions and Indications:

- Regulates and harmonizes the Qi of Spleen and Stomach for all types of digestive disturbances, indigestion, abdominal fullness, distention, belching, nausea, vomiting. Improves appetite, digestion, and absorption of nutrients.
- Warms the chest, transforms dampness, mucus and phlegm encumbering the Lung.

- Resolves coughing with phlegm.
- Strengthens movement of smooth muscle tissue.
- Increases peristalsis.
- Increases contractility of heart muscle and cardiac output.

APPLICATION AND BLENDS:

- Add Chen Pi to blends addressing digestion, especially when there is deficiency and dampness, poor appetite, loose stools, flatulence, malabsorption. Blend Chen Pi 30% with Bi Cheng Qie (Litsea) 30%, Mu Xiang (Saussurea) 25%, and Gan Jiang 15% (Dry Ginger) as a 10% dilution in black cumin seed oil (2% for kids seven to fourteen years, 0.5% to 1% for age two to seven). Apply a few drops over the abdomen and/or on acupoints such as ST25, ST42, SP3, CV12.
- For Heart blood deficiency and insufficiency of the Heart and Spleen Qi with mental emotional disturbance, palpitations, insomnia, anxiety, depression, fatigue, create an aromatic blend of Chen Pi 30% with Qi Li Xiang (Orange Jessamine) 40%, Bai Zi Ren (Biota Seed) 15%, and Ren Shen (Ginseng) 15%, for deep inhalation of the aroma and application on acupoints such as BL15, BL17, BL20, CV14, PC6, SP4.
- To warm the chest and transform dampness encumbering the Lung, blend Chen Pi 20% with Gan Jiang (Dry Ginger) 20%, Hou Po (Magnolia Bark) 20%, and Song Zhen (Pine) 40%. Use neat to diffuse into the air or inhale the steam from a pint of hot water with 3-5 drops of the blend. Dilute to 4-6% in almond oil for application over the chest.

Chuan Xiong 川芎

SICHUAN LOVAGE ROOT

Ligustici wallichii Rhizoma, Ligusticum chuanxiong

Chuan Xiong essential oil is a super fast-acting pain reliever for any type of sinew (muscle, tendon, ligament) including the smooth muscle lining of internal organs. It can be applied directly and undiluted to areas of tension or injury for fast relief and repair. It relaxes spasm in the uterus for menstrual cramping and in the lungs to relax spasm of the bronchi and tight chest causing coughing and wheezing. Chuan Xiong is also famous for treating anything on or inside of the head. It is indispensable as a single oil or an addition to blends for headaches, migraines, blood clots, brain tumors, and to restore brain function. Inhalation of its aroma is helpful to directly affect the brain, as is topical application on the head above the affected areas of the brain. Recently research has found that Chuan Xiong has beneficial effects for the immune system and production of blood cells.

Aroma: Rich, herbaceous, fresh celery and chive.

Note: Middle/Base.

Part of Plant: Rhizome.

Extraction Method: CO2 extraction.

Color: Rust (red-brown).

Growing Region: Sichuan province, China. Harvested May - June.

Major Chemical Components: Phthalides (lactone esters): ligustilide [8], senkyunolide. Monoterpenes: sabinene, limonene. Sesquiterpene: selinene.

CM Category: Invigorating Blood.

Nature and Taste: Pungent, warm.

Affinities: Liver, Pericardium.

Average Dilution: 20-50%. Gentle, may be applied neat.

Pharmacological Actions: Circulatory, antiplatelet, anticoagulant, antispasmodic, smooth muscle relaxant, sedative, analgesic, anti-angiogenesis, radioprotective, hematopoietic.

Actions and Indications:

- Frees the movement of blood and Qi.
- Stops pain.
- Relaxes muscles, tendons, and ligaments.
- Fast-acting on sprains, strains, and muscle tension.

- Moves blood to expel wind, for spasm or numbness.
- Recovers post-stroke difficult movement.
- Relaxes smooth muscle tissue.
- Gynecology: pain, cramping, irregular bleeding, uterine fibroids, ovarian cysts.
- Benefits the head and brain: treats all types of headache, thrombosis, restores cognitive function, treats brain cancer, tumors, glioblastoma.
- Breaks up angiogenesis, starves a tumor (especially head, brain areas).
- Protects against radiation damage.
- According to modern research, it potentiates the immune system, increases blood cells, and enhances the response of Qi tonics.

CM CONCEPTS, CHANNEL SYSTEMS, AND PATTERNS:

- Regulate blood to facilitate Divergent Meridian treatment strategy.
- Resolve physical manifestations of Luo Vessels.
- Facilitate Sinew Meridian treatment.

APPLICATION AND BLENDS:

For gynecological conditions such as dysmenorrhea, uterine cramping and pain, due to Qi stagnation and blood stasis, a blend of Dang Gui (*Angelica sinensis*) with Chuan Xiong is very effective and can be applied neat over the lower abdominal/uterine area for acute, short-term use, or dilute 50% in black cumin seed or safflower oil. Gentle moxibustion or a warm compress may also be applied.

Add Chuan Xiong to blends for treatment of all types of headaches. For example:

- Wind-cold and Yang Ming channel with Bai Zhi (*Angelica dahurica*); Shao Yin channel with Xi Xin (Asarum); wind-heat with Ju Hua (Chrysanthemum) or Bo He (Peppermint); Shao Yang channel with Chai Hu (Bupleurum); Tai Yang channel with Du Huo (Angelica pubescentis).
- Migraine with stabbing pain due to blood stasis with E Zhu (*Curcuma zedoaria*).
- Neurogenic migraine with Du Huo (*Angelica pubescentis*) and Chai Hu (Bupleurum).
- Blood deficient wind with Dang Gui.

In all cases, may be applied neat for acute, short-term use or diluted for chronic longer-term use.

- To recover post-stroke where there has been loss of sensory motor function, paralysis, difficult movement, numbness, or to restore lost cognitive function, blend equal parts Chuan Xiong with Bi Cheng Qie (Litsea) and Du Huo (*Angelica pubescentis*), dilute 15% in walnut or sesame oil and apply to related channels, points and/or associated brain motor areas on the head three days on and three days off for one to three months. If the patient is weak, Huang Qi (*Astragalus*) and Gou Qi Zi (Goji Berry) may be added to the blend or ingested daily as a warm drink, one drop of each mixed with a little honey in water, tea, milk or soy milk.
- To facilitate Sinew Meridian treatment, Chuan Xiong may be applied topically, neat or diluted, together with gua sha or massage techniques.

NOTES:

DANG GUI 當歸

ANGELICA SINENSIS ROOT

Angelicae sinenis Radix

THE CHINESE NAME OF *ANGELICA SINENSIS*, DANG GUI 當歸, means "Protect and Return." Historically, it was worn as a protective amulet. *Angelica sinensis,* like other Angelicas, invokes the presence of angels. It moves the Qi, which in turn restores proper circulation of the blood by way of the dynamic relationships between the Spleen, Lungs, Liver, and Heart to produce, oxygenate, store, and circulate the blood.

Dang Gui essential oil, with its nourishing, earthy quality, has its primary focus on the blood and consequently on menstruation. Applied topically, it is indispensable to bring back the periods when they have stopped, to regulate the cycles when they have become irregular, and to relieve cramping when they are painful. Regulating the menses is a prerequisite to achieving fertility and Dang Gui is an important ingredient in blends when getting pregnant is the goal. It also provides circulation of the Qi and blood to promote healing of injuries. Dang Gui addresses issues that have as their cause insufficiency or "dryness" of the blood which can manifest as skin conditions.

In *The Shen Nong Ben Cao Jing/Divine Farmer's Materia Medica Classic,* Dang Gui is considered a superior grade herb, and was said to treat "mainly cough and counterflow Qi ascent, malaria with fever, leaking causing infertility in females, various malign sores, and incised wounds."

Aroma: Sweet, earthy, musky.

Note: Middle/Base.

Part of Plant: Root.

Extraction Method: CO2 extraction.

Color: Rust (red-brown).

Growing Region: Gansu Province, China. Harvested December - January.

Major Chemical Components: Phthalides (lactone esters): ligustilide [8], cinidilide. Phenols: safrole, ferulic acid. Diterpenes. Phytosterols. Monoterpene: cymene. Coumarin.

CM Category: Tonifying Blood.

Nature and Taste: Sweet, pungent, warm.

Affinities: Heart, Liver, Spleen. As essential oil, also Lung.

Average Dilution: 6-10%.

Pharmacological Actions: Analgesic, anti-inflammatory, antispasmodic, smooth muscle relaxant, antiplatelet, circulatory, anti-arrhythmia, immunostimulant, hepatoprotective, antibiotic.

Actions and Indications:

- Nourishes, invigorates, warms, and harmonizes the blood.
- Gynecology: regulates menses, amenorrhea, dysmenorrhea, infertility.
- Phytoestrogenic, controversial in cases of estrogen receptive cancers.
- Supplements blood to benefit anemia.
- Benefits the immune system.
- Regulates counterflow and descends Lung Qi, to stop cough.
- Speeds recovery from injuries.
- Treats blood deficient wind: rashes, itching, dryness, psoriasis, numbness, spasm, or pain.

CM Concepts, Channel Systems, and Patterns:

- Regulate Dai Mai/Belt Vessel.
- Regulate Bao Mai.
- Facilitate Luo Vessel treatment.

Application and Blends:

To regulate the menses, blend Dang Gui 35% with Chuan Xiong (*Ligusticum wallichii)* 35%, Ai Ye (*Artemisia argyi*) 20%, and Xiang Fu (*Cyperus*) 10%. If there is more Liver Qi constraint with PMS, add Chai Hu (Bupleurum) 5% and Bo He (Peppermint) 5%. May also be applied on acupoints chosen to promote the phases of the cycle. Apply three days on and three days off for one to three months.

For dysmenorrhea, uterine cramping and pain, Dang Gui with Chuan Xiong (*Ligusticum wallichii*) is very effective and can be applied directly over the lower abdominal/uterine area. For acute, short-term use, may dilute 50% in black cumin seed oil. Lower dilutions for repeated use. Gentle moxibustion or a warm compress may also be applied for more cold conditions.

For difficulty with conception and infertility due to cold in the uterus causing obstruction in the Chong/Thoroughfare Vessel and Ren/Conception Vessel, combine Dang Gui 40% with Ai Ye (*Artemisia argyi*) 40%, Rou Gui (Cinnamon Bark) 10%, and Mei Gui Hua (Rose) 10% as a 4-6% dilution in sesame oil. Apply as a warm compress with a hot water bottle or gentle indirect moxibustion to warm the area. May also include placement on distal acupoints such as KI2,

SP8, CV7, KI13, SP4, LU7. Once or twice per day, three days on, three days off for one to three months.

- Cough and counterflow Qi: Historically, before it became mainly associated with gynecology, Dang Gui's main function was to treat counterflow Qi ascent, which is a way to describe what happens when the Lung Qi loses its descending function resulting in cough and difficult breathing. Dang Gui's antispasmodic effect also helps to relax bronchospasm in the case of wheezing and dyspnea. Blend Dang Gui 30% with Yun Shan (Black Spruce) 30%, Wu Wei Zi (*Schisandra Fruit*) 20%, and Zi Su Zi (Perilla Seed) essential oil 20%, blended to 10% in Zi Su Zi (Perilla Seed) cold-pressed carrier oil and applied on BL13 BL17 BL23, and LU9 as well as on the area of Kidney channel points on the chest that affect the lung such as KI24 to 27. Also diffuse the oils into the air.
- To treat signs of blood deficient wind such as rashes, itching, dryness, psoriasis, numbness, or spasm where blood is not nourishing the skin, nerves, or sinews, make a topical application of Dang Gui alone with olive oil as the carrier or combine with other essential oils depending on the presentation, such as: Jing Jie (*Schizonepeta*) for itching, Bai Zi Ren (Biota Seed) for dryness, Ju Hua (Chrysanthemum) for redness and inflammation, Du Huo (*Angelicae pubescentis)* for numbness, Chuan Xiong (*Ligusticum wallichii*) and Xun Yi Cao (Lavender) for spasm.
- Add Dang Gui to topical applications for recovery from injuries to increase blood circulation to nourish the injured area in order to speed recovery and decrease pain. For example, combine Dang Gui with Ru Xiang (Frankincense) and Mo Yao (Myrrh) in equal parts diluted to 10% in safflower oil. Apply on the affected area.

Ding Xiang 丁香

CLOVE BUD

Caryophylli aromaticus Flos, Eugenia caryophyllata

Ding Xiang is a top note essential oil whose warming, spicy, Yang energy benefits all three levels: Wei, Ying, and Yuan. It is an overall tonic with strong antipathogenic as well as pain and spasm relieving properties. It benefits the Wei Protective Qi by boosting the immune system. It works on the Ying Nutritive Qi level mainly by improving digestion and metabolism, and on the Yuan Source level it supports the constitution, mental, reproductive, and sexual function. Clove Bud's strong, spice aroma awakens the senses and appetite for food and for life. Applied topically or ingested, a little goes a long way as it is highly stimulating. Its prominent phenolic content, specifically eugenol, has many beneficial properties but is best used in small doses for limited periods of time.

Aroma: Strong, true clove spice.

Note: Top.

Part of Plant: Flower bud.

Extraction Method: Distillation.

Color: Light yellow.

Growing Region: Indonesia.

Dilution Percentage: 1-2%. May irritate skin. Recommended for short-term use topically, inhaled or ingested.

Major Chemical Components: Phenol (phenylpropanoid): eugenol [9]. Sesquiterpene: caryophyllene. Ester: eugenyl acetate.

CM Category: Warming the Interior and Expelling Cold.

Nature and Taste: Hot and spicy.

Affinities: Kidney, Spleen, Stomach.

Pharmacological Actions: Antiviral, preventative, immune enhancing, antioxidant, anti-aging, anti-inflammatory, antiparasitic, antifungal, anti-infectious, anticancer, analgesic, antispasmodic, carminative.

Actions and Indications:

- Warms and restores Kidney and Spleen Yang deficiency: fatigue, poor appetite and digestion, weak sore low back and knees, cold extremities, memory loss, loose stools, frequent urination, impotence, clear vaginal discharge.
- Boosts reproductive energy.
- Eliminates cold and strengthens deficiency in Stomach and Spleen: vomiting, hiccups, flatulence, abdominal pain, diarrhea.

- Improves immune function, boosts white blood cells.
- Elongates shortened telomeres.
- Improves thyroid function and metabolism.
- Strong muscle relaxant, releases the sinews.
- Treats toothaches.
- Eliminates worms.

CM Concepts, Channel Systems, and Patterns:

- Warm Spleen and Kidney Yang.
- Warm and release in Sinew Meridian treatment.
- Divergent Meridian strategy for Kidney and Bladder. Superficial-deep-superficial (SDS) needling technique to release Yuan to Wei level. Pushes latent heat and dampness out while the phenol content (eugenol) stimulates the immune system.

Application and Blends:

- To warm and strengthen the Kidney and Spleen Yang, blend Ding Xiang 30% with Hu Lu Ba (Fenugreek) 70% as a 4-6% dilution in black cumin seed oil. Apply to KI8, SP15, BL23, BL20, and/or on the navel with gentle, indirect moxibustion.
- To boost the immune system and increase white cells, combine Ding Xiang with Huang Qi (*Astragalus*), Chuan Xiong (*Ligusticum wallichii)*, and Dang Gui (*Angelica sinensis*). Dilute 3% in almond oil and massage into areas that tend to sweat a lot such as the soles of feet and on the middle of the chest around the thymus gland.
- To improve sexual function and libido, blend Ding Xiang 10% with She Chuang Zi (Cnidium Fruit) 35%, Hu Lu Ba (Fenugreek) 25%, Xiao Hui Xiang (Fennel) 25%, and Rou Gui (Cinnamon Bark) 5%, as a 5% dilution in sesame oil. Apply to acupoints such as: KI3, BL23, BL35, ST29, CV4, LR5, three days on and three days off for one month. Wear a drop of Mo Li Hua (Jasmine) as an aphrodisiac perfume.
- As a digestive aid for acute symptoms due to cold, such as vomiting, hiccups, flatulence, abdominal pain, and diarrhea, apply a warm compress over the abdomen with Ding Xiang, Gan Jiang (Dry Ginger), and Bi Cheng Qie (Litsea) diluted 4% in black cumin seed oil. If necessary, to relieve acute symptoms, Ding Xiang can be ingested, 1 drop in 1 tsp of coconut or black cumin seed oil or mixed with a little honey in 1/2 cup warm water, tea, milk or soy milk.

- To eliminate intestinal worms in children, as a topical application around the navel and ST25 area, dilute Ding Xiang and Qing Hao (*Artemisia annua*) with one drop of Long Nao (*Borneolum*) or Zhang Nao (White Camphor). 0.5% dilution for children up to two years old. Can be increased to 1%-2% for those two to seven years old. May dilute in black cumin seed oil or apple cider vinegar.
- For children and the elderly to nourish and support bones and teeth, or to address issues pertaining to growth or deterioration, Ding Xiang may be combined with Hu Lu Ba (Fenugreek). Dilute in sesame oil, 0.5% dilution for children up to two years old. Can be increased to 1% for those between two and seven, 2% for seven to fourteen or for the elderly. Apply topically on areas or acupoints related to the Kidneys once per day, three days on and three days off.
- For teeth and gums: Apply a 1% dilution of Clove in sesame or coconut oil on a small wad of cotton or swab directly on the painful area of gums or teeth for toothaches. *Add:* Mo Yao (Myrrh) to benefit the gums, a citrus peel essential oil such as Chen Pi (Aged Tangerine Peel) and Hu Lu Ba (Fenugreek) for tooth decay. For oil pulling to remove bacteria or draw out toxins, dilute 10 drops of Clove in 1 oz of sesame oil and swish 1 tbsp for 5 to 15 minutes then spit the oil out and rinse with water.
- For memory loss, create an aromatic blend of Ding Xiang with Wu Wei Zi (*Schisandra Fruit*), Du Huo (*Angelica pubescentis*), Shi Chang Pu (Acorus), and Chuan Xiong (*Ligusticum wallichii*) for direct inhalation or diffusion. Dilute 5% in sesame or walnut oil for application on LI20, GV20, GV26, and points or areas of Governing Vessel and Bladder channel on the head over the brain's prefrontal lobe, which deals with short-term memory, and the hippocampus (occipital region), which receives scent messages directly from the olfactory bulb and deals with longer term memory.

Du Huo 獨活

ANGELICA PUBESCENTIS ROOT

Angelicae pubescentis Radix

THE NAME DU HUO 獨活 means "Self-Reliant Existence." Its aroma embodies a rich, nourishing sweetness with an invigorating pungency. Its color is like blood. Du Huo essential oil is deeply supportive as an aid to overcome disability. It seems to have a special affinity for the spine and brain. Applied topically, it relieves pain and benefits neurological conditions. It strengthens the will and builds self-reliance, overcomes fear and the feeling of insignificance. *Angelicae pubescentis,* like other Angelicas, invokes the presence of angels and may be used as an anointment during prayer for healing. Du Huo is quite gentle and can be applied neat, short-term, for fast relief of pain and to speed recovery in the treatment of injuries to the muscles, tendons, joints, and nerves.

Aroma: Heavy, sweet with a spicy edge.

Note: Base.

Part of Plant: Root.

Extraction Method: CO2 extraction.

Color: Deep rusty red.

Growing Region: Hubei and Sichuan provinces, China.

Major Chemical Components: Phenols: angelol [10], drynol. Coumarins: osthole. Monoterpenes: pinene, cedrene, silvestrene, cryptone.

CM Category: Dispelling Wind-Damp and Relieving Pain.

Nature and Taste: Bitter, pungent, warm.

Affinities: Kidney, Bladder, Heart, Liver.

Average Dilution: 10-20%. Gentle, may be used neat for limited time.

Cautions and Contraindications: Can be photosensitive, caution on exposed skin.

Pharmacological Actions: Analgesic, antispasmodic, anti-inflammatory, restorative, neuroprotective and regenerative, vulnerary, circulatory stimulant, disinfectant, antibiotic.

ACTIONS AND INDICATIONS:

- Warms and invigorates Qi and blood.
- Stimulates and strengthens spine, back, and legs.
- Benefits joints, chronic arthritic conditions.
- Increases mobility and relieves pain.
- Restores lost or limited function.
- Releases common cold with dampness, heaviness, muscle aches, fever, headache.

- Relieves toothaches.
- Benefits the brain and central nervous system, memory, cognition, vascular dementia and Alzheimer's.
- Regulates the Qi and nervous system to calm seizures, epilepsy, tetany.
- Eliminates blood stasis, resolves hematoma and breaks up blood clots.
- Promotes wound healing.

CM Concepts, Channel Systems, and Patterns:

- Support Du Mai/Governing Vessel.
- Dispel wind-damp Bi painful obstruction syndrome.
- Relieve Shao Yin Stage headache and toothache.
- Release Exterior wind-cold-damp.
- Treat Running Piglet Qi.

Application and Blends:

For acute or chronic spinal injuries or dysfunction due to neurological or structural disorders, Du Huo may be applied as a single oil, neat, for a limited time. For extended use, dilute 10%. Or blend Du Huo 50% with Bi Cheng Qie (Litsea) 40% and Rou Gui (Cinnamon Bark) 10%. Prepare a 1-4% dilution, depending on age and skin sensitivity (0.5% to 1% for children under 7 years old). Dilute in a gentle carrier oil and apply along the spine, on each side, with massage using a glass rod. Three days on, three days off, once per day for one to three months. Apply to the opening points of Du Mai/Governing Vessel and Yang Qiao Mai/Yang Heel Vessel: SI3 and BL62 and GV20.

To benefit the joints and treat chronic arthritic conditions, make a liniment for topical application on the joints, consisting of Du Huo 30%, Xi Xin (Asarum) 15%, Chuan Xiong (*Ligusticum wallichii*) 25%, and Yi Yi Ren (Coix) 30% as a 10% dilution in ethyl alcohol.

To strengthen the will, help to build self reliance and overcome fear, inhale the aroma, and apply Du Huo, neat, on BL52.

To regulate the Chong Mai/Thoroughfare Vessel when symptoms of Running Piglet Qi arise, defined as a powerful feeling of the Qi rushing upward usually accompanied by a sense of extreme anxiety, apply neat on SP4 and ST30, and inhale with deep breaths.

For acute headaches or toothaches, especially when caused by wind-cold, or when accompanying Shao Yin stage illness, combine Du Huo 80% with Xi Xin (Asarum) 20% and apply directly on the painful areas and associated channel points. Dilute 10% in almond oil for longer term use or sensitive skin.
Dilute 1% if applied inside the mouth for toothache.

E Zhu 莪術

CURCUMA ZEDOARIA

Curcumae zedoaria Rhizoma

E ZHU IS A POWERFUL ESSENTIAL OIL. Its aroma is sharp and penetrating. It is applied topically to break up serious blood stagnation that has resulted in the formation of masses. At the same time, studies into some of its chemical components find it to have anticancer properties.

The Chinese character for zhu/shu 術 in E Zhu, refers to artistry and skill. The essential oils of plants with this name, such as Cang Zhu (Atractylodes), can be an ally, used to transmit the intention of the practitioner and of a blend. E Zhu is an adaptogen, meaning it helps to adapt to stressors which may be physical pathogenic factors or emotional challenges. Interestingly, Cang Zhu essential oil also has these adaptogenic qualities. On the psycho-emotional level, E Zhu is a warrior. It supports the stance of the "heroic journey," the struggle to fight perceived perversity in the world or in one's life.

Aroma: Strong, sharp, earthy, penetrating.

Note: Middle.

Part of Plant: Rhizome.

Extraction Method: Distillation.

Color: Red-orange.

Growing Region: Sichuan, Guangdong, and Guangxi provinces, China. Native to tropical and subtropical, wet forest regions.

Major Chemical Components: Sesquiterpenes [11]: beta-elemene, curzerene, furanodiene. Sesquiterpenoids: curzerenone, germacrone [12], curcumenol, eudesmol. Monoterpene ether oxide: 1-8 cineole (eucalyptol).
Monoterpene: phellandrene, cymene. Monoterpene ketone: camphor <1.5%.

CM Category: Invigorating Blood, Removing Stasis.

Nature and Taste: Pungent, bitter, warm.

Affinities: Liver, Spleen.

Average Dilution: 6-8%.

Pharmacological Actions: Adaptogenic, anticancer, antitumor, anticoagulant, antiplatelet, antimicrobial.

Actions and Indications:

- Resolves chronic blood and Qi stasis, breaks up accumulations, palpable masses and hardenings.
- Resolves swelling of liver or spleen, ascites.
- Anticancer effects from research: small cell carcinoma, solid cancers, cervical cancer, gastric cancer, breast cancer.
- Breaks up phlegm and food stagnation.
- Prolongs platelet aggregation, prevents blood clots.
- Eliminates bacterial infections: staph, strep, salmonella, E. coli.

Application and Blends:

- As a poultice to break up masses, hardenings, tumors, blend E Zhu 60% with Qing Pi (Green Tangerine Peel) 20% and Chai Hu (Bupleurum) 20%. Dilute 8% in castor oil or calophyllum (tamanu) oil and apply over the area. Cover and keep in place for 60 minutes. May be done twice per day three days on and three days off for one month as one course of treatment. Consider Divergent meridian strategy according to the location and diagnosis.

- For dysmenorrhea or amenorrhea due to Liver Qi and blood stasis with fixed abdominal masses, emotional pain, and depression, blend E Zhu with Chuan Xiong (*Ligusticum wallichii*), Xiang Fu (*Cyperus*), Dang Gui (*Angelica sinensis*), and Qi Li Xiang (Orange Jessamine) as an 8% dilution in safflower oil. Compress over the lower abdominal area. Source Luo and Luo Vessel treatments may be helpful. Three days on and three days off or as needed for pain.

- In the case of skin cancers, a blend of E Zhu 25%, Ru Xiang (Frankincense) 25%, Qing Pi (Green Tangerine Peel) 25%, She Chuang Zi (Cnidium Fruit) 20%, and Xing Ren (Bitter Almond) 5%, diluted to 3% in calophyllum (tamanu) oil may be applied topically, directly onto lesions, twice per day, three days on and three days off. Keep covered during the day to avoid sun exposure.

- As a treatment and preventative for blood clots and plaque buildup in the blood, blend E Zhu 20% with Jiang Xiang (*Dalbergia*) 20%, Ru Xiang (Frankincense) 20%, Mo Yao (Myrrh) 20%, Rou Gui (Cinnamon Bark)10%, and Fo Shou (Buddha's Hand) 10% as an 8% dilution in safflower oil for application on acupoints, choosing from Luo Connecting points of the Heart, Pericardium, Liver and Spleen channels: HT5, PC6, LR5, SP4 and their blood harmonizing points: HT2, P2, LR9, SP10 as well as on visible signs along the Luo Vessels such as dark spider veins or nodules. Treat every other day for three weeks as one course of treatment.

Fo Shou 佛手

BUDDHA'S HAND, FINGER CITRON

Citri sarcodactylis Swingle Fructus

Fo Shou 佛手 means "Buddha's Hand", named for its shape, a golden hand with finger-like projections, as well as for its ability to be an ally, in meditation or spiritual practice. Fo Shou lifts and brightens the spirit. Its fruity, tart aroma is literally mouth-watering. It gets the digestive juices flowing and moves the Qi of the Stomach and Intestines. It is also good at smoothing the flow of the Liver Qi when pent up emotions such as anger and frustration have affected the Stomach. Its nature as the essential oil of a fruit with peel is to bring things to the surface to be released, like suppressed emotion, and to allow one's true nature and inner beauty to shine forth.

Like other citrus essential oils with their high limonene content, Fo Shou is an effective antiseptic and is a great addition to hand and surface sanitizers and to diffusion blends for cleaning the air of pathogens.

Aroma: Light and fruity, sweet, slightly pungent with a tart citrus peel overtone.

Note: Top/Middle.

Part of Plant: Fruit and Peel. Harvested in summer when the fruit turns yellow and starts to wrinkle.

Extraction Method: Distillation.

Color: Pale yellow.

Growing Region: Jinhua, Zhejiang Province, and Guangzhou, Guangdong Province, China.

Major Chemical Components: Monoterpenes: d-Limonene [13], y-terpinene, dipentene, ocimene, pinene, thujene. Monoterpene alcohols: linalool, terpineol, geraniol, nerol. Monoterpene aldehyde: citral. Coumarins [14]. Flavonoids.

CM Category: Regulating Qi.

Nature and Taste: Acrid, bitter, warm.

Affinities: Liver, Lung, Stomach, Spleen.

Average Dilution: 4-6%.

Cautions and Contraindications: Photosensitive, caution on exposed skin.

Pharmacological Actions: Digestive stimulant, antacid, mucolytic, antidiabetic, antimicrobial, astringent.

Actions and Indications:

- Digestive: Relieves abdominal discomfort, belching, vomiting, poor appetite, neutralizes gastric acid, heartburn, GERD, and supports normal peristalsis.
- Relieves morning sickness.
- Regulates and spreads Liver Qi, resolves emotional indigestion.
- Breaks up phlegm, expands the chest, and stops coughing and wheezing.
- Reduces water retention and swollen joints.
- Alleviates pain.
- Reduces blood glucose levels and thickening of blood.
- Breaks down plaque and cholesterol.

CM Concepts, Channel Systems, and Patterns:

- Regulate Qi as part of Divergent Meridian treatment strategy.
- Harmonize Wood overacting on Earth.

Application and Blends:

To relieve digestive discomfort and dysfunction caused by emotion, create an aromatic blend of Fo Shou, with other essential oils such as Mu Xiang (Saussurea), Xiang Fu (*Cyperus*), Chai Hu (Bupleurum), and a floral such as Qi Li Xiang (Orange Jessamine), Mo Li Hua (Jasmine), or Mei Gui Hua (Rose). Deeply inhale and wear as perfume. May also dilute 4-6% and spread a few drops on the upper abdomen and lower ribs.

Add Fo Shou as the top note in blends for breaking up phlegm, freeing the Lung Qi and respiration. For example: Fo Shou with Song Zhen (Pine Needle), An Shu Ye (Eucalyptus), and Zi Su Ye (Perilla Leaf). Diffuse neat, 15-20 drops in a diffuser, or inhale the steam directly by placing 3-5 drops in a pint of steaming water. May also be diluted 4% and applied on the chest.

To help reduce blood glucose levels and the consequential thickening of the blood, make a blend for internal ingestion with Fo Shou 20%, Wu Wei Zi (*Schisandra Fruit*) 35%, Hu Lu Ba (Fenugreek) 30%, Mo Yao (Myrrh)10%, and Rou Gui (Cinnamon Bark) 5%. Dilute 4% in pomegranate seed oil. 3 drops per dose, twice per day.

Gan Jiang 乾姜

DRY GINGER ROOT

Zingiberis officinale Rhizoma

Gan Jiang essential oil with its fresh, sharp, spicy aroma is extracted from the dried, mature, hearty *Zingiberis* rhizomes collected in the winter when their energy to generate heat and counteract cold and damp is strongest. The yellow and white color of the root at this time affirms its affinity with the Earth and Metal Elements and its beneficial effects on digestion and respiration. Dry Ginger oil is a warming, strengthening tonic. It is an excellent choice whenever there is a need to restore the Yang, increase metabolic and functional aspects of the body, and as an addition to blends when cold and damp conditions need to be addressed. Gan Jiang essential oil's buttressing quality applies on the mental emotional level as well where it helps to reinforce "intestinal fortitude," self-control and the ability to deal with the shame of addictive behaviors.

Aroma: Spicy, sharp.

Note: Middle/Base.

Part of Plant: Rhizome.

Extraction Method: CO2 extraction.

Color: Deep reddish brown.

Growing Region: Guangxi province, China. Harvested November – December

Major Chemical Components: Monoterpene alcohols: gingerol [15], cineole, geraniol, borneol, linalool. Sesquiterpenes: zingiberene, farnesene, curcumene, sesquiphellandrene, bisabolene. Monoterpenes: phellandrene, camphene, terpinene.

CM Category: Warming the Interior and Expelling Cold.

Nature and Taste: Spicy, hot.

Affinities: Lung, Spleen, Stomach, Kidney.

Average dilution: 2-4%.

Cautions and Contraindications: Photosensitive, caution on exposed skin. Spicy, may irritate skin.

Pharmacological Actions: Antioxidant, anti-aging, anti-inflammatory, antiemetic, stomachic, carminative, analgesic, mucolytic, expectorant.

Actions and Indications:

- Strengthens Yang Qi.
- Treats cold and damp conditions with cold limbs, aching joints, and lethargy.
- Prevents motion sickness and relieves morning sickness.

- Harmonizes and warms the middle burner, for cold or deficiency of Spleen Qi causing nausea, poor appetite and digestion, abdominal discomfort, gas, bloating, loose stools, and constipation.
- Warms the lungs and expectorates phlegm for colds, coughs, and congestion.
- Breaks up mucus and phlegm in respiratory and lymphatic systems.
- Decreases swelling, stiffness and pain of cold Bi Obstruction, arthritis, and rheumatism.
- Promotes anti-aging effect.

CM Concepts, Channel Systems, and Patterns:

- Break up Yin stasis with excess fluid and phlegm accumulation.
- Clear Ren Mai/Conception Vessel stagnation of Yin due to Yin deficiency.

Application and Blends:

As a warming liniment for cold Bi Obstruction, Gan Jiang may be applied to the painful areas alone as a 4% dilution or with other essential oils such as Yun Shan (Black Spruce) and Yi Yi Ren (Coix) as an 8% dilution in ethyl alcohol.

To harmonize and warm the middle burner and improve digestion, blend Gan Jiang 10% with Huo Xiang (Patchouli) 35%, Chen Pi (Aged Tangerine Peel) 20%, and Bai Dou Kou (Cardamom), or Rou Dou Kou (Nutmeg) 35%, as a 4% dilution in black cumin seed oil to gently apply over the abdominal area. Light moxibustion may be applied. May also be applied on acupuncture points of the Stomach and Spleen channels.

To prevent motion sickness, inhale the aroma of Gan Jiang with Bo He (Peppermint) directly from the bottle as needed before and during travel. Place a 2% dilution directly on PC6 and apply acupressure. Do not rub into the skin; ginger is spicy and may cause irritation.

For morning sickness, inhale the aroma.

To warm the lungs when wind-cold has caused cough, congestion, or phlegm, blend Gan Jiang with An Shu Ye (*Eucalyptus globulus*), Song Zhen (Pine Needle), and Fo Shou (Buddha's Hand). Diffuse 10 to 15 drops in a diffuser or place 5 drops in a pint of steaming water and inhale. Dilute 4-6% in Zi Su Zi (Perilla Seed) carrier oil for application over the chest and upper back.

For breaking up Yin stasis in Ren Mai/Conception Vessel, Gan Jiang may be diluted and applied alone or with Nan Mu (Cedarwood), on points along the trajectory such as CV3, CV9, CV12, and the opening point LU7, three days on and three days off for one to three months. May add other essential oils depending on the case.

GOU QI ZI 枸杞子

GOJI BERRY

Lycii barbarum Fructus

GOU QI ZI ESSENTIAL OIL, with its mild, fruity, nutty aroma and taste, is gentle enough to apply neat. It can be used either as an essential oil, nutritional oil or as a carrier oil for blends. Gou Qi Zi is one of the rare essential oils that is said to be able to nourish Jing Essence and assist in building up a weakened constitution. It may be ingested daily as a restorative tonic for issues commonly related to aging, depletion due to chronic illness, or recovery after an acute illness that has depleted the body fluids, Yin essences, or blood.

Benefitting the eyes is one of Gou Qi Zi's main functions because it nourishes Liver blood. The Liver opens to the eyes. Liver Yin, along with the circulation of Liver blood, is essential to provide the moisture and nutritive substance that maintains eye health and vision.

Aroma: Mild, nutty.

Note: Middle/Base.

Part of Plant: Seed.

Extraction Method: CO2 extraction.

Color: Yellow-green.

Growing Region: Ningxia Province, China. Harvested in October.

Major Chemical Components: Sesquiterpene: beta-elemene. Fatty acid esters: hexadecanoic (palmitic) acid, linoleic acid, cinnamic acid, ferrulic acid, myristic acid. Ethyl ester: ethyl hexadecanoate. Coumarin: lycibaracoumarin. Monoterpenoid: geranylacetone. Diterpenenoids. Phenols (Phenylpropanoids).

CM Category: Tonifying Yin.

Nature and Taste: Sweet, neutral.

Affinities: Liver, Kidney, Lung.

Average Dilution: 20-100%. Very gentle, may be ingested and applied neat.

Pharmacological Actions: Restorative, antioxidant, anti-aging, neuroprotective, anxiolytic, antiglaucoma, antitussive, expectorant, adaptogenic, metabolic, hematopoietic (red and white blood cells), immunoregulatory, antidiabetic, hydrating.

Actions and Indications:

- Supplements Liver and Kidney Yin and blood, with signs of deficiency such as dizziness, blurry vision, tinnitus, nocturnal emissions, impotence, infertility, weakness of lower back and knees, prematurely gray hair, emaciation, wasting and thirsting (diabetes), insomnia, night sweats, and dryness.
- Benefits the eyes and vision, diminished visual acuity, blurry vision, or dryness of the eyes caused by insufficient Liver Yin and blood.
- Moistens Lung Yin for chronic respiratory disorders and pulmonary tuberculosis, with such symptoms as dry cough with little or no sputum that is difficult to expectorate, blood in sputum, afternoon fevers, sensation of steaming bones.
- Regulates blood sugar.

CM Concepts, Channel Systems, and Patterns:

- Supplement Liver and Kidney Yin and blood.
- Benefit Jing Essence.
- Enrich Lung Yin.

Application and Blends:

For internal ingestion, the average dosage is 1/4 to 1/3 tsp per day, three days on and three days off, as a single oil. May also be used as the carrier oil in a blend with other edible essential oils that supplement the Qi and blood.

For diminished visual acuity, a blend of Gou Qi Zi either as one of the essential oils or as the carrier oil, with Ju Hua (Chrysanthemum), Ho Luo Bo Zi (Carrot Seed), Man Jing Zi (Vitex), Wu Wei Zi (*Schisandra Fruit Fruit*), Du Huo (*Angelica pubescentis*), and a small percentage of Xi Xin (Asarum) diluted to 4-6%, may be applied on acupoints around the eyes, being careful not to let the oil drip into the eyes. Can also be applied on distal channel points that benefit the eyes such as ST36, ST41, LR1, GB7, GB8, GB20, GB37, with gentle moxibustion on the Liver's Shu point BL18 in the case of deficiency and for those over fifty years old. Apply three days on and three days off. A warm compress with a few drops of Gui Zhi/Gui Ye (Cinnamon Twig and Leaf) diluted in almond oil applied on the neck and occipital region may help to open the channels to the head and eyes.

To strengthen or release the lower back, blend equal parts Gou Qi Zi with Du Huo (*Angelica pubescentis*), Hu Lu Ba (Fenugreek), and Chuan Xiong (*Ligusticum wallichii*) as a 10% dilution in sesame oil and apply as a massage oil over the area as needed.

GUI ZHI / GUI YE 桂枝

CINNAMON TWIG AND LEAF

Cinnamomi cassia Ramulus et Folium

WHETHER INHALED OR APPLIED TOPICALLY, Gui Zhi/Gui Ye is very warming and stimulating. Its aroma enlivens the heart and mind and brightens the spirit. Deep inhalation warms and comforts the chest. Application on the skin produces a tingling sensation. Aromatic sweetness and spice together balance Ying Nutritive and Wei Protective Qi, interior and exterior. This makes Gui Zhi/Gui Ye effective to resolve conditions that are affecting either or both levels at the same time. It addresses the skin, nerves, and sinews, as well as the channels, blood vessels, and waterways.

Aroma: Sweet, herbaceous, and spicy.

Note: Middle.

Part of Plant: Twig and Leaf.

Extraction Method: Distillation.

Color: Golden.

Growing Region: Guangxi Province, China. Harvested March to June.

Major Chemical Components: Coumarin [14]. Phenols (phenylpropanoids): eugenol, trans-cinnamaldehyde. Esters: cinnamyl acetate, benzyl benzoate [16]. Monoterpene: camphene. Sesquiterpene: beta caryophyllene.

CM Category: Releasing the Exterior.

Nature and Taste: Acrid, sweet, warm.

Affinities: Heart, Lung, Bladder.

Average Dilution: 2-3%.

Cautions and Contraindications: Very spicy, will irritate the skin if applied neat. Photosensitive, caution on exposed skin.

Pharmacological Actions: Anti-inflammatory, anti-infectious, Cox-2 inhibitor, analgesic, circulatory and respiratory stimulant, emmenagogue.

ACTIONS AND INDICATIONS:

- Expels wind-cold conditions by warming the Yang Qi and releasing the muscle layer.
- Releases constraint in the upper back and occipital region which inhibits the free movement of Qi, blood, and fluids to the eyes and upper orifices.
- Prevents and treats frequent colds, too much or too little perspiration, and skin conditions.

- Frees the Yang function of Heart and Lungs with symptoms such as chest pain, irregular pulse, shortness of breath, cough with thin mucus, or phlegm.
- Disperses blood stagnation, pain, masses.
- Moves water and resolves edema, dysuria.
- Warms and unblocks the channels and collaterals to relieve wind-cold-damp related muscle and joint pain, stiffness.
- Frees the movement of Yang Qi through the back and spine to benefit neurological or structural disorders.
- In gynecology, warms the uterus and blood circulation to relieve abdominal pain, dysmenorrhea, as well as regulate menstruation and promote fertility. For men, warms, stimulates and circulates the Yang Qi to assist treatment of erectile dysfunction.

CM Concepts, Channel Systems, and Patterns:

- Open Du Mai/Governor Vessel.
- Open Yang Qiao Mai/Yang Heel Vessel.
- Warm Chong Mai/Thoroughfare Vessel and Ren Mai/ Conception Vessel.
- Harmonize Ying and Wei.

Application and Blends:

Dilute 3% in almond oil and compress over the upper back and occipital region to expel wind-cold, warm, and release the muscles, channels, and vessels. Cupping may be applied.

To warm and relieve menstrual pain and cramping, blend Gui Zhi/Gui Ye 20% with Wu Zhu Yu (Evodia) 20%, Chuan Xiong (*Ligusticum wallichii*) 30%, and Dang Gui (*Angelica sinensis)* 30%. Prepare a 4% dilution in safflower oil to move blood and ease pain. Gently spread over the lower abdomen as a warm compress once or twice per day or gentle moxibustion may be used to further warm the area.

Add Gui Zhi/Gui Ye to liniments for wind-cold-damp Bi Obstruction causing muscle or joint pain and stiffness. Use alone, diluted to 2%, or with equal parts Du Huo (*Angelica pubescentis*), Chuan Xiong (*Ligusticum wallichii*), and Song Zhen as a 4-6% dilution in ethyl alcohol to massage into the affected areas.

To free the back and spine and open Du Mai/Governor Vessel and Yang Qiao Mai/Yang Heel, Motility Vessel, blend Gui Zhi/Gui Ye with Du Huo (*Angelica pubescentis*). Prepare a 0.5-3% dilution, depending on age and skin sensitivity in a gentle carrier oil to be applied along the spine, on each side, with massage using a glass rod. Three days on, three days off, once per day for one to three months. Apply to the opening points, SI3 and UB62.

- To promote fertility by warming the Chong Mai/Thoroughfare Vessel and Ren Mai/Conception Vessel, blend Gui Zhi/Gui Ye 10% with Ai Ye 20% (*Artemisia argyi*), Dang Gui (*Angelica sinensis*) 20%, and Mei Gui Hua (Rose) 50%. Dilute 2% in sesame oil. Gently spread over the lower abdomen once per day, and place on opening points of Chong and Ren Mai: LU7 and SP4, three days on and three days off.

NOTES:

Hou Po 厚朴

MAGNOLIA BARK

Magnoliae officinalis Cortex

Hou Po is derived from the bark of the Magnolia tree. Good quality magnolia bark sparkles with resin. Its essential oil not only expresses the attributes of a bark, which represents protection and hiding or numbing of pain, but also that of a resin, which represents wound healing for both physical and emotional trauma. Hou Po, with its affinity to the Metal and Earth elements and its complex bitter, pungent, and sweet aroma helps to unravel and heal old issues around guilt and forgiveness. It is a gentle bark to gradually peel off layers of protective guarding, which hide painful memories.

Aroma: Bitter and sharply pungent with a deep, syrupy-sweet undertone.

Note: Middle.

Part of Plant: Bark.

Extraction Method: CO2 extraction.

Color: Rust red.

Growing Region: Hunan province, China. Harvested April - June.

Major Chemical Components: Phenols: magnolol, honokiol [17]. Sesquiterpene alcohol: eudesmol. Sesquiterpenes.

CM Category: Aromatic Transforming Dampness.

Nature and Taste: Bitter, pungent, warm.

Affinities: Lung, Large Intestine, Stomach, Spleen.

Average Dilution: 4-6%.

Pharmacological Actions: Neuroprotective, antidepressant, sedative, antihypertensive, gastrointestinal relaxant, mucolytic, respiratory, antiparasitic, antifungal, antibiotic, vulnerary, anticoagulant.

Actions and Indications:

- Regulates digestive stagnation and accumulation, as well as sluggishness and constipation.
- Decongests the lungs and regulates the Lung Qi for coughing, wheezing, and phlegm.
- Eliminates parasites, worms, funguses, and yeast.
- Regenerates dead tissue (necrosis) for wound care.
- Resolves mood swings, fright palpitations, depression, grief, shame, and pain.

- Frees the Lungs and anchors the Lung Qi to the Kidneys to help get to the root of difficult issues and find the will to start over with a clean slate.

CM CONCEPTS, CHANNEL SYSTEMS, AND PATTERNS:

- Descend rebellious Lung and Stomach Qi.
- Transform dampness.

APPLICATION AND BLENDS:

- To regulate digestive sluggishness and constipation combine Hou Po and Zhi Ke (*Citrus aurantium*). If there is more damp stagnation, add Cang Zhu (Atractylodes). If more Qi stagnation add Mu Xiang (Saussurea). Dilute 4-6% in black cumin seed oil and gently spread a few drops over the abdomen. May also apply on acupoints that move and descend the digestive Qi such as SP3, SP15, CV6, CV12, TH6.

- To open the Lung Qi and transform dampness for congestion, coughing, wheezing, and phlegm, blend Hou Po with An Shu Ye (*Eucalyptus globulus*) and Zhi Ke (*Citrus aurantium*), neat, for diffusing into the air with 15 drops in a diffuser or inhaling 5 drops in a pint of steaming water.

- To kill intestinal yeast, parasites, or worms, Hou Po 80% may be ingested as a short, five-day course of treatment together with Ding Xiang (Clove) 20%, in a 4% dilution in black cumin seed oil for adults, 2% for kids seven to fourteen years, and 0.5% to 1% for younger, as a drink in apple cider vinegar and water, 1-2 tbsp of vinegar in 1/2-1 cup water per dose. Take three times per day on an empty stomach.

- To resolve mood swings, depression, grief, and to foster forgiveness and acceptance, create an aromatic blend of Hou Po with Xiang Fu (*Cyperus*) and Mo Li Hua (Jasmine) for deep inhalation. Wear as a perfume on Yuan Source and Luo Connecting points like HT5, LR5, LU9, CV17.

Hu Lu Ba 葫蘆巴

FENUGREEK SEED

Trigonellae foenum-gracum Semen

FENUGREEK SEED IS ONE OF THE STAPLE DIGESTIVE SPICES used in Indian cooking. Both in taste and smell, it is sweet and nutty. As an essential oil, when inhaled, the aroma stimulates saliva and takes on the bitterness of the raw seed. Its nourishing warmth descends and spreads throughout the lower body.

Hu Lu Ba essential oil works with the Kidney system, supporting its Yang function by turning up the Ming Men Life Gate fire, which is the pilot light that warms the body and makes digestion, metabolism, growth, circulation, and movement possible. As an example, this quality can help in the recovery of children who exhibit failure to thrive or developmental issues. Hu Lu Ba also helps with colicky and gassy pain in the intestines.

In the realm of the temperament and Shen Spirit, Hu Lu Ba supports the Kidney's attribute of the Zhi Will which helps to deal with issues of fear, loss of will power, and motivation.

Aroma: Soft, nutty, herbaceous, bitter.

Note: Middle.

Part of Plant: Seed.

Extraction Method: CO2 extraction.

Color: Golden yellow.

Growing Region: Guangzhou, China.

Major Chemical Components: Monoterpene: pinene. Sesquiterpenes: caryophyllene, a-selinene. Sesquiterpene alcohol: farnesol. Terpene aldehyde: geranial. Ester: neryl acetate. Trigonelline [18]. Monoterpene ketone: camphor.

CM Category: Tonifying Yang.

Nature and Taste: Bitter, warm.

Affinities: Kidney, Liver. As essential oil, also Spleen.

Average Dilution: 8-10%. Gentle, may be applied neat.

Cautions and Contraindications: Estrogenic, contraindicated during pregnancy.

Pharmacological Actions: Analgesic, emmenagogue, galactagogue, antidiabetic, antifungal, antibacterial, diuretic, hypoglycemic, neuroprotective, anti-invasive, estrogenic.

ACTIONS AND INDICATIONS:

- Warms and supplements Kidney Yang with symptoms such as: cold limbs, coldness affecting the lower abdomen, genitals, lower back and legs, or cold causing pain, edema, hypothyroid, impotence, or low libido.
- Promotes kidney diuresis.
- Warms the Liver channel and treats pain and accumulation in lower burner such as hernias and fibroids.
- Reduces blood sugar, thickening of the blood, cholesterol, and hypertension.
- Breaks down fatty deposits, belly fat and cellulite.
- Chelates oxalates, oxalic acid to treat gout.
- Mineralizes bone.
- For children, it activates the Du/Governing Vessel to support the spine and posture, and it warms the Spleen Yang to treat colicky or difficult digestion and absorption.
- Promotes lactation and menstruation.
- Balances adrenals and thyroid.

CM CONCEPTS, CHANNEL SYSTEMS, AND PATTERNS:

- Tonify Kidney Yang.
- Treat Bulging Disorders.

APPLICATION AND BLENDS:

To warm and supplement the Kidney Yang, blend Hu Lu Ba 45% with She Chuang Zi (Cnidium Fruit) 30%, Rou Gui (Cinnamon Bark) 15%, and Ding Xiang (Clove) 10%. Dilute 4-6% in sesame seed or black cumin seed oil and spread 3 drops across the kidney treatment area of the lower back and around the navel with light moxibustion, once per day, three days on and three days off for one to three months.

For children, to activate the Du Mai/Governing Vessel to support the spine and posture for developmental issues, dilute 0.5% to 2% (0.5% to 1% up to age seven to eight years old) in untoasted sesame oil and apply along both sides of the spine with a glass rod or smooth stone and on SI3, three days on and three days off, once per day for one to three months.

To strengthen Spleen Yang for children who tend to be colicky and have difficulty with digestion, combine Hu Lu Ba 60% with Xiao Hui Xiang (Fennel) 20% and Chen Pi (Aged Tangerine Peel) 20%. Dilute 0.5% to 2% (0.5% to 1% up to age seven to eight years old) in black cumin seed oil. Gently spread 3 drops over the abdomen and apply to Shu Transport points of Spleen and Stomach, BL20 and BL21, once per day, three days on and three days off as needed.

- Promote lactation, a drink with 3 drops of Hu Lu Ba in warm honey water, milk or soy milk may be taken twice per day. May also apply to acupoints local to breast area such as ST18 and CV17, on Stomach channel points such as ST36 and ST42, and on SI1 three days on and three days off.
- To break down fatty deposits, belly fat and cellulite, combine essential oils of Hu Lu Ba 50% (Fenugreek), Zhi Zi (Gardenia Fruit) 25%, and Wu Wei Zi (*Schisandra Fruit*) 25% diluted to 2% in cod liver or castor oil and vigorously apply over the area, then compress with a hot washcloth to insulate the heat. Once per day, three days on and three days off.
- For inguinal hernia and bulging disorders of the lower abdomen apply a warm compress of essential oils Hu Lu Ba 40%, Xiao Hui Xiang (Fennel) 40%, and Wu Zhu Yu (Evodia) 20% as a 4% dilution in castor oil. Soak a flannel cloth in the oil and compress the affected area with heat for 20 minutes, twice per day, three days on three days off for one month as one course of treatment.

NOTES:

Hu Luo Bo Zi 胡蘿蔔子

CARROT SEED

Daucus carota Semen

THE AROMA OF DEEPLY ORANGE-COLORED CARROT SEED ESSENTIAL OIL is softly spicy and sweetly nutty. Upon inhalation, it brings cool soothing water to the eyes, while awakening and calming the mind. Carrot Seed is nutritious and can be ingested when diluted in a nutritional carrier oil. It is rich in Vitamin A, an important antioxidant essential for the health of the eyes, skin, bones, growth, and the immune system. The main action of Carrot Seed essential oil in the context of Chinese medicine is to nourish the Liver blood, and consequently the eyes and vision. Carrot Seed essential oil is a natural sunscreen and repairs damaged skin.

Aroma: Softly spicy with a sweet, nutty undertone.

Note: Middle.

Part of Plant: Seed.

Extraction Method: CO2 extraction.

Color: Orange.

Growing Region: Inner Mongolia. Harvested in November.

Major Chemical Components: Sesquiterpenol: carotol. Sesquiterpene: bisabolene. Monoterpenes: pinene, sabinene, camphene, myrcene, terpene, limonene. Monoterpenoid acetate ester: geranyl acetate.

CM Category: Tonifying Blood.

Nature and Taste: Spicy, sweet and cool.

Affinities: Liver, Kidney.

Average Dilution: 8-10%.

Pharmacological Actions: Hepatoprotective, hemotonic, antioxidant, anti-inflammatory, antifungal, antiviral.

ACTIONS AND INDICATIONS:

- Nourishes the Liver blood to treat dry eyes, poor vision, brittle nails, dizziness, scanty menses, PMS, and mood swings.
- Supplements Liver and Kidney Yin, reduces insomnia, agitation, dryness, and heat.
- Benefits the hormonal system and reduces menopausal symptoms.
- Regulates thyroxine, hypothyroid, progesterone.
- Clears heat and toxins.

CM Concepts, Channel Systems, and Patterns:

- Supplement Liver blood deficiency.
- Tonify Liver and Kidney Yin deficiency.
- Clear fire toxins.

Application and Blends:

- For eye and vision problems due to deficient Liver blood, blend equal parts Carrot Seed with Dang Gui (*Angelica sinensis*), Gou Qi Zi (Goji Berry), Chuan Xiong (*Ligusticum wallichii*), and Ju Hua (Chrysanthemum) as a 10% dilution in olive oil. Apply to channel points such as LR3, GB1, GB37 (empirical point for vision), LR14, BL18, ST36.

- To supplement Liver and Kidney Yin, blend Carrot Seed 40% with Mei Gui Hua (Rose) 20% and Wu Wei Zi (*Schisandra Fruit*) 40% as a 10% dilution in sesame oil. Apply to the Liver and Kidney Shu Transport points BL18, BL23, and their Yuan Source points LR3, KI3 as well as CV4, CV12, CV15, and CV24.

- As a natural sunscreen and to protect and repair damaged skin, dilute Carrot Seed 4% in coconut oil and apply on the skin as needed.

- For regulating production of thyroxine and to address hypothyroid, blend Carrot Seed with other essential oils that help to stimulate and regulate the pituitary/hypothalamus/adrenal/thyroid (HPA) axis such as: Song Zhen (Pine) or Yun Shan (Black Spruce), Ai Ye (*Artemisia argyi*), and Hu Lu Ba (Fenugreek). Dilute 10% in pomegranate seed oil. Depending on the case, choose among the oils and apply on related local and distal acupuncture points.

Hu Po 琥珀

AMBER

Succinum

THE CHINESE NAME FOR AMBER, HU PO 琥珀, translates as "Tiger Soul". The traditional legend about Hu Po is that, when a tiger dies, its soul enters the earth and transforms into stone. Amber originates from the resins of ancient trees, which have been buried and hardened underground. Pine trees are a primary source. The White Tiger is a symbol for the Lung and Metal element. As an essential oil, the resinous, pine-like aroma of Hu Po has a deep affinity with the Lung including its spirit aspect, the Po (corporeal earthbound soul), which can refer to ghosts, whether they be literal, or figurative as the things that "haunt" one. Resins heal physical and emotional wounds. Pine-like essential oil aromas free the Lung Qi and treat respiratory illnesses. The thick, resinous substance of this oil, having been extracted from something buried in the earth, has a grounding, stabilizing effect. Hu Po treats neurological, mental, and emotional disturbances by calming the nervous system, opening the senses and quieting the spirit. Amber eases pain and has a regulating effect on the heart and blood circulation as well as on the bladder and movement of water.

Aroma: Resinous, balsamic, pine, sweet, pungent.

Note: Base.

Part of Plant: Fossilized pine resin.

Extraction Method: CO2 extraction.

Color: Amber-orange.

Region: Yunnan province, China.

Major Chemical Components: Diterpene: cembrene. Sesquiterpenes: longipinene, caryophyllene, longifolene. Monoterpenic alcohol: terpineol. Monoterpenes: alpha pinene, camphene, beta pinene, delta 3 carene.

CM Category: Substances that Calm the Spirit.

Nature and Taste: Sweet and neutral.

Affinities: Heart, Liver, Bladder. As essential oil, also Lung, Kidney.

Average Dilution: 4-6%.

Pharmacological Actions: Sedative, CNS suppressant, analgesic, vulnerary, circulatory, emmenagogue, diuretic.

ACTIONS AND INDICATIONS:

- Tranquilizes the mind and nervous system. Subdues fright, palpitations, restlessness, insomnia, forgetfulness.

- Arrests tremors, seizures, or infantile convulsions.
- Unblocks the senses.
- Gets rid of ghosts (literal or metaphorical).
- Breaks up phlegm and Yin stasis.
- Promotes circulation.
- Breaks up blood stasis and angina.
- Treats injuries, pain, swelling, and promotes wound healing.
- Cools blood and stops bleeding.
- Regulates menstrual disorders.
- Breaks up palpable masses.
- Promotes urination, regulates urinary dysfunction with pain, blood, kidney stones.
- Dermatological use: resolves ulcers, boils, swellings, promotes tissue regeneration.

CM Concepts, Channel Systems, and Patterns:

- Quiet the Qi of the Five Zang.
- Settle the Hun and Po (ethereal and corporeal souls).
- Eliminate Jing level infestations.
- Open orifices as part of Divergent Meridian treatment strategy.
- Open and clear Yin stasis in Ren Mai.
- Treat the Five Lin syndromes.

Application and Blends:

- To calm the nerves, the heart, and the mind, create an aromatic blend with Hu Po, Bai Zi Ren (Biota Seed), and a floral oil such as Xun Yi Cao (Lavender) or Mo Li Hua (Jasmine). Use neat, for direct inhalation or diffusion and in the bath as a bath salt, with 15-20 total drops of essential oils emulsified in salt before adding to bath water.

- To arrest tremors, seizures, or convulsions, use Hu Po as a single oil or blend Hu Po 25% with Shi Chang Pu (Acorus) 25% and Long Nao (*Borneolum*) 50%, neat, as a smelling salt and direct application on Jing Well points at the corners of the fingernails.

- To break up palpable masses and relieve pain, combine Hu Po with E Zhu (*Curcuma zedoaria*) and Qing Pi (Green Tangerine Peel) as a 4-6% dilution in safflower oil. Gently spread a few drops over the affected area twice per day, three days on and three days off. May be compressed with heat.

HUANG QI 黄芪 / BEI QI 北芪

Astragalus, MILK-VETCH ROOT

Astragali membranaceus Radix

ASTRAGALUS ROOT IS A POWERFUL TONIC. It has become quite well known as an adaptogen and is in common use in natural immune-boosting products. Its essential oil shares this attribute with the added benefits of being able to reach from the level of the Wei Protective Qi to Ying Nutritive Qi to the deepest level of Yuan Source. It strengthens the Lung in its roles of defense against illness, respiration, and oxygenation of the blood. It improves digestion and absorption of nutrients which produce the blood and Qi, and it restores the root Yuan Source Qi which can be depleted or corrupted due to chronic, degenerative illness, age and genetic changes. Huang Qi is also regenerative for the flesh. Topically it is helpful to heal chronic ulcers and sores such as the type that might be seen in diabetes or to restore healthy skin after a serious burn. On an emotional level, the strong, earthy, woody sweetness of Huang Qi essential oil gives one a feeling of hope, restores self-esteem, and provides faith in one's ability to overcome obstacles and forge ahead.

Aroma: Strong, rich, earthy, woody, sweet.

Note: Base.

Part of Plant: Root.

Extraction Method: CO2 extraction.

Color: Dark brown.

Growing Region: Gan Su Province, native to Northeastern China. Harvested spring and autumn.

Major Chemical Components: Triterpenoid saponins: astragalosides, lanosterol, γ-sitosterol. Triterpenes: lupenone triterpene [19]. Monoterpene alcohol: eucalyptol, linalool. Linoleic acid methyl ester.

CM Category: Tonifying Qi.

Nature and Taste: Sweet, slightly warm.

Affinities: Spleen, Lung.

Average Dilution: 4-6%. May be ingested, 1 drop per dose, as a restorative nutritional supplement.

Pharmacological Actions: Immunopromotive, adaptogenic, restorative, metabolic, anti-inflammatory, antiviral, antidiabetic, anticancer (recent research).

ACTIONS AND INDICATIONS:

- Improves digestion and absorption when insufficiency has led to fatigue, weakness of the extremities, poor appetite, diarrhea, or prolapse.

- Strengthens the constitution.
- Boosts the immune system.
- Restorative for conditions that have severely weakened the body.
- Preventative for chronic, recurring illness. Strengthens the Wei Protective Qi to stop sweating.
- Generates flesh and discharges pus for non-healing wounds, ulcers, sores, burns.
- Treats aftereffects of chemotherapy and radiation leading to insufficient white and red blood cells and overall depletion.

CM Concepts, Channel Systems, and Patterns:

- Strengthen the Righteous Zheng Qi.
- Raise the Yang Qi.
- Fortify Spleen Qi and Spleen Yang.
- Tonify Yuan Source Qi.
- Fortify the Wei Protective Qi.

Application and Blends:

To treat the aftereffects of chemotherapy and radiation, to nourish Qi and blood, strengthen the immune system, and as a preventative or restorative, take by internal ingestion, one drop of Huang Qi added to one gram (1/3 tsp) of Ling Zhi/Ganoderma spore oil three times per day.

To boost the immune system and increase white blood cells, combine Huang Qi with Chuan Xiong (*Ligusticum wallichii*) and Dang Gui (*Angelica sinensis*). Dilute 4% in almond oil and massage into areas that tend to sweat, such as the soles of feet and on the center of the chest around the thymus gland.

To strengthen the exterior and fortify the Wei Protective Qi with tendency to easily catch colds or flus, have allergies, or spontaneous sweating, blend Huang Qi 20% with Wu Wei Zi (*Schisandra Fruit*) 30%, Chen Pi (Aged Tangerine Peel) 15%, and Zi Su Ye (Perilla Leaf) 35%. Diffuse into the air daily, or as needed in order to directly affect the Wei Qi via the breath entering the lungs. May be applied neat to the Yuan Source and Luo Connecting points of the Lung and Large Intestine channels, three days on and three days off once per day.

To fortify Spleen Qi and Spleen Yang, strengthen digestion and absorption to treat fatigue, weakness of the extremities, poor appetite, diarrhea, or prolapse, blend Huang Qi 35% with Bi Cheng Qie (Litsea) 35%, Gan Jiang (Dry Ginger) 15%, and Chen Pi (Aged Tangerine Peel) 15%, diluted 4% in black cumin seed oil. Take three drops as a warm drink in acidophilus milk or honey water twice per day after meals. May also be applied to source points of the Spleen and Stomach channels SP3 and ST42 with gentle moxibustion around the navel CV8. For prolapse, add Chai Hu (*Bupleurum*) to the blend, and apply on Bai Hui / GV20.

Huo Xiang 藿香 / Guang Huo Xiang 廣藿香

PATCHOULI

Pogostemonis cablin Herba

Patchouli goes through an alchemical transformation in the process of becoming an essential oil involving fermentation of the leaves before distilling, which brings out its characteristic aroma. This process potentiates the energy of its transformational actions. Patchouli's strong, musky spice aromatically transforms damp accumulation which is both a cause and effect of sluggishness of the digestive function to break down food and turn it into useable energy. On the psycho-emotional level, the aroma transforms pent up emotions and dampness inhibiting the ability to change and breaks up stuck patterns of thinking and behavior. Patchouli's powerful aroma may be used as an aid during the process of death and dying. It helps to orient and integrate Hun and Po (ethereal and corporeal Souls). It can open the portals to summon the Po back in and restore consciousness when near death, but the chest is still warm. As a topical application or diffused into the air, Patchouli is strongly antifungal and antibacterial.

Aroma: Musky, woody, spicy.

Note: Middle/Base.

Part of Plant: Leaf and Twig.

Extraction Method: Fermentation prior to distillation.

Color: Amber.

Growing Region: Guangzhou, Guangdong province, China. The variety from Guangzhou has been considered to have the greatest medicinal potency since ancient times. Harvested from May to June.

Major Chemical Components: Sesquiterpene alcohol: patchoulol. Sesquiterpenic lactone: pogostone. Sesquiterpenes: a-guaiene, a-bulnesene, caryophyllene, a-farnesene.

CM Category: Aromatic Transforming Dampness.

Nature and Taste: Pungent, slightly warm.

Affinities: Spleen, Stomach, Lung. As essential oil, also Heart, Bladder.

Average Dilution: 4-6%.

Pharmacological Actions: Stomachic, digestive, vascular decongestant, anti-inflammatory, antifungal, antiviral, antibacterial, anti-infectious, preventative, nervine.

Actions and Indications:

- Harmonizes upward and downward movement of the Qi and draws it into the center.

- Transforms dampness and harmonizes the middle burner and digestion for nausea, vomiting, diarrhea, fullness, lethargy, and discomfort.
- Increases secretion of gastric acid and promotes digestion.
- Releases exterior wind-damp conditions with digestive flu-like symptoms of fever, chill, headache, fatigue, heaviness, chest and abdominal discomfort, nausea, vomiting, and diarrhea.
- Eliminates fungal, viral, or bacterial infections.
- Breaks up vascular congestion, hemorrhoids, varicose veins.
- Releases entrenched emotions and thought patterns.

CM Concepts, Channel Systems, and Patterns:

- Harmonize Spleen and Stomach.
- Open the Chong Mai/Thoroughfare Vessel.
- Treat emptiness of Spleen's Luo.
- Orient and integrate Hun and Po.

Application and Blends:

To break up vascular congestion and treat varicose veins or hemorrhoids, blend Huo Xiang 60% with Mo Yao (Myrrh) 30% and Qi Li Xiang (Orange Jessamine) 10% as a 4-6% dilution in witch hazel and apply to the affected areas. If hemorrhoids are internal, dilute 3% with coconut oil, form into boluses, and keep refrigerated to solidify for anal insertion.

To harmonize digestion, blend Huo Xiang 40%, Bi Cheng Qie (Litsea) 20%, Mu Xiang (Saussurea) 20%, and Chen Pi (Aged Tangerine Peel) 20%. Dilute 4-6% in black cumin seed oil. Gently spread a few drops over the abdomen and place on acupoints of Stomach and Spleen channels such as ST36 and SP3. For digestive symptoms due to an exterior syndrome like a digestive flu virus, replace Mu Xiang with Bai Dou Kou (Cardamom) and add LI4 and LU7 to the point prescription.

To transform stuck emotional patterns, blend Huo Xiang 50% with Hou Po (Magnolia Bark) 30% and Qing Pi (Green Tangerine Peel) 20%. Use neat for inhalation or in the bath. Yuan Source, Luo Connecting points, and Luo Vessel treatment, depending on the case may be helpful.

Place Huo Xiang, neat, on SP4 to open the Chong Mai/Thoroughfare Vessel or to address emptiness of Spleen's Luo.

For fungal infections on the skin such as athlete's foot, Huo Xiang may be applied as a wash using 20% dilution of Huo Xiang in apple cider vinegar and water directly on the affected areas daily until resolved.

JIANG XIANG 降香

ROSEWOOD

Dalbergiae odoriferae Lignum

THE CHINESE NAME JIANG XIANG 降香 means "Descending Fragrance." The effect of this essential oil and its aroma is grounding and soothing. An alternate name is "Heart Wood" or "Wood of the Heart." As an essential oil, Jiang Xiang focuses on the Heart, both the physical heart residing in the chest with its relationship to the blood and vessels, and the ethereal Heart Mind with its relationship to the emotions and Shen Spirit. Physically, Jiang Xiang relaxes the vessels and descends the Qi and blood to lower blood pressure. Psycho-emotionally, its grounding energy helps one reconnect to one's foundation when trauma or mental illness has severed the connection, giving a new lease on life. In the case of severe depression, it stimulates renewed interest in life. It is stabilizing and healing for the wounds of post traumatic stress. Its aroma opens the consciousness and draws the soul back down. Spiritually, it can be used in meditation practice as incense to invoke the divine.

Aroma: Sweet, woody, leather, with a hint of spice.

Note: Base.

Part of Plant: Wood.

Extraction Method: Distillation or CO2 extraction.

Color: Distilled – clear. CO2 – deep red brown.

Growing Region: Hainan Island, China.

Major Chemical Components: Sesquiterpenes: myrrhene and farnesene >35%. Monoterpene alcohol: linalool. Lactones. Phenols.

CM Category: Regulating Blood.

Nature and Taste: Pungent, slightly warm.

Affinities: Liver, Spleen, Stomach, Heart.

Average Dilution: 8-15%.

Cautions and Contraindications: Caution during menstrual bleeding.

Pharmacological Actions: Hypotensive, nervine, anxiolytic, analgesic, antitussive, antiplatelet, vulnerary, anti-inflammatory, hemostatic.

ACTIONS AND INDICATIONS:

- Relaxes and descends rebellious Qi and blood of head, shoulders, chest, and stomach to treat headache, hypertension, cough, nausea, and vomiting.
- Disperses blood stasis and regulates bleeding.

- Stops bleeding due to blood stasis or clots.
- Breaks up blood stasis due to heat.
- Inhibits platelet aggregation, prevents and breaks up embolisms, clots, and cholesterol.
- Resolves chest Qi stagnation and relieves angina.
- Promotes the healing of injuries, eases pain and generates flesh for wound healing.
- Stabilizes panic attacks, anxiety, personality disorders, mania, PTSD, OCD, and ADD.

CM Concepts, Channel Systems, and Patterns:

- Descend Qi and blood to the Lower Dan Tian.
- Ground and consolidate to promote latency.

Application and Blends:

To lower blood pressure, apply neat, as a single oil or with Wu Wei Zi (*Schisandra Fruit*) on the bottom of the feet. Deeply inhale the aroma directly or diffuse.

Heart pain and wounds may be physical or emotional as the blood is an extension of the Heart Mind and carries the emotions and memories.

- To regulate the blood and break up blood stagnation in the case of emotional wounds and trauma, create an aromatic blend of Jiang Xiang with Qi Li Xiang (Orange Jessamine), Tan Xiang (Sandalwood), and Chen Pi (Aged Tangerine Peel).
- To regulate the blood, break up blood stagnation and resolve chest Qi stagnation with physical pain, angina, or blood clots, blend Jiang Xiang with Zhi Ke (*Citrus aurantium*), and E Zhu (*Curcuma zedoaria*).
- In either case, applying essential oils on Yuan Source Luo Connecting point combinations and along Luo Vessels may be appropriate as well as Yin Wei Mai/Yin Link Vessel. Dilute 10% in pomegranate seed oil to benefit the heart or safflower oil to vitalize the blood. Apply three days on and three days off. Deeply inhale the aroma.

To relax abdominal discomfort with sluggish digestion and short temper caused by Liver Qi constraint stemming from long term suppressed emotion, create an aromatic blend of Jiang Xiang, Mu Xiang (Saussurea), and Zhi Ke (*Citrus aurantium*). Dilute 4-6% in black cumin seed oil and gently spread over the diaphragm and abdomen. Directly inhale the aroma.

JIN YIN HUA 金銀花

HONEYSUCKLE

Lonicerae Japonica Flos

THE CHINESE NAME JIN YIN HUA 金銀花 means "Gold and Silver Flower," referring both to Yang and Yin as well as to the alchemical transmutation of precious metals. Jin Yin Hua essential oil is the sweetest way to clear heat and eliminate toxicity from the body. Its aroma is strong yet pleasantly sweet and floral. It can detoxify without harshness or harm. It is antiviral and antibacterial and is the main ingredient in the popular herbal formula, Yin Qiao San, for treating colds and flus. Applied topically, it is gentle on the skin even though it is powerful enough to eliminate infections, dark spots, and scars. Emotionally, it reduces the intensity of fear and fire, relieving anxiety and insomnia. It purifies the mind and spirit, providing a clean slate, the chance for renewal, and an opening to the spirit as an aid to meditation.

Aroma: Intense, sweet floral.

Note: Middle/Base.

Part of Plant: Flower.

Extraction Method: CO2 extraction.

Color: Golden yellow.

Growing Region: Guilin, Guangxi province, China. Harvested mid-June.

Major Chemical Components: Monoterpene alcohol: linalool. Esters: benzyl acetate, hexenyl acetate. Sesquiterpenes: caryophyllene, humulene. Monoterpenes: ocimene, limonene, alpha-pinene. Phenol (Phenylpropanoid): methyl eugenol.

Average Dilution: 2-4%.

CM Category: Clearing Heat, Resolving Toxicity.

Nature and Taste: Sweet and cold.

Affinities: Lung, Large Intestine, Stomach.

Pharmacological Actions: Anti-inflammatory, antipyretic, antipathogenic, antimicrobial, anticancer, anxiolytic, prebiotic.

ACTIONS AND INDICATIONS:

- Draws toxins out of the body.
- Resolves childhood fire toxins as in the aftereffects of inoculations or infectious and inherited diseases.
- Eliminates wind and fire syndromes.
- Detoxifies the liver.

- Acts as preventative for breast cancer, prostate cancer, and viral infections.
- Treats wind-heat type colds and flus with fever, sore throat, congestion, cough, headache, body aches, and thirst.
- Reduces blood sugar.
- Relaxes, cools, and descends to reduce blood pressure.
- In the digestive tract, acts as prebiotic, supporting microbial flora in the gut, colonization of good bacteria in support of gut flora. It eliminates harmful intestinal bacterial or fungal infections, dysentery, and damp terrain.
- Promotes elimination and diuresis, clears urinary tract infections.
- In OB/GYN it benefits delivery and postpartum, relaxes the uterus and the mind to smoothe labor, delivery, and postpartum recovery.
- In dermatology, it eliminates skin infections, fibrotic tissue, scarring, keloids, boils, pustules, abscesses, and reduces hyperpigmentation (age spots, liver spots, sun damage).

CM Concepts, Channel Systems, and Patterns:

- Clear damp-heat as part of Divergent Meridian treatment strategy.
- Facilitate Yang Qiao Mai/Yang Heel Vessel treatment.
- Benefit the Career Palace of the Nine Palaces.

Application and Blends:

- Blend with Huo Xiang (Patchouli) to promote probiotic terrain in the gut and eliminate harmful bacterial or fungal infections. Dilute equal parts Jin Yin Hua and Huo Xiang 4-6% in black cumin seed oil and take 3 drops with 1 tbsp of yogurt once per day between meals. Three days on, three days off.
- As a preventative, take by internal ingestion with Ling Zhi/Ganoderma spore oil, 1 drop of Jin Yin Hua in 1/3 tsp Ling Zhi spore oil twice per day. Take three days on and three days off for three weeks with a break for one week and then continue the pattern.
- To reduce age spots and reduce hyperpigmentation, blend Jin Yin Hua with Bai Zhi (*Angelica dahurica*), equal parts diluted to 2% in milk and coconut oil. Keep refrigerated. Apply directly on the dark spots once per day at night. Cover and keep overnight.
- For wind-heat illnesses, combine Jin Yin Hua with Lian Qiao (Forsythia) and Bo He (Peppermint), equal parts, and dilute to 4-6% in almond oil, grapeseed oil, or ethyl alcohol and apply to the upper back area around GV12, 13, 14, on the forehead and on acupoints LI20, LI11, LU11, and LI1. If gua sha is going to be used, apply oils afterward. Add 3-5 drops neat to a pint of steaming hot water and inhale the steam with eyes closed.

- To relax the uterus and the mind to smooth labor and promote delivery, use Jin Yin Hua as aromatherapy with deep breathing, or diffuse in the birthing room. Take 1 drop neat by mouth. May also apply on acupoints such as LI4, SP6, GB21, LR5, GB41, BL67 to promote labor and delivery.
- To slow labor and allow for a short break in contractions when the mother is exhausted, apply Jin Yin Hua with Wu Wei Zi (*Schisandra Fruit*) on HT7, PC6, KI4, GB34, LR3, CV17. Restart labor when ready with Jin Yin Hua alone on LI4, SP6, and UB60.
- To ease recovery and treat postpartum depression, add 12 drops of Jin Yin Hua and Bai Zi Ren (Biota Seed) to the daily bath water. Mix first in full fat milk or cream to emulsify the oils. Combine Jin Yin Hua with Ru Xiang (*Boswellia sacra*) in the bath to help heal episiotomy or surgical wounds and prevent scarring.
- To lower blood pressure, blend equal parts Jin Yin Hua 20% with Jiang Xiang (*Dalbergia*) 60%, and Ju Hua 20% (Chrysanthemum). Diffuse or inhale neat. Dilute 10% in Bai Zi Ren (Biota Seed) or black cumin seed cold-pressed carrier oil and apply to the bottom of the feet. May also apply on other acupoints appropriate to the case.

NOTES:

Jing Jie 荊芥

SCHIZONEPETA, NEPETA

Schizonepetae tenuifolia Herba

An interesting thing about Jing Jie essential oil is that it equally affects both Wei Qi exterior and Ying Qi interior levels of the body. On the surface, its strong herbaceous pungency disperses and resolves skin, eye, ear, and nose conditions, as well as common colds. On the level of muscle tendons and joints, it warms, relaxes, and relieves pain. Deeper, it regulates the digestive Qi and moves blood and fluids. It is a wonderful multipurpose addition to activate blends and is useful both diffused for inhalation as well as applied for topical application. Another interesting note is that Nepeta is related to catnip. The two plants share the same chemical component that makes cats euphoric.

Aroma: Strong, fresh, herbaceous, peppery.

Note: Top/middle.

Part of Plant: Leaf, Bud, and Twig.

Extraction Method: Distillation.

Color: Pale yellow.

Growing Region: Jiangxi and Hubei provinces, China. Harvested in September.

Major Chemical Components: Monoterpene ketones: nepetalactone [20], menthone, pulegone, isomenthone, isopulegone. Monoterpene: limonene. Monoterpene alcohol: schizomedol. Monoterpene glycoside: schizonepetoside. Flavonoids. Phenolic acids.

CM Category: Releasing the Exterior.

Nature and Taste: Pungent, slightly warm.

Affinities: Lung, Liver.

Average Dilution: 2-3%. Jing Jie contains a number of ketone chemical constituents. Safe for external use, not recommended for internal ingestion.

Pharmacological Actions: Antispasmodic, bronchodilating, antipyretic, diaphoretic, antibiotic, antipruritic.

Actions and Indications:

- Expels wind-cold or wind-heat type common colds.
- Eliminates congestion, opens the nasal and bronchial passages, relieving chest tightness.
- Vents wind, moves blood, relaxes muscles and tendons, muscular spasms, and bronchospasm.

- Treats damp Bi syndrome joint pain and stiffness.
- Regulates the middle burner, resolves dampness, abdominal swelling, borborygmus.
- Use in dermatology: moves blood in order to expel wind manifesting on the skin with rashes, itching, hives, fistulas, boils.
- Clears phlegm, lymphatic swelling, turbid fluids.
- Promotes diuresis.
- Promotes menstruation and stimulates ovulation.
- Breaks up blood stasis.
- Opens the sensory orifices.
- Clears eye screens and membranes.

CM Concepts, Channel Systems, and Patterns:

- Divergent Meridian SDS treatment strategy (superficial-deep-superficial needling technique for releasing from deep level out to the surface).
- Stimulate release of stagnant Yin.

Application and Blends:

Include in blends to expel exterior wind-cold or wind-heat type common cold. To clear congestion, add 3-5 drops of Jing Jie, neat to 1 pint of hot water and inhale the steam. To release the chest and upper back, dilute 3% in almond oil and apply topically.

For dermatological use:

- For itching, rashes, or hives, blend Jing Jie 25% with Bo He (Peppermint) 25% and Ju Hua (Chrysanthemum) 50% as a 3% dilution in almond oil and apply to the affected areas.
- For fistulas, boils, and pustular sores, blend Jing Jie 25% with Bai Zhi (*Angelica dahurica*) 25%, Ye Ju Hua (Wild Chrysanthemum) 25%, and Qing Pi (Green Tangerine Peel) 25%. Dilute 3% in calophyllum (tamanu) oil and make a paste with green clay powder for application directly over the lesions.

Steam the eyes to dissolve screens or membranes caused by dampness and phlegm accumulation with 3-5 drops combined of Jing Jie and Bai Yu Lan Ye (Magnolia Leaf) equal parts in 1-2 pints of hot, steaming water. Allow the steam to rise from the water to the eye area for 5 to 10 minutes, once or twice per day. If a stinging sensation occurs, increase distance from the water. Three days on and three days off.

Lian Qiao 連翹

FORSYTHIA FRUIT

Forsythiae suspensa Fructus

LIAN QIAO IS EXTRACTED FROM THE WHOLE FORSYTHIA FRUIT along with the seeds within the fruit's shell. Its shape, with its chamber-like interior structure, represents its affinity with the Heart. In Chinese medicine, the heart and mind are one and the same. The Heart belongs to the Fire element with its expressions of joyful enthusiasm, love, and warmth. But Heart fire can flare up requiring moderation, either due to internal causes like strong emotion, or to external causes like an infection that has gone into the blood. In either case, irritability, restlessness, and signs of heat such as fever or skin conditions are likely to occur. Lian Qiao's fresh menthol and camphor aroma produces a cooling, calming, and cleansing effect. Applied topically it clears heat from the blood and the skin.

Aroma: Fresh, herbaceous with menthol-like overtones and camphorous, sharp, bitter undertones.

Note: Middle.

Part of Plant: Fruit.

Extraction Method: Distillation.

Color: Clear.

Growing Region: Shanxi province, China.

Major Chemical Components: Monoterpenes: pinene, sabinene, thujene, camphene, cymene, limonene, terpinene. Monoterpene ether oxide: 1-8 cineole (eucalyptol). Monoterpene alcohols: geraniol, borneol, terpineol, safrole, linalool. Triterpenes. Coumarins.

CM Category: Clearing Heat, Resolving Toxicity.

Nature and Taste: Bitter, slightly acrid, cool.

Affinities: Heart, Lung, Gallbladder.

Average Dilution: 2-3%. May be sun sensitive, caution on exposed skin.

Pharmacological Actions: Mucolytic, antibacterial, antiviral, antipyretic, analgesic, nervine.

Actions and Indications:

- Clears heat and toxins for both interior and exterior syndromes.
- Resolves exterior wind-heat illnesses with fever, thirst, sore throat, swollen glands, headache, body aches, red eyes, cough, congestion.
- Clears exterior heat that has gone deeper, entering the level of Ying and blood with high fever, irritability, restlessness, and impaired consciousness.

- Cools interior heat and heat in the blood expressing as skin lesions, sores, rashes, abscesses, or swollen lymph nodes.
- Clears heat from the Heart and Pericardium.
- Cools Heart fire disturbing the mind to calm agitation, anxiety, and insomnia with heat signs.

CM Concepts, Channel Systems, and Patterns:

- Clear damp-heat as part of Divergent Meridian SDS treatment strategy (superficial-deep-superficial needling technique to draw from deep in the interior out to the surface for release).

Application and Blends:

To treat agitation, anxiety, or insomnia with heat signs, blend Zhi Zi (Gardenia Fruit) 20%, Bai Zi Ren (Biota Seed) 25%, Bo He (Peppermint) 5%, Xun Yi Cao (Lavender) 25%, and Tan Xiang (Sandalwood) 25%. Diffuse or directly inhale neat. May also dilute 4% in Bai Zi Ren (Biota Seed) cold-pressed carrier oil and apply on acupoints that calm the Heart and clear Heart fire.

For wind-heat illnesses combine with Jin Yin Hua (Honeysuckle) and Bo He (Peppermint), equal parts, and dilute to 4-6% in almond oil, grapeseed oil, or ethyl alcohol and apply to the upper back area, and on the forehead. If gua sha is going to be used, dilute to 4% and apply the oils afterward. Add 3-5 drops neat to a pint of steaming hot water and inhale the steam with eyes closed.

To treat skin lesions, sores, rashes, abscesses, or swollen lymph nodes, combine Lian Qiao 30% with Ye Ju Hua (Wild Chrysanthemum) 50%, and Jing Jie (*Schizonepeta*) 20% as a 3% dilution in grapeseed or calophyllum (tamanu) oil. Apply to the affected areas three days on and three days off. Apply as a paste with green clay powder to dry and draw out.

Long Nao 龍腦

BORNEOL

Dryoblanops aromatica, Borneolum

Long Nao 龍腦,the Chinese name of this essential oil, means "Dragon's Brain," indicating the powerful effect it has on the brain and nervous system. Its aroma is piercing, and upon inhalation it travels upward, stimulating and enlivening the senses and the mind. It wakes one up and improves concentration. Long Nao has a smelling salt effect for emergencies to bring one back from a sudden state of shock, delirium, loss of consciousness, or heart failure.

Applied topically, it benefits the nerves, relieves pain, and treats various types of hot skin conditions. The major monoterpene alcohol in Long Nao, borneol, is found in many essential oils and is a natural insect repellant. It has been shown to be a mast cell stabilizer inhibiting allergic reactions. It is a natural antihistamine and anti-inflammatory.

Aroma: Piercing, resinous, acrid.

Note: Top.

Part of Plant: Leaves, twigs, and sap.

Extraction Method: Distillation.

Color: Clear.

Growing Region: Jiangxi province, China.

Average Dilution Percentage: 4-6%.

Major Chemical Components: Monoterpene alcohols: borneol, terpinen-4-ol [21], terpineol. Sesquiterpene: caryophyllene. Monoterpenes: pinene, terpinene, limonene, myrcene.

CM Category: Aromatic Substances that Open the Orifices.

Nature and Taste: Pungent, bitter, slightly cold.

Affinities: Heart, Liver, Lung.

Average Dilution: 4-6%.

Cautions and Contraindications: Contraindicated in pregnancy.

Pharmacological Actions: Analgesic, anti-inflammatory, antihistamine, antifungal, antiviral, antibacterial, neurotonic, antiseizure, insecticide.

Actions and Indications:

- Opens the senses, resuscitates consciousness, awakens the spirit for fainting, loss of consciousness, stroke, convulsions, seizures, dizziness, or sudden loss of Heart Qi.

- Mitigates neurological conditions.
- Use in dermatology for heat, inflammation, pain, itching, swelling, congestion, hot skin sores, herpes zoster, or herpes simplex.
- Eliminates fungal, viral, bacterial infections.
- Repels insects.

CM Concepts, Channel Systems, and Patterns:

- Calm and relax Yin Wei Mai.
- Eliminate fetal toxins.
- Open orifices as part of Divergent Meridian treatment strategy.

Application and Blends:

- To make a smelling salt, mix 5-10 drops in 1/2 oz of salt and keep in a closed container for use as needed.
- On acupuncture points to open the sensory portals and restore consciousness place neat, directly on the Jing Well points, and on either side of the nose at LI20. For wind stroke or epilepsy, place on GV25, GV24, and KI1.
- To treat active or prodromal herpes zoster or simplex and other hot type skin sores or fungal infections, blend Long Nao 15%, Qing Hao 70% (*Artemisia annua*), and 15% of Huo Xiang (Patchouli) or Yin Chen Hao (*Artemisia scoparia*) as a 4-6% dilution in calophyllum (tamanu) carrier oil. May be directly applied on the affected area two to three times per day until resolved.
- To treat allergic reactions, combine with Zi Su Ye (Perilla Leaf). Dilute 4% in coconut oil. Apply topically for symptoms on the skin. Diffuse neat or inhale the steam of 3-5 drops in 1 pint of hot water for allergic sinus or respiratory reactions.
- Add to liniments for pain alone or with other essential oils as a 4% dilution in ethyl alcohol to massage into the painful area.
- To benefit central nervous system disorders, and for nerve or spinal pain, combine with Du Huo (*Angelica pubescentis*) in a 4% dilution as a plaster using egg white as the carrier and apply along the spine or affected areas.

Man Jing Zi 蔓荆子

VITEX, CHASTETREE FRUIT

Viticis agnus castus Fructus

In modern times, Vitex has become a popular supplement for reducing menopausal symptoms. In classical Chinese medicine this can be partially explained by its heat clearing effects. It also calms the Liver which in turn improves mood and balances hormones. It is this association with the Liver that accounts for Man Jing Zi's beneficial effects on the eyes. It is helpful alone or added to blends for treatment of all kinds of eye diseases. Man Jing Zi essential oil's herbaceous spice aroma cools, rises upward, and disperses. Its ascending energy relieves headaches, especially in the area of the temples, including migraines. This essential oil is generally analgesic and anti-inflammatory. For example, it is also helpful when added to blends to treat pain in the muscles and joints.

In *The Shen Nong Ben Cao Jing/Divine Farmer's Materia Medica Classic*, Man Jing Zi is considered a superior grade herb. It says, "It mainly treats cold and heat in the sinews and bones, damp impediment, and hypertonicity. It brightens the eyes, fortifies the teeth, disinhibits the nine orifices and eliminates white worms (pin worms)."

Aroma: Herbaceous, spicy.

Note: Middle/Top.

Part of Plant: Leaf.

Extraction Method: Distillation.

Color: Transparent, pale greenish-yellow.

Growing Region: Native to China's Himalayan Mountain slopes. Cultivated in Bosnia Herzegovina.

Major Chemical Components: Monoterpene ether oxide: 1-8 cineole (eucalyptol). Sesquiterpenes: farnesene, caryophyllene. Monoterpenes: pinene, sabinene. Monoterpene ester: alpha-terpinyl acetate.

CM Category: Releasing Wind-Heat.

Nature and Taste: Acrid, bitter, cool.

Affinities: Liver, Stomach, Bladder.

Average Dilution: 4-6%.

Pharmacological Actions: Antipyretic, anti-inflammatory, analgesic, sedative, antibiotic, antimicrobial, hormone modulatory.

Actions and Indications:

- Dispels wind-heat from the head for dizziness, headache, swelling and pain on the face or gums.
- Cools and relaxes the Liver.
- Balances estrogen and progesterone and relieves menopausal symptoms.
- Treats eye disorders with redness, swelling, pressure, tearing, floaters.
- Relieves aching pain of the muscles, tendons, and joints with spasms and cramps.
- Clears and detoxifies hot skin conditions, abscesses, ulcerations, and carbuncles.

CM Concepts, Channel Systems, and Patterns:

- Brighten the eyes.
- Treat Bi Zheng painful obstruction syndrome.
- Dispel wind and heat in the Liver channel. Drain Liver fire.

Application and Blends:

- For eye disorders with signs of wind and heat in the Liver channel such as redness, swelling, and irritability, blend Man Jing Zi with Ju Hua (Chrysanthemum). Dilute 2% in almond oil and apply as a cool compress over closed eyes, being careful to thoroughly wring out the cloth and do not let the oil drip into the eyes. Additionally, apply a few drops over the occipital area of the back of the neck and on acupoints such as GB37, LR3.

- For menopausal hot flashes, blend Man Jing Zi 25% with Tan Xiang (Sandalwood) 50% and Mei Gui Hua (Rose) 25%. Dilute 4-6% in Bai Zi Ren (Biota Seed cold-pressed) carrier oil and apply on acupoints such as BL23, CV4, KI3, ST42. If there is sweating, add Wu Wei Zi (*Schisandra Fruit*) for application on additional points LI4 and KI7.

- For headaches, facial swelling, and pain, dilute Man Jing Zi with Bo He (Peppermint) 3% in almond oil and apply directly on the painful area.

- To treat arthritis or painful joints with spasm and cramping due to wind and damp blend Man Jing Zi 20% with Yun Shan (Black Spruce) 30%, and Chuan Xiong (*Ligusticum wallichii*) 50% as a 6-8% dilution in ethyl alcohol to make a liniment for application with massage on the affected areas. Cupping after application may be helpful.

Mei Gui Hua 玫瑰花

DAMASCUS ROSE

Rosa damacena Flos

Authentic 100% steam-distilled Damascus Rose is considered one of the "precious" florals. Its aroma is strong and long-lasting. The effect is deeply penetrating, positively influencing both Jing Essence and Shen Spirit. It inspires feelings of beauty, love, and transcendence. Rose essential oil helps one deal with the struggles associated with the cyclical transitions of life: birth and death, puberty, menarche, fertility, menopause, and andropause. It benefits the hormonal system. Rose increases libido and sexual arousal as well as sperm and egg counts. It is calming and mildly sedating. Rose oil is also a great addition to skin care, nourishing, moisturizing, brightening the skin and evening skin tone. Rose oil nourishes the blood.

In Chinese medicine, emotions and memories are stored in the blood as an extension of the Heart Mind. Rose's beneficial effects on the blood lead to a sense of being emotionally nourished. Plants with thorns in Chinese herbal medicine are used to treat nervous system disorders referred to as wind such as tremors. In a positive sense, wind is also a force that enables one to change. Rose addresses wind and its ability to foster change as well as to calm the impact of wind on the nervous system.

Aroma: Sweet, floral, true rose with delicate citrus overtones.

Note: Middle/Base.

Part of Plant: Flower.

Extraction Method: Distillation. Harvested several times per year beginning in May. Flowers are picked on sunny days when in full bloom for maximum aroma and distilled immediately.

Color: Transparent pale yellow.

Growing Region: Shanxi province, China.

Major Chemical Components: Monoterpene alcohols: citronellol, geraniol, nerol, linalool. Alcohol: phenethyl alcohol. Sesquiterpene: caryophyllene. Ester: benzyl acetate. Monoterpenes: pinene, myrcene. Phenols (Phenylpropanoids): eugenol, methyl eugenol.

CM Category: Nourishing Yin.

Nature and Taste: Sweet, slightly bitter and warm.

Affinities: Heart, Liver, Kidney.

Average Dilution: 2%.

Pharmacological Actions: Hormone modulatory, hydrating, hemopromotive (red cells), antidepressant, anxiolytic, nervine, CNS modulatory.

ACTIONS AND INDICATIONS:

- Nourishes the Yin and the Jin Ye body fluids, including hormonal secretions.
- Benefits estrogen, promotes fertility, increases sperm and egg counts.
- Promotes lactation.
- Regulates menses, eases menstrual pain and PMS.
- Regenerates and relaxes the Liver.
- Calms the nervous system. Treats PTSD.
- Eases pain relaxes spasms.
- Regenerates tissue, repairs skin and wounds.
- Benefits the blood, increases blood clotting factor, and generates red blood cells.

CM CONCEPTS, CHANNEL SYSTEMS, AND PATTERNS:

- Regulate and Tonify Liver blood. Nourish Yin.
- Course Liver wind.
- Benefit the Relationship Palace of the Nine Palaces.

APPLICATION AND BLENDS:

- To nourish the Yin, Jin Ye body fluids, and hormonal secretions, dilute 2% in sesame oil. Apply on acupoints of Ren Mai/Conception Vessel, Stomach and Kidney channels that help to generate Yin such as: CV12, ST42, KI6, CV4, CV15.

- To increase sperm and egg counts, dilute Rose alone to 2% in sesame oil and apply to points of Chong and Ren Mai (Thoroughfare and Conception Vessels) such as KI13 (especially for women), KI8, KI11, and KI12 (especially for men), along with ST30 and CV4. Apply three days on and three days off for one to three months. At the woman's mid-cycle ovulation time add 3 drops each of Song Zhen (Pine) and Wu Wei Zi (*Schisandra Fruit*) in order to encourage and hold on to conception by benefiting the Lung Qi. Finish the treatment with LU7 (opening point of Ren Mai/Conception Vessel and Luo of the Lung). Deeply inhale the aroma.

- For promoting lactation, blend 50% Rose and 50% Xiao Hui Xiang (Fennel) in a 4% dilution and apply directly on acupoints such as SI1, ST18, CV17, BL17.

- To relax and regenerate the liver, combine Rose 25% with Chai Hu (Bupleurum) 35% and Xun Yi Cao (Lavender) 40%. Dilute to 4% in jojoba or rapeseed oil and gently spread over the liver area of the right ribs, and on LR8 twice per day, three days on and three days off.

To help regulate the menses, ease PMS and menstrual pain, especially when there is an emotional component affecting the Liver Qi with symptoms such as bloating, breast distention and emotional lability, create an aromatic blend of Rose 20% with Xiang Fu (*Cyperus*) 30%, Dang Gui (*Angelica sinensis*) 25%, and Chuan Xiong (*Ligusticum wallichii*) 25%. Dilute 4% in safflower oil and apply a few drops on LR14, the Mu Accumulation point of the Liver, and over the lower abdomen for three consecutive days at the beginning of each phase of the menstrual cycle and during the first three days of the menstrual flow.

NOTES:

MO LI HUA 茉莉花

JASMINE SAMBAC FLOWER

Jasminum sambac Flos

AUTHENTIC 100% CO2-EXTRACTED JASMINE is considered one of the "precious" florals. Its aroma is a strong and long-lasting base note and the effect is deeply penetrating and elevating, powerfully influencing both Jing Essence and Shen Spirit, body and mind.

The Jasmine plant itself is water-loving and blooms at night. These indicate the nourishing qualities of Yin and its hydrating and hormonal effects. Applied topically, it is gentle, regenerative, and moisturizing for mature skin. Upon inhalation the heady Jasmine aroma immediately affects the pineal gland which balances circadian rhythm, calms the mind, and can have the effect of expanding consciousness. In this way, it can be used to treat insomnia and restlessness or as an aid to meditation, spiritual transformation, and connection to the divine. Jasmine's affinity to the Liver, Lung, and Kidney explains its ability to lift depression, release feelings of grief and loss, and raise self-esteem. Its effect inspires forgiveness, acceptance, and graceful comfort with the aging process. It opens a door to possibilities of completion and new beginnings.

Aroma: Strong, sweet floral, hypnotic.

Note: Base.

Part of Plant: Flower.

Extraction Method: CO2 extraction.

Color: Golden.

Growing Region: Hengxian, Guangxi province, China. Fresh flowers are harvested from May to October on dry days and taken immediately to the factory for extraction.

Major Chemical Components: Monoterpene alcohol: linalool [2]. Esters: benzyl acetate, cis-3-hexenel acetate, methyl anthranilate. Alcohols: cis-3-hexanol, phenethyl alcohol. Sesquiterpene: caryophyllene. Monoterpene: a-farnesene. Phenol (Phenylpropanoid): eugenol. Aldehydes.

CM Category: Nourishing Yin.

Nature and Taste: Sweet and cool.

Affinities: Liver, Kidney, Lung. As essential oil, also Heart, Pericardium.

Average Dilution: 2-4%.

Pharmacological Actions: CNS protective, sedative, anti-inflammatory, antimicrobial, analgesic, antihyperalgesic, antinociceptive, hormone modulatory, anxiolytic, galactagogue, hydrating.

Actions and Indications:

- Nourishes water and clears fire.
- Clears Yin deficiency heat, reduces nighttime heat, sweat, agitation, and insomnia.
- Opens the Heart and Mind and calms the Shen Spirit.
- Strengthens Kidney Qi, nourishes Kidney Yin and Jing Essence.
- Promotes the Ye Thick fluids including hormonal and enzymatic secretions.
- Balances hormones, estrogen, benefits the breasts, ovaries, and testicles and is an aphrodisiac.
- Relieves pain.
- Promotes childbirth and is a uterine tonic and stimulant.
- Eases the stress of prolonged labor.
- Promotes lactation.
- Promotes menstruation.
- Treats sexually transmitted diseases (STD)s.
- Benefits and regenerates mature skin.
- Breaks up scar tissue.
- Mucolytic, breaks up phlegm stasis.
- Clears heat and inflammation from the eyes, treats conjunctivitis.
- Treats dysentery and abdominal pain.
- Opens the lungs and sinuses.
- Relaxes spasms.

CM Concepts, Channel Systems, and Patterns:

- Support the Creativity Palace of the Nine Palaces.
- Open the Yin Qiao Mai/Yin Heel Vessel.
- Break up excess Yin Stasis in Ren Mai/Conception Vessel.

Application and Blends:

- To relax muscular spasms and the mental state causing the tension at the same time, dilute 2% in jojoba or rapeseed oil and use as an aromatic massage oil.
- To open the Lungs and ease the grieving process, diffuse neat 10 drops in the diffuser.
- As an aphrodisiac for low libido, blend Jasmine 50% with She Chuang Zi (Cnidium Fruit) 25% and Xiao Hui Xiang (Fennel) 25% as a 4% dilution in sesame oil. Gently spread over the area of CV2 with light, indirect moxibustion, and apply on LR5. Deeply inhale the aroma.

- During labor to promote childbirth and ease the stress of prolonged labor, deeply inhale the aroma, and take 1 drop neat on the tongue. May also dilute 2-4% in safflower oil, apply a few drops over the abdomen and sacrum, or apply on acupoints such as LI4, SP6, GB21, and BL67.
- To nourish Kidney Yin, promote Ye Thick fluids and hormonal secretions, dilute 4% in sesame oil and apply on acupoints such as: ST42, KI6, CV7, CV12, CV15, and BL23.
- If Yin stasis in Ren Mai is blocking the free distribution of Yin, pair Jasmine with Nan Mu (Cedarwood) and place on LU7 to open the Ren Mai/Conception Vessel and on its trajectory points such as CV3, 4, 9, 17, and 22.
- As an aid to meditation to open the consciousness and a connection to the divine, anoint Yin Tang (Third Eye), and GV20. Deeply inhale the aroma or diffuse in the meditation space.

NOTES:

Mo Yao 沒藥

MYRRH

Commiphorae myrrhae Resina

The character for Mo 沒 (or Mei) in Mo Yao translates as "Not, None, or Without." It is a medicine of nothingness which also means it has great potential. Its color is dark, and its aroma is a deep, complex balsamic. Myrrh is one of the aromatic resins considered holy fragrances that have been used for millennia as incense and anointments in religious rites and rituals to assist healing and spiritual transformation. Being a resin, one of Mo Yao essential oil's most important attributes is that it promotes wound healing for both physical and emotional trauma. Frankincense and Myrrh are traditionally often paired together as they were among the precious gifts given to the baby Jesus Christ by the three wise men from the East.

Aroma: Balsamic, with a piercing, spicy, bitter edge.

Note: Base.

Part of Plant: Resin.

Extraction Method: CO2 extraction or Distillation.

Color: Deep red-brown.

Growing Region: Oman, Somalia.

Major Chemical Components: Sesquiterpenes: curzerene, elemene, germacrene, lindestrene, selinene. Sesquiterpenoids [22]: furanoeudesma, eudesmol. Sesquiterpene ether: heerabolene. Aldehyde: cuminaldehyde. Phenols (Phenylpropanoids): eugenol, eudesmol. Ester: a-elemyl acetate.

CM Category: Invigorating Blood and Dispelling Stasis.

Nature and Taste: Spicy, bitter, neutral.

Affinities: Heart, Liver, Spleen. As essential oil, also Lung, Stomach.

Average Dilution: 4-6%.

Cautions and Contraindications: Contraindicated during uterine bleeding or pregnancy.

Pharmacological Actions: Analgesic, vulnerary, expectorant, anti-inflammatory, antiviral, antifungal, antihyperlipidemic, hormone modulatory.

Actions and Indications:

- Invigorates blood and disperses blood stasis.
- Reduces swelling, pain, bruising, and varicose veins.
- Generates new tissue and promotes wound healing of sores, skin lesions, ulcerations, injuries.

- Repairs mucus membranes and gut mucosa, Crohn's disease, ulcerative colitis.
- Clears Lung and Stomach heat causing cough with thick yellow phlegm, gum swellings, toothaches, laryngitis, or hyperthyroidism.
- Activates blood circulation.
- Promotes and increases menstrual flow and therefore contraindicated during uterine bleeding or pregnancy.

CM Concepts, Channel Systems, and Patterns:

- Break up blood stasis in Luo Vessel treatment strategy.
- Generate flesh.

Application and Blends:

For wound healing, to generate new tissue, or break up scar tissue, combine Mo Yao (Myrrh) and Ru Xiang (Frankincense) in equal parts. If there is redness and inflammation add a small percentage of an essential oil which has heat clearing and antimicrobial properties such as Ju Hua or Ye Ju Hua (Chrysanthemum or Wild Chrysanthemum). If there is swelling or pus, add Yi Yi Ren (Coix) or Bai Zhi (*Angelica dahurica*). For scars or burns, add Ce Bai Ye (Biota Leaf). Dilute the blend to 3-4% in calophyllum (tamanu) or almond carrier oil. If the wound is not completely closed, apply around the borders.

To treat emotional wounds and scars, create an aromatic blend of Mo Yao and Ru Xiang (Frankincense) with floral aromas such as Qi Li Xiang (Orange Jessamine), Bai Yu Lan Ye (Magnolia Leaf), Mo Li Hua (Jasmine), or Mei Gui Hua (Rose) along with Xiang Fu (*Cyperus*). Neat or diluted, deeply inhale the aroma directly from the bottle or diffused and wear as perfume. Place on case appropriate acupoints, for example on the Yin Wei Mai/Yin Link Vessel opening and trajectory points, once per day, three days on, and three days off.

To invigorate blood and disperse blood stasis, relieve pain, resolve bruising, and varicose veins, apply Mo Yao and Ru Xiang (Frankincense) with Chuan Xiong (*Ligusticum wallichii*), equal parts, as a liniment on the affected areas. Make a 4-6% dilution in ethyl alcohol or safflower oil. For varicose veins use witch hazel as the carrier.

For inflammation of the gums, blend Mo Yao with Ding Xiang (Clove) and a citrus oil such as Qing Pi (Green Tangerine Peel) or Zhi Ke (*Citrus aurantium*). Dilute the blend 1% in sesame oil to swoosh in the mouth as oil-pulling.

Mu Xiang 木香

SAUSSUREA, COSTUS ROOT

Aucklandiae lappa Radix

Mu Xiang 木香 means "Wood Fragrance" and this essential oil's aroma is distinctly woody. Whereas modern Chinese medicine focuses Mu Xiang's activity on the Earth element as an aid to digestion, its main affinity as an oil is with the Wood element, most especially the Gallbladder. Gallbladder is one of the Extraordinary Fu, with an intimate association with the brain. Its attributes are courage and decision-making, maintaining harmony between opposing forces and coordination of right and left sides of body and brain. A manifestation of this is found in the Chinese name of the Gallbladder channel's Mu Accumulation point which is Ri Yue 日月, meaning Sun and Moon. The essence of Mu Xiang, with its woody aroma, is an ally to resolve inner conflict and to cultivate the Wood temperament. When the Qi of the Gallbladder—with its effect on the Stomach and Spleen—is not functioning well, dampness can accumulate, clouding the mind and upsetting digestion. Mu Xiang regulates the Qi and transforms the dampness. This can help to resolve depression, anxiety, foggy mind, or mental and personality disorders that may result.

The *Shen Nong Ben Cao Jing/Divine Farmer's Materia Medica Classic* gives Mu Xiang the distinction of an upper-grade herb and says that it "gets rid of evil, worms, ghosts, strengthens discipline and will power." Sun Si Miao, an influential Tang dynasty physician and writer also used Mu Xiang to get rid of ghosts.

Aroma: Woody, bitter and spicy.

Note: Middle/base.

Part of Plant: Root.

Extraction Method: CO2 extraction.

Color: Dark brown.

Growing Region: Yunnan Province, China.

Major Chemical Components: Sesquiterpene lactones: costunolide [23] (woody lactone dehydrogenase) > 60%, eremanthin. Sesquiterpenes: guaiene, himachalene, caryophyllene.

CM Category: Regulating Qi.

Nature and Taste: Pungent, bitter, warm.

Affinities: Spleen, Stomach, Large Intestine, Gallbladder.

Average Dilution: 2-4%.

Pharmacological Actions: Anti-inflammatory, antioxidant, antifungal, antibiotic, antiulcer, cholagogue, smooth muscle relaxant, neuroprotective, antidepressant, anxiolytic.

Actions and Indications:

- Regulates the movement of Qi throughout the middle burner.
- Unblocks Qi stagnation of Spleen, Stomach, Gallbladder and Liver.
- Promotes the food transforming and transporting functions of the Stomach, Spleen, and regulates bowel elimination.
- Alleviates all kinds of digestive dysfunction and discomfort: poor appetite, indigestion, food stagnation, diarrhea, abdominal fullness, pain, spasms, and colitis.
- Protective effect for gastric ulcers.
- Regulates digestive disharmony caused by strong emotion as when Liver Qi stagnation is affecting the Stomach.
- Clears damp heat accumulation, jaundice, gallstones, damp heat diarrhea, and dysentery.
- Transforms dampness and phlegm.
- Antibiotic against strep, staph, and E. coli.
- Antifungal against candida.

CM Concepts, Channel Systems, and Patterns:

- Regulate middle burner Qi.
- Harmonize Liver and Spleen.

Application and Blends:

- For signs of dampness due to sluggish and stagnant Qi affecting mind and body, causing symptoms as bloating, diarrhea, candida, foggy mind, fatigue, and depression, blend equal parts Mu Xiang with Huo Xiang (Patchouli), Cang Zhu (Atractylodes), and Chen Pi (Aged Tangerine Peel) as a 4-6% dilution in black cumin seed oil. Deeply and often inhale the aroma and apply to acupoints such as SP4, ST40, and GB24. Point application three days on, and three days off.

- To ease abdominal fullness and pain, blend Mu Xiang 70% with Fo Shou (Buddha's Hand Fruit) or Zhi Ke (*Citrus aurantium*) 30% as a 4% dilution in black cumin seed oil and apply a few drops gently spread over the area of discomfort as well as on acupoints of Stomach and Large Intestine channels. Apply two to three times per day, three days on, and three days off.

- To clear damp-heat accumulation, jaundice, or gallstones, blend a 4-6% dilution in castor oil with Mu Xiang 20%, Yin Chen Hao (*Artemisia scoparia*) 30%, Qing Pi (Green Tangerine Peel) 20%, and Zhi Zi (Gardenia Fruit) 30%. Apply as a compress over the liver and gallbladder area of the right ribs twice per day for three days, then take three days off and repeat the cycle for one month or as needed.

- Diffuse to clear the air of unwanted entities with 10 to 15 drops of Mu Xiang, neat, in the diffuser.

NAN MU 楠木

SOUTHERN CHINESE CEDARWOOD

Cupressus funebris Lignum

THE DISTINCTIVE, SMOKY, EVERGREEN AROMA of Southern Chinese Cedarwood essential oil takes one on a journey from high treetops, down straight, strong trunks to roots buried deep in the moist earth of a dense forest. It inspires freedom to extend upward and outward while keeping a sense of grounded quietude. The bright, balsamic evergreen aspect of the aroma connects with the Lungs and Wei Protective Qi while the dark, mysterious smoky quality connects with the Kidneys, and the Yuan Source Qi. Medicinally, Nan Mu's effects reach from the skin on the exterior to the deepest interior level, preserving and protecting the constitution against environmental factors. The prominent sesquiterpene content of Nan Mu essential oil means that it is gentle on the skin, calming, grounding, regulates the Qi, reduces pain, and relaxes spasm.

Aroma: Smoky, woody, balsamic.

Note: Base.

Part of Plant: Wood.

Extraction Method: Distillation.

Color: Clear, slightly yellow.

Growing Region: Southern China.

Major Chemical Components: Sesquiterpenes: cedrene, thujospene, funebrene, caryophyllene, himachalene, cuparene, chamigrene, cuprenene. Sesquiterpene alcohols: cedrol, widdrol.

CM Category: Phlegm and Damp-Heat Resolving.

Nature and Taste: Spicy, cool.

Affinities: Lung, Kidney, Bladder.

Average Dilution: 6-8%.

Pharmacological Actions: Antifungal, antiyeast, antiviral, antibacterial, mucolytic, insect repellant, anti-inflammatory, analgesic, antispasmodic, nervine,

ACTIONS AND INDICATIONS:

- Clears Lung heat and phlegm, breaks up mucus and phlegm, prevents pneumonia and chest congestion.
- Descends and anchors the Lung Qi to the Kidneys.
- Clears the lymphatic system.

- Promotes urination and clears lower burner damp-heat conditions, burning, painful urination, yellow discharge with foul odor, genital sores, warts, HPV, and gout.
- Breaks down gallstones and polyps.
- Eliminates yeast and fungal infections.
- Repels insects and soothes bug bites.
- Prevents decay and damage due to insects and environmental factors.
- Protects and purifies through diffusion to clear the air.

CM Concepts, Channel Systems and Patterns:

- Open Dai Mai/Belt Vessel, Ren Mai/Conception Vessel, Du Mai/ Governing Vessel.
- Break up Yin stasis.
- Affinity to Ren 15 (source point of Yin).
- Facilitate KI/BL Divergent Meridian treatment strategy.

Application and Blends:

As an insect repellant and treatment for bug bites, combine Nan Mu 40% with Ai Ye (*Artemisia argyi*) 30% and Bo He (Peppermint) 30% in a 4-6% dilution of equal parts ethyl alcohol and water as a spray to apply topically or 12-15 drops of the blend, neat, in a diffuser to affect the environment.

To clear the lungs, respiratory infections, asthma, break up mucus and phlegm, or to prevent pneumonia, blend Nan Mu 40%, An Shu Ye (Eucalyptus) 20%, Song Zhen (Pine Needle) 20%, Xing Ren (*Prunus armeniaca*) 5%, and Zhi Ke (*Citrus aurantium*) 15% as a 4-6% dilution in Zi Su Zi (Perilla Seed) or almond carrier oil and apply over the chest and upper back two to three times per day, three days on and three days off. Diffuse 10-15 drops of the essential oil blend, neat, in a diffuser to open the breathing passages and to disinfect the air.

To break down gallstones or polyps, prepare a 4-6% dilution of Nan Mu 60%, Yin Chen Hao (*Artemisia scoparia*) 20%, and Qing Pi (Green Tangerine Peel) 20% in castor oil for compress directly over the affected area, twice per day, three days on and three days off.

For genital sores, warts, or HPV, blend Nan Mu 60% with She Chuang Zi (Cnidium Fruit) 30%, and Qing Hao (*Artemisia annua*) 10% as a paste made from 3% total essential oils with calophyllum oil and green clay powder. Apply topically, cover and leave in place overnight, three days on, three days off.

For gout, a topical application with 60% Nan Mu and 40% Hu Lu Ba (Fenugreek Seed) as an 8% dilution with calophyllum (tamanu) or castor oil. Apply to the affected area three times per day, three days on and three days off.

Qi Li Xiang 七里香

ORANGE JESSAMINE FLOWER

Murraya paniculata Flos

The beautiful and complex floral scent of Qi Li Xiang is calming and vitalizing. Its name 七里香 means "Seven Mile Fragrance," so named because the enduring fragrance of its blossoms are said to waft for miles. Upon inhalation it can immediately change a mood from stuck and dark to free and bright. In traditional medicine Qi Li Xiang essential oil is used as an analgesic, to treat injuries and to clear toxins. Its aroma brings these affects to the level of the mind and spirit as well, transforming entrenched psycho-emotional pain and toxic thoughts that result from injury due to post traumatic stress. Additionally, this oil's chemistry, which exhibits an immune system boosting effect, translates emotionally as giving one the strength to defend oneself and to stand up against adversity.

Aroma: Soft, floral, heady, jasmine-like with a sweet, citrus tone and light spice.

Note: Middle.

Part of Plant: Flower.

Extraction Method: CO2 extraction.

Color: Orange.

Growing Region: Guangxi province, China. A tropical evergreen with small, white, sweet-scented flowers which are harvested from April to August.

Major Chemical Components: Esters: benzyl acetate, linalyl acetate. Phenethyl alcohol.* Phenol (phenylpropanoid): eugenol. Monoterpene alcohol: linalool. Sesquiterpene: caryophyllene.

CM Category: Invigorating Blood.

Affinities: Heart, Pericardium, Liver.

Average Dilution: 2-4%.

Pharmacological Actions: Antioxidant, anti-inflammatory, analgesic, nervine, sedative, antinociceptive, preventative, immunostimulant.

Actions and Indications:

- Vitalizes the blood.
- Benefits the heart and cardiovascular system.
- Resolves injuries, swelling, bruising, and inflammation.

---

* *Phenethyl alcohol, widely occurring in nature and responsible for a certain floral scent, prevents bacteria growth and acts as a natural preservative. The scent attracts bees for pollination.*

- Calms the spirit.
- Relieves physical and psycho-emotional pain, as well as PTSD on account of its antinociceptive properties—a term in psychology, meaning it increases tolerance for, or reduces sensitivity to, perceived dangerous or harmful stimuli.
- Clears toxins.
- Benefits immunity by boosting white blood cell production.

CM Concepts, Channel Systems, and Patterns:

- Tonify Heart Qi.
- Nourish the Heart calm the Shen Spirit.
- Open Yin Wei Mai/Yin Link Vessel.
- Balance Fire and Water relationship.
- Benefit the Prosperity Palace of the Nine Palaces.

Application and Blends:

To ease emotional pain or trauma, treat PTSD, and to calm the spirit, wear Qi Li Xiang alone as a perfume, deeply inhale the aroma directly from the bottle, diffuse, or add to the bath as a bath salt. An aromatic blend can be created with Qi Li Xiang, Xiang Fu (*Cyperus*), Bai Zi Ren (Biota Seed), Jiang Xiang (*Dalbergia*), and Mei Gui Hua (Rose) as a choice of possible ingredients for these purposes. Consider placement on opening and trajectory points of the Yin Wei Mai/Yin Link Vessel.

As a cardiovascular tonic, blend essential oils of Qi Li Xiang 40%, Ren Shen (Ginseng) 10%, Rou Gui (Cinnamon Bark) 10%, Bai Zi Ren (Biota Seed) 20%, and Dang Gui (*Angelica sinensis*) 20%. Dilute 4-6% in safflower carrier oil and apply to acupoints such as Yuan Source and Luo Connecting points of the Heart, Pericardium, and Lung: LU9, PC6, and HT7 plus Back Shu Transport and Front Mu Accumulation points of the Heart BL15, CV14.

As a topical liniment to promote healing and relieve pain for injuries with bruising, inflammation, swelling make a 4-6% dilution in ethyl alcohol or safflower oil with essential oils of Qi Li Xiang 30%, Ru Xiang (*Boswellia sacra*) 40%, Mo Yao (Myrrh) 20%, and Fo Shou (Buddha's Hand Fruit) 10%. Apply to the affected area on unbroken skin.

Qing Hao 青蒿

SWEET WORMWOOD

Artemisiae annuae Herba

The aroma of Qing Hao is complex, both sharply bitter and softly sweet, expressing its dual natures of detoxifying and nourishing. It exudes the cleansing, renewal of springtime, season of the Wood element, as well as the restorative quiet of winter, the season of the Water element. Inhaling clears and cools the eyes, the forehead, and the mind while also vibrating deeply into the level of blood and bone. In the body it works through the Liver and Gallbladder, whose natures are Yang and whose actions are on the Qi and blood, as well as through the Kidney, whose nature is Yin and whose action is on the bones and joints.

Qing Hao is powerfully detoxifying. At the same time, it cools heat due to deficiency of Yin and replenishes the fluids. Water, the source that engenders all life, nourishes Wood's attributes of growth and change. Qing Hao restores a feeling of faith in oneself, and trust as one moves through life's difficulties that everything will become clear and work out the way it is meant to.

Aroma: Sharp, herbaceous, bitter, sweet.

Note: Top/Middle.

Part of Plant: Leaf and Twig.

Extraction Method: Distillation.

Color: Golden yellow.

Growing Region: Guangxi province, China. Harvested in autumn.

Major Chemical Components: Sesquiterpenes <33%: caryophyllene, copaene, serinene, beta-elemene. Sesquiterpene lactone: artemisinin [24]. Monoterpene ketone: camphor ~22%. Sesquiterpene alcohols: a-bisabolol. Monoterpene alcohol: eucalyptol, borneol.

CM Category: Deficiency Heat Clearing.

Nature and Taste: Bitter, pungent, cold.

Affinities: Liver, Gallbladder, Kidney. As essential oil, also Lung.

Average Dilution: 4-6%.

Pharmacological Actions: Antiviral, antibacterial, antimalarial, antiparasitic, insecticide, antipyretic, expectorant, hydrating.

Actions and Indications:

- Clears heat toxin type skin sores, resolves herpes zoster and simplex.
- Nourishes yin, hydrates, and cools heat.

- Treats steaming bone syndrome, a deep pervasive heat and dryness caused by insufficient Yin with chronic low-grade or tidal fevers, irritability, thirst.
- Clears accumulation, congestion, inflammation and heat from the Liver and Gallbladder.
- Eliminates worms, intestinal parasites, ringworms.
- Kills head lice, insect infestation, bed bugs.
- Benefits and clears the lung, respiratory infections, cough, asthma, expectorates mucus and phlegm.

CM Concepts, Channel Systems, and Patterns:

- Treat steaming bone syndrome.
- Clear Liver/Gallbladder damp-heat.
- Break up Yin stasis.
- Facilitate Yin Qiao Mai/Yin Heel Vessel treatment.

Application and Blends:

As a topical application to resolve active herpes simplex or zoster outbreak, prodromes, or as a preventative in chronic cases. A 4-6% dilution of Qing Hao alone in calophyllum (tamanu) carrier oil or as a blend of Qing Hao 70%, Long Nao (*Borneolum*) 15%, and Huo Xiang (Patchouli) or Yin Chen Hao (*Artemisia scoparia*) 15%, may be directly applied on the affected area two to three times per day during the prodromal or active phase until resolved. For prevention, apply three days on and three days off.

Qing Hao's common name, Wormwood, refers to its property to eliminate worms. It may be ingested as a short, five-day course of treatment, Qing Hao 50% together with Hou Po (Magnolia Bark) 30% and Ding Xiang (Clove) 20% as a 4% dilution in black cumin seed oil for adults, 2% for kids seven to fourteen years, 0.5% to 1% for age two to seven. Take 1-3 drops of the oil blend with 1 tsp of apple cider vinegar prepared as a drink in 1/2 cup of water. Take one to three times per day on an empty stomach.

As part of a blend to nourish Yin, clear deficiency heat and treat steaming bone syndrome, blend Qing Hao 30%, Wu Wei Zi (*Schisandra Fruit*) 50%, and Mei Gui 20% (Rose) as a 4-6% dilution in pomegranate seed carrier oil. Deeply inhale the aroma and apply to acupoints such as KI6, HT6, TH4, BL43, and CV7. Apply twice per day, three days on and three days off.

Qing Hua Jiao 青花椒

GREEN SICHUAN PEPPER

Zanthoxyli schinifolium Pericarpium

Qing Hua Jiao essential oil has a very pleasant and fresh green pepper aroma which conceals its intense pungency and powerful germ and parasite-killing properties. In its concentrated essential oil form, it is most effective and safe when used as a diluted, topical application. The stagnating nature of cold causes pain and interruption of the normal movement of Qi, blood, and fluids. The hot, spiciness of Qing Hua Jiao is numbing on the surface, warming, and dispersing internally.

Aroma: Fresh, herbaceous, peppery, citrus.

Note: Top.

Part of Plant: Peel.

Extraction Method: CO2 extraction.

Color: Dark olive-brown.

Growing Region: Sichuan Province, China.

Major Chemical Components: Monoterpenes: myrcene, limonene, phellandrene, pinene. Monoterpene ether oxide: 1-8 cineole (eucalyptol). Phenolic ketone: xanthoxylin. Furoquinaline alkaloids: skimmianine, kokusaginine. Coumarin: herniarin [25] (methoxycoumarin).

CM Category: Warming the Interior and Expelling Cold.

Nature and Taste: Acrid, hot.

Affinities: Kidney, Spleen, Stomach, Bladder.

Average Dilution: 1-2%. Very hot and acrid. Will irritate the skin if insufficiently diluted.

Pharmacological Actions: Anesthetic, analgesic, antibiotic, antiparasitic.

Actions and Indications:

- Warms and relieves excess cold accumulation in stomach or abdomen with pain, vomiting, diarrhea, or toothache.
- Eliminates intestinal parasites and parasitic skin infections, pruritis, eczema, and itching.
- Regulates water circulation to relieve edema, or water accumulation in the lungs with dyspnea and wheezing.
- Numbs pain.

APPLICATION AND BLENDS:

- For coldness and pain in the epigastric and abdominal areas with digestive disharmony, mix 20 drops of Qing Hao in 4 cups of hot water, soak a cotton cloth in the dilution and apply to the painful area as a warm compress.
- As a topical application for parasitic skin infections such as scabies, tinea, and funguses, combine 50% Qing Hua Jiao with 50% She Chuang Zi (Cnidium Fruit) essential oil. Make a wash or a spray as a 2% dilution with apple cider vinegar and water to apply to the affected areas three times per day for one week.
- For toothache, a 1% dilution of Qing Hua Jiao with sesame oil may be applied neat directly on the painful area with a small wad of cotton or swab as an anesthetic and antibiotic acute care remedy.

NOTES:

Qing Pi 青皮

GREEN MANDARIN TANGERINE PEEL

Citri reticulatae viride Pericarpium

Qing Pi, with its bright, tart aroma, is very good at cutting through and breaking up emotional or tangible accumulations that get in the way of the free and easy flow of one's life and Qi. Holding on to long-term, unexpressed, unresolved emotions and frustrations can manifest physically as hard lumps, fibroids, or masses, or may simply cause the stomach to back up resulting in discomfort and digestive problems. In Chinese medicine, the Liver is responsible for the smooth flowing of the Qi and blood throughout the body. Anger, frustration, resentment, and suppressed emotions injure the Liver. Qing Pi regulates the Liver Qi and promotes the ability to move, change, and grow. It facilitates letting go of imposed social constructs that inhibit self-expression.

Aroma: Bright, fruity, with tart and slightly bitter tones.

Note: Top.

Part of Plant: Peel.

Extraction Method: Cold-pressed.

Color: Light golden-yellow.

Growing Region: Guangdong Province, China.

Major Chemical Components: Monoterpenes: limonene, terpinene, pinene, myrcene, cymene, sabinene, thugene. Monoterpene alcohols: linalool, terpineol, citronellol. Methyl esters. Phenol: thymol.

CM Category: Regulating Qi.

Nature and Taste: Bitter, acrid, warm.

Affinities: Gallbladder, Liver, San Jiao, Stomach.

Average Dilution: 4-6%.

Pharmacological Actions: Antimicrobial, antiseptic, mucolytic, expectorant, astringent.

Actions and Indications:

- Breaks up accumulations, clumping, and masses.
- Unbinds the chest and abdomen.
- Spreads Liver Qi and breaks up stagnant Qi.
- Decongests fatty liver and gallbladder.
- Dissipates stones, clumping, hardenings, masses, accumulations, and food stagnation.

- Releases distention and pain of chest, breast, hypochondriac, and epigastric regions.
- Descends rebellious Stomach and Liver Qi causing digestive disturbances.
- Alleviates emotional stagnation, repression, anger, resentment, and frustration.
- Safe for children's stomach "bugs," as well as digestive flu.
- Guides blends to the surface for discharging and dispersing.

CM Concepts, Channel Systems, and Patterns:

- Liver Qi Stasis.
- Dredge the Liver.
- Regulate Liver overacting on the Stomach.
- Regulate Rebellious Stomach and Liver Qi.
- Regulate Qi as part of Divergent Meridian treatment strategy.

Application and Blends:

When there are digestive disturbances due to strong or suppressed emotion causing rebellious Stomach and Liver Qi, create an aromatic blend of Qing Pi, Chai Hu (Bupleurum), and Mu Xiang (Saussurea) as a 4-6% dilution in black cumin seed oil. Compress over the upper abdominal and ribs area.

To alleviate emotional stagnation, formulate an aromatic blend of Qing Pi 20%, Chai Hu (Bupleurum) 20%, and Huo Xiang (Patchouli) 60% to use neat as direct inhalation with deep breaths as needed. Place on acupoints such as the Pericardium Yuan Source point P7, Liver Luo Connecting point LR5, and GB12. Three days on, three days off.

For long term Qi stagnation leading to blood stagnation, fixed pain, palpable masses, and breast lumps, combine Qing Pi with E Zhu (*Curcuma zedoaria*), Xiang Fu (*Cyperus*), and Chuan Xiong (*Ligusticum wallichii*) essential oils. Dilute to 4-6% in calophyllum (tamanu) or safflower carrier oil. Apply over the affected area and on associated channel points twice per day, three days on, three days off.

Ren Shen 人参

Bai Shen 白参 / Ji Lin Shen 吉林参

WHITE GINSENG ROOT

Panax ginseng Radix

Ginseng's Chinese name, Ren Shen 人参, means "Humanity Root." Its shape typically looks like a human body reflecting its benefits to the entire body and the whole person, body, mind, and spirit. As a root, it works on the deep, Yuan Source level. Ren Shen tonifies Yuan Source Qi by strengthening the Spleen/Stomach's digestion and absorption of vital nutrients, along with the Lung's role of oxygenating the blood and maintaining protective immune mechanisms. These are the foundations of postnatal Qi and blood which in turn support the constitutional, prenatal Yuan Source Qi.

Ginseng essential oil powerfully promotes the recovery and maintenance of physical and mental vitality. The sweet, earthy aspect of its aroma and taste attests to its blood nourishing and Qi boosting qualities while the concentrated bitter aspect reflects its primary focus on the Fire element's Heart Mind. This is in keeping with *The Shen Nong Ben Cao Jing/Divine Farmer's Materia Medica Classic* which distinguishes Ren Shen as a superior grade herb, saying: "It mainly supplements the five viscera, it quiets the essence spirit, settles the ethereal and corporeal soul, checks fright palpitations, eliminates evil Qi, brightens the eyes, opens the Heart, and sharpens the wits."

Aroma: Earthy, sweet, bitter.

Note: Base.

Part Of Plant: Root.

Extraction Method: CO_2 extraction.

Color: Dark brown.

Growing Region: Changbai Mountains, Jilin Province, China. Must grow in very cold climate. Will go dormant if temperature rises above 30 degrees Celsius. Harvested in late September when the temperature is around 15 degrees Celsius at least six years after planting. Sun dried.

Major Chemical Components: Sesquiterpenes: pansinsene, farnesene, caryophyllene, elemene, neodovene, selinene, humelene, patchoulene. Sesquiterpene alcohols: spathulenol, sanatalol, eudesmol. Triterpene saponin: ginsenosides.

CM Category: Tonifying.

Nature and Taste: Sweet, slightly bitter, slightly warm.

Affinities: Lung, Spleen. As essential oil, also Heart.

Average Dilution: 20%-50%. Gentle and nutritional. May be ingested, 1 drop per dose.

Pharmacological Actions: Adaptogenic, anti-aging, restorative, antidiabetic, antioxidant, antiplatelet, antiulcer, anxiolytic, cardiotonic, cognitive, antifatigue, endocrine (pituitary, adrenal), metabolic, hypotensive, immunostimulant, radioprotective.

Actions and Indications:

- Benefits the Heart Qi, calms the Shen Spirit, palpitations, anxiety, insomnia, restlessness, and improves mental faculties and memory.
- Restores and revitalizes the body after severe depletion due to loss of Yin fluids, blood, or chronic illness.
- Promotes the generation of body fluids and relieves thirst.
- Benefits marrow and enhances blood cell production.
- Tonifies Spleen and Stomach functions of transformation as well as transportation of food and fluids.
- Strengthens the Lung, treats deficiency of Lung Qi, benefits respiration especially in the case of chronic respiratory illness such as tuberculosis.
- Boosts the Wei Protective Qi, immune system, and resistance.

Application and Blends:

- To improve mental function and memory, combine Ren Shen with Shi Chang Pu (Acorus) and Wu Wei Zi (*Schisandra Fruit*), neat, for diffusion or by direct inhalation several times per day. Additionally, hydrosols of Ren Shen and Yuan Zhi (*Polygala tenuifolia*) as a spray over the face and head are beneficial.

- To benefit and calm the Heart and Spirit, create an aromatic blend of Ren Shen with Bai Zi Ren (Biota Seed) and Qi Li Xiang (Orange Jessamine Flower) or Mei Gui Hua (Rose) for inhalation, in the bath and to apply on points of the Heart or Pericardium channels.

- Ren Shen essential oil may be ingested as a restorative, nutritional supplement. 1 drop of Ren Shen with 1/3 tsp of a nutritional oil such as Ling Zhi (Ganoderma) spore, may be taken two to three times per day, three days on and three days off.

- To tonify Yuan Source and Postnatal Qi, dilute Ren Shen as a single oil or with other essential oils that benefit the Jing Essence, Qi, and blood, such as Gou Qi Zi (Goji Berry) and Wu Wei Zi (*Schisandra Fruit*), and apply to Yuan Source and Shu Transport points, especially those associated with Kidney, Spleen, and Lung channels. Three days on and three days off.

Rou Dou Kou 肉豆蔻

NUTMEG

Myristicae fragrans Semen

Rou Dou Kou is one of the essential oils extracted from what are commonly used as kitchen spices, in this case, nutmeg. Not only do these spices share sweet, pungent aromas that stimulate the appetite, but they are also digestives, cooked with food to warm and settle the stomach and improve the digestive function. They tend to be helpful to condition the environment in the gut, making it inhospitable to yeast, bacterial, or parasitic infections. Rou Dou Kou in particular has an astringent nature which makes it especially helpful to stop diarrhea.

Aroma: Strong, spicy, sweet.

Note: Middle.

Part of Plant: Seed.

Extraction Method: CO2 extraction.

Color: Golden yellow.

Growing Region: Guangdong and Yunnan Provinces, China.

Major Chemical Components: Monoterpenes: sabinene, camphene, pinene. Phenols (phenylpropenes): myristicin [26], elemicin [27], (phenylpropanoids): eugenol, safrole. Monoterpene ether oxide: 1-8 cineole (eucalyptol). Alcohols. Esters. Oxides.

CM Category: Stabilizing and Binding.

Nature and Taste: Acrid, warm.

Affinities: Large Intestine, Spleen, Stomach.

Average Dilution: 2%.

Cautions and Contraindications: Contraindicated for internal ingestion, psychotropic and toxic if ingested.

Pharmacological Actions: Stomachic, astringent, analgesic, antibiotic, antifungal, antiparasitic, antioxidant, anti-inflammatory, psychedelic.

Actions and Indications:

- Warms the center, strengthens the functions of the Spleen and Stomach and binds the intestines to stop chronic diarrhea, cold abdominal discomfort, indigestion, flatulence, nausea, vomit, and poor appetite.
- Eases tension and pain.
- Warms and circulates the sinews to relieve cold-damp joint pain, soreness, numbness, and heavy sensations of the limbs and joints.

CM Concepts, Channel Systems, and Patterns:

- Warm and tonify Spleen Yang.
- Treat cold-damp Bi Obstruction.
- Bind the Intestines.

Application and Blends:

- To warm the center and regulate the digestive Qi, blend Rou Dou Kou with equal parts Gan Jiang (Dry Ginger), Mu Xiang (*Saussurea*), and Chen Pi (Aged Tangerine Peel) as a 2% dilution in black cumin seed carrier oil. Apply to the abdomen as a warm compress.
- To bind the intestines for chronic diarrhea due to Spleen and Kidney Yang deficiency, blend Rou Dou Kou with equal parts Ding Xiang (Clove), Xiao Hui Xiang (Fennel), and Wu Wei Zi (*Schisandra Fruit*) as a 2% dilution in black cumin seed carrier oil. Apply to the lower abdomen and navel area as a warm compressor with moxa cones burned on a slice of ginger on the navel. May be placed on acupoints such as KI8, SP4, BL21, BL23, three days on, three days off.
- May be added to blends for cold-damp Bi Obstruction, with soreness, pain, numbness and heavy sensations of the limbs and joints. For example: Rou Dou Kou 20%, Gui Zhi/ Gui Ye (Cinnamon Twig and Leaf) 10%, Du Huo *(Angelica pubescentis)* 20%, Yi Yi Ren (Coix) 20%, and Song Zhen (Pine Needle) 30%, as a 3% diluted blend in safflower carrier oil or ethyl alcohol and applied as a liniment.

NOTES:

Rou Gui 肉桂

CINNAMON BARK

Cinnamomi cassia Cortex

The characteristic strong and spicy aroma of Cinnamon has a stimulating effect on the brain, the spine, and the nervous system. At the same time, it is warming and grounding for the Kidneys at the root, as well as fortifying for the Heart. In the Chinese model, the Heart and Mind are inseparable. Good communication between the Heart (the Fire element) and the Kidneys (the Water element) is essential for mental, emotional, neurological, and physiological balance. Cinnamon facilitates the connection among all of these systems and frees any blockage in their pathways. On an emotional level, by anchoring the root, and strengthening the Heart Mind, Rou Gui helps to overcome fear and anxiety, giving one a feeling of warmth and security.

Aroma: Sharp, spicy, sweet.

Note: Base.

Part of Plant: Bark.

Extraction Method: CO2 extraction.

Color: Red-brown.

Growing Region: Guangxi Province, China. Harvested February – March.

Major Chemical Components: Phenols (Phenylpropanoids): cinnamaldehyde [28] > 80%, eugenol 5-10%. Aldehydes 65-75%. Coumarin [14].

CM Category: Warming the Interior.

Nature and Taste: Pungent, sweet, hot.

Affinities: Kidney, Bladder, Spleen, Heart, Liver.

Average Dilution: 1-2%.

Cautions and Contraindications: Hot and pungent, will irritate the skin if insufficiently diluted. Photosensitive, caution on exposed skin.

Pharmacological Actions: Cardiovascular tonic, neurotonic, anti-infectious, preventative, antifungal, antioxidant, anti-inflammatory, antidiabetic, antimicrobial, anticancer, antihyperlipidemic.*

---

* *Numerous studies have confirmed that in addition to being an antioxidant, anti-inflammatory, antidiabetic, antimicrobial, anticancer, lipid-lowering and cardiovascular-disease-lowering compound, cinnamon has also been reported to have therapeutic activities against neurological disorders.*

Actions and Indications:

- Warms and eliminates cold blockage and relieves pain of the joints and lower back.
- Opens the spine and regulates nervous system for epilepsy, seizures, convulsions, and Down's syndrome.
- Anchors the root for grounding, stabilizing fear and chaotic Qi.
- Strengthens Kidney Yang to treat impotence, lumbar pain, frequent clear urination.
- In OB/GYN it warms the uterus, promotes menses and fertility, relieves cold-induced cramping or stabbing pain, and increases uterine contractions during childbirth.
- Harmonizes the digestion and the emotions.
- Benefits the cardiovascular system and opens blocked blood vessels.
- Reduces blood sugar levels.
- Eliminates fungal and candida infections.

CM Concepts, Channel Systems, and Patterns:

- Fortify Kidney and Heart Yang.
- Promote Heart and Kidney communication.
- Treat cold-damp Bi syndrome.
- Warm middle and lower burners.
- Harmonize Spleen/Stomach.
- Supplement and awaken Yang in Du Mai/Governor Vessel treatment strategy.

Application and Blends:

To open the spine and regulate nervous system for children with congenital or developmental delay, a 0.5%-1% dilution (0.5% for children under twelve years) of Rou Gui combined with Du Huo (*Angelica pubescentis*) and Nan Mu (Cedarwood) in a gentle carrier oil can be applied along both sides of the spine, with gentle massage using a glass rod. Three days on, three days off, once per day.

To increase uterine contractions during labor, apply directly on BL67. For difficult labor apply on LI1.

For use in OB/GYN to warm the uterus in order to promote menstruation and fertility or to relieve cold-induced pain, apply a 4% diluted blend with Rou Gui 10%, Ai Ye (*Artemisia argyi*) 45%, and Dang Gui (*Angelica sinensis*) 45%. For infertility, add Mei Gui Hua (Rose). For cramping pain add Chuan Xiong (*Ligusticum wallichii*). Apply as a warm compress with a hot water bottle. Gentle, indirect moxabustion may be used to warm the area.

- To promote Heart and Kidney communication and to anchor the root for grounding, to overcome fear and chaotic Qi, create an aromatic blend of Rou Gui 10%, Jiang Xiang (*Dalbergia*) 30%, Bai Zi Ren (Biota Seed) 30%, and Qi Li Xiang (Orange Jessamine) 30% for inhalation and direct application on acupoints such as the Yuan Source and Luo Connecting points of the Kidney and Heart channels, on KI1, CV14, and CV7. Once or twice per day three days on, three days off.

NOTES:

RU XIANG 乳香

FRANKINCENSE

Olibanum Gummi, Boswellia carterii

AS A CHINESE MEDICINE, THE RESIN OF THE *BOSWELLIA CARTERII* tree is focused on vitalizing the blood to relieve pain and to generate new tissue for the healing of wounds. As an essential oil, applied topically it shares these attributes. Especially the CO2 extraction, with its thick and sticky consistency, is well suited to bind wounds and sores which are slow to heal. Frankincense essential oil's healing attributes apply equally to emotional trauma as well. Its aroma is deeply relaxing and revitalizing for body and mind.

Like other aromatic resins and woods such as Myrrh and Sandalwood, Frankincense has been used in the rituals and religious ceremonies of diverse cultures throughout the ages as an incense and anointment to purify the soul, lift the spirit, and invoke the presence of the divine. It stimulates the pineal gland in the brain, sometimes called "the seat of the soul."

Frankincense resins may be obtained from different species of Boswellia trees, each with their own unique qualities but similar in most of their therapeutic properties. Chemically their essential oils are very similar, with differences in the percentages of components. Much recent research into its chemistry has focused on anticancer, antitumor effects.

Aroma: Rich, balsamic, sweet, with a sharp edge.

Note: Base.

Part of Plant: Sap resin.

Extraction Method: CO2 extraction or Distillation.

Color: CO2 – Gold. Distilled – Clear.

Growing Region: Egypt, Puntland area of Somalia (sustainably sourced).

Major Chemical Components: Triterpenic acids: boswellic acids [29], 11 keto-B-boswellic acid [30]. Monoterpenes: pinene, dipentene, camphene, a-thujene, limonene, sabinene, myrcene, phellandrene, cadinene. Sesquiterpenes: caryophyllene, caryophyllene oxide, cadinene. Sesquiterpenic alcohols: muurolol, cadinol, cubelol. Monoterpene alcohol: terpinen-4-ol. Monoterpene ether oxide: 1-8 cineole (eucalyptol).

CM Category: Invigorating Blood, Removing Blood Stasis.

Nature and Taste: Pungent, bitter, warm.

Affinities: Liver, Heart, Spleen.

Average Dilution: 8-10%.

Pharmacological Actions: Vulnerary, analgesic, antinociceptive, antispasmodic, anticoagulant, anti-inflammatory, antioxidant, anticancer, chemopreventative, antitumor, mucolytic, immunostimulant, antifibrotic, anti-ulcer, sedative.

Actions and Indications:

- *Boswellia carterii* is the type of Frankincense most commonly used in Chinese medicine.
- It invigorates the blood, relaxes the sinews, and smoothes the movement of the Qi and blood.
- It unbinds the chest and releases the diaphragm.
- Topically, treats acute swelling and pain, and in wound care, speeds healing, generates new tissue, and breaks up scar tissue.
- Internally promotes repair of mucus membranes and gut mucosa, Crohn's disease, ulcerative colitis.
- Initiates the healing response for stubborn chronic illnesses such as chronic lung conditions or chronic fatigue syndrome.
- Boosts platelets.
- Enhances the immune system.
- Has a tonic effect on the adrenal glands.
- Breaks up phlegm accumulation, masses, and tumors.

CM Concepts, Channel Systems, and Patterns:

- Luo Vessel treatment – Break up blood stasis, accumulation, or nodules along Luo Vessels.

Application and Blends:

For both *Boswellia carterii* and *Boswellia sacra*:

- To treat emotional trauma, wounds, and scars, create an aromatic blend of Frankincense with floral aromas such as Qi Li Xiang (Orange Jessamine), Bai Yu Lan Ye (Magnolia Leaf), Mo Li Hua (Jasmine) or Mei Gui Hua (Damascus Rose), along with Xiang Fu (*Cyperus*). Deeply inhale the aroma directly, diffuse, or wear as perfume. A healing bath salt can be made with 15-20 drops of the blend. May be placed on case appropriate acupoints, for example Yin Wei Mai/ Link Vessel opening and trajectory points once per day, three days on, and three days off.

- As a liniment or massage oil to relax the sinews, and to smooth the movement of blood and Qi, blend a 4-6% dilution in ethyl alcohol or safflower oil with equal parts essential oils of Chuan Xiong (*Ligusticum wallichii*) and Xun Yi Cao (Lavender) for topical application on affected areas as needed.

- For wound healing, to generate new tissue, and break up scar tissue, combine equal parts Ru Xiang with Mo Yao (Myrrh). If there is redness and inflammation add a small percentage of an essential oil which has heat clearing and antimicrobial properties such as Ju Hua or Ye Ju Hua (White or Wild Chrysanthemum). If there is swelling or pus, add Yi Yi Ren (Coix Seed) or Bai Zhi (*Angelica dahurica*) to draw it out. For scars or burns add Ce Bai Ye (Biota Leaf). Dilute the blend to 3-4% in calophyllum (tamanu) or almond carrier oil. If the wound is not completely closed, apply around the borders.
- To repair mucus membranes and gut mucosa, Crohn's disease, or ulcerative colitis, internal ingestion of a 3% dilution of Ru Xiang 30%, Mo Yao (Myrrh) 20%, Jin Yin Hua (Honeysuckle) 25%, and Chen Pi (Aged Tangerine Peel) 25%, with coconut oil as the carrier. Three drops three times per day in yogurt, kefir, or coconut milk for one month.
- To free the movement of Qi and blood in the chest and diaphragm, blend Ru Xiang 35% with Tan Xiang (Sandalwood) 35%, Xiang Fu (*Cyperus*) 25%, and Bo He (Peppermint) 5% as a 4% dilution in almond or safflower oil and apply topically over the area of constraint. Deeply inhale the aroma.

NOTES:

Ru Xiang 乳香

SACRED FRANKINCENSE

Olibanum Gummi, Boswellia sacra

The word sacra in the species name of this Boswellia tree distinguishes its resin as Sacred Frankincense. The magic of its essential oil's heavenly aroma transports one to an elevated state. *Boswellia sacra* has been prized as an incense and anointment in rituals and religious ceremonies throughout the ages for its transformative healing properties, both physically and spiritually. It works miraculously quickly when applied topically for the pain, bruising, swelling of acute injuries. It gradually heals the scars of old wounds and breaks up masses and tumors.

Although this essential oil shares many of the same medicinal attributes as *Boswellia carterii,* the aroma of Sacred Frankincense more specifically elicits awareness of the spiritual side of healing, the deeper meanings behind our pain and wounds. Where the heavy, resinous nature of CO2 *Boswellia carterii* can bind a physical wound, *Boswellia sacra*'s focus is on healing wounds of the Heart and Spirit. It connects us to the divine.

Aroma: Bright resinous, balsamic with light citrus and floral tones.

Note: Base.

Part of Plant: Sap resin.

Extraction Method: Distillation.

Color: Clear.

Growing Region: Oman.

Major Chemical Components: Triterpenic acids: boswellic acids [29], 11 keto-B-boswellic acid [30]. Monoterpenes: pinene, dipentene, camphene, a-thujene, limonene, sabinene, myrcene, phellandrene, cadinene. Sesquiterpenes: caryophyllene, caryophyllene oxide, cadinene. Sesquiterpenic alcohols: muurolol, cadinol, cubelol. Monoterpene alcohol: terpinen-4-ol. Monoterpene ether oxide: 1-8 cineole (eucalyptol).

CM Category: Invigorating Blood, Removing Blood Stasis.

Nature and Taste: Resinous, pungent, bitter, warm.

Affinities: Liver, Heart, Spleen.

Average Dilution: 8-10%. Gentle but powerful. May be applied neat for short-term use.

Pharmacological Actions: Vulnerary, analgesic, antinociceptive, antispasmodic, anticoagulant, anti-inflammatory, antioxidant, anticancer, chemopreventative, antitumor, mucolytic, immunostimulant, antifibrotic, anti-ulcer, sedative.

ACTIONS AND INDICATIONS

(also see *Boswellia carterii*)

- Speeds recovery from injury, bruising, swelling, blood stasis, pain, burns, and generates tissue to promote wound healing.
- Breaks up tumors, masses, and fibroids.
- Speeds cancer cell death.

CM CONCEPTS, CHANNEL SYSTEMS, AND PATTERNS:

- Luo Vessel treatment – Break up blood stasis, accumulation, or nodules along Luo Vessels.
- Generate flesh.

APPLICATION AND BLENDS

(also see *Boswellia carterii*)

- Apply neat for short-term use as topical application to treat acute symptoms of injury, bruising, swelling, blood stasis, pain, or burns. Dilute for longer term recovery.
- Make a bath salt to assist with healing the wounds of emotional trauma.

NOTES:

She Chuang Zi 蛇床子

CNIDIUM FRUIT

Cnidium monnieri Fructus

She Chuang Zi essential oil's musky, salty aroma warms the lower back and abdomen and stimulates the genital region. The translation of She Chuang Zi 蛇床子, "Snake's Bed Seed," refers to the observation that snakes often rest under this plant and eat its seeds which symbolically illustrates its benefits to sexual and reproductive function. Snakes also shed their skin, which metaphorically refers to She Chuang Zi's ability to treat skin problems. Many of the benefits of She Chuang Zi are related to its special relationship to the Kidneys, some of whose attributes, according to Chinese medicine, include maintaining the strength of the bones, and supporting will power and motivation. This essential oil gives one "backbone."

She Chuang Zi is categorized in CM as an herb for topical application. The CO2-extracted essential oil adapts well to treatment for skin conditions such as weeping, itchy skin lesions, parasites, scabies, ringworm, tinea, trichomonas, fungal infections, chronic eczema, or rashes, as well as swelling and pain of the groin and genital region, and hemorrhoids.

Aroma: Musky, earthy, salty, with sharp bitter overtones.

Note: Base.

Part of Plant: Seed.

Extraction Method: CO2 extraction.

Color: Light golden-brown.

Growing Region: Shandong Province, China.

Major Chemical Components: Coumarin: osthole [31], Monoterpenes: limonene, pinene. Sesquiterpenes: farnesene, himachalene. Monoterpene ester: bornyl acetate.

CM Category: Topical Application.

Nature and Taste: Pungent, bitter, warm.

Affinities: Kidney.

Average Dilution: 2-4%.

Cautions and Contraindications: Photosensitive, caution on exposed skin.

Pharmacological Actions: Antifungal, antipruritic, antiparasitic, pro-libido, osteopromotive, immunomodulatory, anti-inflammatory, analgesic, antitumor, anticancer.

ACTIONS AND INDICATIONS:

- Treats dermatological conditions.
- Stops itching.
- Kills parasites on the skin.
- Resolves fungal infections, chronic eczema, and rashes.
- Benefits the groin and genital region to treat pain, swelling, itching, trichomoniasis, hemorrhoids, and STDs.
- Benefits and warms Kidney Yang to improve libido, sexual, and reproductive function.
- Engenders bone and benefits joints to improve osteopenia, osteoporosis, low back pain, swollen painful joints.
- Draws heat and toxins from the deep level outward.

CM CONCEPTS, CHANNEL SYSTEMS, AND PATTERNS:

- Open the Eight Extraordinary Vessels as part of a blend.
- Fortify Kidney Yang.
- Assist Kidney Yang to drain Dai Mai/Belt Vessel.

APPLICATION AND BLENDS:

- Use in dermatology: To treat itchy skin lesions caused by parasites or fungal infections, make a wash or spray with 2 tbsp apple cider vinegar and 1 quart of water. Or can be prepared as an oily application with calophyllum (tamanu) carrier oil. 2% dilution with She Chuang Zi alone or together with essential oils of Long Nao (*Borneolum*), Zhang Nao (White Camphor), Ye Ju Hua (Wild Chrysanthemum), or Wu Zhu Yu (Evodia). Apply directly over the affected area three times per day for one to three weeks.

- For genital region conditions, make a 1% dilution of She Chuang Zi as a salve with coconut oil to apply on the affected area. Or prepare as a vaginal douche in vinegar and water, 3-5 drops of essential oil per quart of water and vinegar (1-2 tbsp white vinegar to 1 quart water). Use one to three times per day, for one to three weeks as needed.

- To fortify and warm Kidney Yang, improve reproductive and sexual function and libido, blend She Chuang Zi 40% with Hu Lu Ba (Fenugreek) 25%, Xiao Hui Xiang (Fennel) 25%, Rou Gui (Cinnamon Bark) 5%, and Ding Xiang (Clove) 5% as a 4-6% dilution in sesame oil. Apply to acupoints such as: KI3, BL23, CV4, or LR5, once per day, three days on and three days off for one month. Include Mei Gui Hua (Rose) to increase sperm and egg counts. Wear a drop of Mo Li Hua (Jasmine) as an aphrodisiac perfume.

- To engender bone and benefit joints, for osteopenia and osteoporosis, chronic low back or joint pain due to deficiency, aging or disability, and to mend broken bones, combine She Chuang Zi 30% with Du Huo (*Angelica pubescentis*) 40%, and Ce Bai Ye (Biota Leaf) 30%, as a 4-6% dilution in sesame oil. Gently spread a few drops over affected areas as well as across the kidney area of the lower back and on acupoints BL11 (the influential point for bone), and SI6, whose point name, Yang Lao, means "Support the Aged;" three days on and three days off for one to three months. Light moxibustion may be applied.

- May be added to blends to assist in opening the Eight Extraordinary Vessels for treatment. An example of essential oils that resonate with each of the 8XV are:

  Ren Mai/Conception Vessel – Nan Mu (Cedarwood)

  Du Mai/Governing Vessel – Rou Gui (Cinnamon Bark)

  Chong Mai/Thoroughfare Vessel – Huo Xiang (Patchouli)

  Dai Mai/Belt Vessel – Qing Hao (*Artemisia annua*) if damp-heat, Ai Ye *(Artemisia argyi)* if damp-cold.

  Yin Wei Mai/Yin Link Vessel – Mei Gui Hua (Damascus Rose)

  Yang Wei Mai/Yang Link Vessel – Xiang Fu (*Cyperus*)

  Yin Qiao Mai/Yin Heel Vessel – Mo Li Hua (Jasmine)

  Yang Qiao Mai/Yang Heel Vessel – Su He Xiang (Styrax)

These may be placed neat on opening points and chosen trajectory points once per day, three days on, and three days off for one to three months.

SHI CHANG PU 石菖蒲

ACORUS, SWEET-FLAG

Acori tatarinowii Rhizoma

SHI CHANG PU ESSENTIAL OIL'S strong, bright, and sharp aroma has an immediate effect on the brain, bringing a heady expansion which sharpens and focuses the mind and the senses. It can bring one back from sudden loss of consciousness or, used over time, it can improve memory and mental capacity. Shi Chang Pu awakens the spirit and expands consciousness. A little goes a long way in this regard and it can even have what might be called a "psychedelic" effect if overused, but when treated with respect, it can be a tool for meditation and spiritual practices.

According to *The Shen Nong Ben Cao Jing/Divine Farmer's Materia Medica Classic*, Shi Chang Pu is classified as a superior grade herb. The text says, "It opens the heart portals, supplements the five viscera, frees the nine orifices, brightens the eyes and sharpens the hearing. Continued use can make the body light, improve memory, prevent confusion, and prolong life. Its other name is Chang Yang (Flourishing Yang)."

Aroma: Bright, sharp, pungent, slightly sweet.

Note: Base.

Part of Plant: Rhizome.

Extraction Method: Distillation.

Color: Copper.

Growing Region: Anhui Province, China. Harvested in mid-summer

Major Chemical Components: Phenols (Phenylpropanoids): β-asarone [32] ~60%-80%, α-asarone ~3-14%, eugenol, elemicin [27], eusarone, sekishone. Sesquiterpenes: caryophyllene, humulene. Aldehyde: asarylaldehyde.

CM Category: Aromatic Substances that Open the Orifices.

Nature and Taste: Acrid, bitter, warm, aromatic.

Affinities: Heart, Stomach. As essential oil, also Bladder, Liver, Gallbladder.

Average Dilution: 3-4%.

Cautions and Contraindications: External use or diffusion is recommended. Internal ingestion of Acorus essential oil is controversial due to its asarone component. Overuse can cause neurological symptoms.

Pharmacological Actions: Sedative, antidepressant, cognitive, CNS suppressant, antiseizure, anticonvulsant, anti-Alzheimer's, psychedelic.

Actions and Indications:

- Pacifies the spirit.
- Harmonizes and promotes digestive function to transform dampness, vaporize phlegm, and remove turbidity.
- Unblocks the senses and revives consciousness as in the case of stroke, seizures, mania, stupor, delirium, and spasms.
- Improves sensory and cognitive functions and treats memory loss, dementia, confusion, dizziness, dulled senses, and aphasia.
- Sharpens the vision and hearing, for tinnitus, deafness, and visual obstruction.

CM Concepts, Channel Systems, and Patterns:

- Harmonize the Middle Jiao.
- Strengthen Spleen and Stomach.
- Transform turbid dampness.
- Transform phlegm obstructing the Heart and sensory portals.
- Benefit the Wisdom Palace of the Nine Palaces.

Application and Blends:

- To unblock the senses and revive consciousness as emergency medicine, use neat as direct inhalation and apply on the Jing Well points (at the corners of the nails), on GV25 and LI20 (at the tip and sides of the nose). A smelling salt can be made with Shi Chang Pu alone or with other essential oils that open the senses such as Long Nao (*Borneolum*) or Zhang Nao (White Camphor). Mix 5 drops neat in 1/2oz of salt and keep in a closed container for use as needed.
- For improved sensory and cognitive functions, combine with essential oils that specifically address the particular function. For example, memory and cognitive functions: Wu Wei Zi (*Schisandra Fruit*) and Chuan Xiong (*Ligusticum wallichii)*; Vision: Gou Qi Zi (Goji Berry), Ju Hua (Chrysanthemum), and Bo He (Peppermint); Aphasia and loss of sensory motor function: Bi Cheng Qie (Litsea). 4% dilutions may be applied on the head over the impaired brain area and on associated channels (0.5%-1% for children). Apply two to three times per day, three days on, and three days off for one to three months. As an example, for aphasia: apply over the affected brain speech area (temporal and/or frontal lobe) and on acupoints: HT5, KI6, GV15, and CV23.
- For memory care, 6-9 drops of Shi Chang Pu can be added to a 2-3oz spray bottle of the hydrosols of Yuan Zhi (*Polygala tenuifolia*) and Bai Ren Shen (White Ginseng), and gently sprayed on the face and head as often as desired. Shake well before each use to distribute the oil. To nourish the Heart and calm the Spirit, add the essential oil of Bai Zi Ren (Biota Seed) together with Shi Chang Pu (a total of 6-9 drops).

SONG ZHEN 松針

PINE NEEDLE

Pinus tabuliformis

THE BRIGHT AND EVERGREEN AROMA OF PINE NEEDLES from high atop a tall tree elicits a feeling of reaching upward to exchange breath with the heavens while being rooted to the earth. Upon inhalation, it opens the senses, frees the breathing passages, expands the chest, and inspires a feeling of ease and quietude. Song Zhen essential oil's primary affinity is to the Lung, including its spirit aspect, the Po (corporeal soul).

Applied as a liniment, Song Zhen essential oil effectively relieves pain. Diffused into the air or applied as a chest rub, it resolves respiratory illness. In the Chinese culture the aroma of Pine is used to aid and ease the dying process by helping the dying person to let go, to release the Po from its earthly attachments and allow the ascension of the Hun (ethereal soul) to move on. The aroma also helps those left behind to process the feelings of grief and loss associated with the Lung.

Aroma: Balsamic, bright, sharp, pungent.

Note: Middle.

Part of Plant: Needle.

Extraction Method: Distillation.

Color: Clear.

Growing Region: Native to northern China.

Major Chemical Components: Monoterpenes: pinene, camphene, phellandrene, limonene, myrcene, ocimene. Monoterpene ether oxide: 1-8 cineole. Monoterpene alcohol: terpineol. Sesquiterpenes: germacrene, caryophyllene, cadinene.

CM Category: Dispelling Wind-Damp and Relieving Pain.

Nature and Taste: Bitter, sweet, warm.

Affinities: Lung, Kidney.

Average Dilution: 8-10%.

Pharmacological Actions: Mucolytic, decongestant, antitussive, respiratory, antibacterial, antiviral, antifungal, disinfectant, analgesic, nervine.

ACTIONS AND INDICATIONS:

- Benefits and warms the joints for arthritis and tendino-muscular pain.
- Anchors the Lung Qi downward to the Kidneys and opens the breathing passages to reduce coughing, wheezing, phlegm, congestion, and upper respiratory infections.

- Opens the sensory orifices.
- Strengthens the lungs and immune system.
- Supports the adrenal glands, adrenal exhaustion, and hormonal secretions.
- Stimulates underactive thyroid and regulates elevated TSH.

CM Concepts, Channel Systems, and Patterns:

- Diffuse and descend Lung Qi.
- Dispel wind-cold-damp Bi Obstruction.
- Aid Kidney to grasp Lung Qi.
- Release the Po (corporeal soul).

Application and Blends:

- Diffuse for upper respiratory infections to open the breathing passages, resolve coughing, wheezing, phlegm, congestion, and to disinfect the atmosphere. Combine Song Zhen, An Shu Ye (Eucalyptus), and Zi Su Ye (Perilla leaf) together with a total of 10-15 drops neat in the diffuser. As a topical application for the chest and upper back, add Bo He (Peppermint) and dilute to 4% in Zi Su Zi (cold-pressed Perilla Seed) or almond carrier oil.

- Add to blends as a topical application to warm the joints and alleviate pain. Make an 8% dilution of Song Zhen in ethyl alcohol as a vitalizing liniment or in safflower oil for massage over affected areas. Other essential oils that may be combined with Song Zhen for this purpose are: Du Huo (*Angelica pubescentis*), Jing Jie (Schizonepeta), Chuan Xiong (*Ligusticum wallichii*). To make the blend more warming, add Gui Zhi/Gui Ye (Cinnamon Twig and Leaf), or Rou Gui (Cinnamon Bark). These last two oils are quite spicy and should not exceed 5% of the total essential oils in the blend.

- To anchor the Lung Qi and strengthen the Kidney's function, to grasp the Lung Qi when there is underlying deficiency or when emotional issues dealing with fear, trauma, or loss cause respiratory distress. Create an aromatic blend of Song Zhen with Mo Li Hua (Jasmine), Zi Su Zi (Perilla Seed), Wu Wei Zi (*Schisandra Fruit*), and Bai Zi Ren (Biota Seed). Diffuse neat and deeply inhale the aroma. Dilute 8% in Zi Su Zi (Perilla Seed) or sesame seed carrier oil for application across the kidney treatment area of the lower back, and on the chest area of the Kidney channel and Ren Mai/Conception Vessel along with its opening point LU7.

- To tonify Kidney Yang and support the adrenal and thyroid glands, blend Song Zhen 20% with essential oils of Ho Luo Bo Zi (Carrot Seed) 20%, Hu Lu Ba (Fenugreek) 40%, and Ai Ye (*Artemisia argyi*) 20% as an 8% dilution in sesame or black cumin seed oil and apply to acupoints BL23 and on Stomach and Large Intestine channels around the thyroid area of the throat. May be applied twice per day, three days on and three days off.

SU HE XIANG 蘇合香

STYRAX

Liquidamber orientalis

SU HE XIANG MEANS "Aroma of Revival and Unification:" revive (su 蘇), indicating to revive consciousness, unify (he 合), indicating the reunification of the mind with the body, which would be needed, for example, to bring someone back from a faint. Or, in a spiritual sense, the merging of the inner Heart Mind with the outer universal consciousness, referred to as the Little Shen and Big Shen Spirit, respectively. Upon inhalation, Su He Xiang's penetrating aroma clears away turbidity clouding the mind. It warms and opens the channels and restores normal circulation. Diffusing it into the air provides the added benefits of reducing electromagnetic radiation and cleansing the aura.

Aroma: Penetrating, heady, resinous, with balsamic, leathery sweetness and sharp, terpenic tones.

Note: Middle.

Part of Plant: Resin.

Extraction Method: CO2 extraction.

Color: Reddish amber.

Growing Region: Central and southern China.

Major Chemical Components: Phenols: 3-phenylpropanol, 3-phenylpropyl cinnamate. Ester: cinnamyl cinnamate. Aldehyde: cinnamyl aldehyde. Monoterpene: pinene. Sesquiterpene: caryophyllene.

CM Category: Aromatic Substances that Open the Orifices.

Nature and Taste: Sweet, acrid, warm, aromatic.

Affinities: Heart, Lung, Spleen.

Average Dilution: 4-6%.

Pharmacological Actions: Antiseizure, antiepileptic, anticonvulsant, mucolytic, analgesic, vasodilator, antiplatelet, antifungal, antiparasitic, stimulant.

ACTIONS AND INDICATIONS:

- Disperses turbidity and expectorates phlegm.
- Resolves cough and congestion.
- Warms the channels and opens the sensory orifices.
- Awakens the senses for cloudiness, depression, and poor concentration.
- Restores Qi collapse as in coma, stroke, heart attack, childhood epilepsy, and convulsions.

- Expels damp-cold Bi Obstruction to relieve joint pain and stiffness, cramps, and spasms.
- Invigorates blood, relieves angina, promotes menstruation, and eases pain.
- Eliminates intestinal worms.

CM Concepts, Channel Systems, and Patterns:

- Treat cold type Bi Zheng/Closed Disorder.

Application and Blends:

- May be inhaled neat for a smelling salt effect and/or placed on GV26 (Ren Zhong), on the Jing Well or Ba Xie points, or on PC8 and KI1 to revive loss of consciousness. To awaken the senses for cloudy-headedness, depression, or poor concentration due to turbid phlegm, blend Su He Xiang 35% with Shi Chang Pu (Acorus) 15%, Cang Zhu (Atractylodes) 35%, and An Shu Ye (*Eucalyptus radiata*) 15% as a 4-6% dilution in a carrier oil for application on acupoints such as ST40, PC5, and CV14, as well as points on the head such as GV20. Use neat for direct inhalation or diffusion.
- To assist unity (he 合) of the Big and Little Shen in spiritual practice, use as an incense alone or with essential oils of sacred resins or woods such as Sacred Frankincense (*Boswellia sacra)*, Tan Xiang (Sandalwood), and Jiang Xiang (*Dalbergia*). Anoint directly on Bai Hui (GV20), Yin Tang (Third Eye), and Tan Zhong (CV17).
- Diffuse 10-15 drops in a diffuser to reduce electromagnetic radiation and cleanse the aura.

NOTES:

TAN XIANG 檀香

INDIAN SANDALWOOD
Santalum album Lignan

DESERT GUANDONG NORTHERN SANDALWOOD
Santalum lanceolatum Lignan

THE CHINESE NAME FOR SANDALWOOD, TAN XIANG 檀香, means "Fragrance of the Altar." Like other fragrant woods and resins that are considered sacred substances long used in religious ceremonies as incense and anointment, Tan Xiang is revered for its aroma. In spiritual practices it is used to invoke a dream state, to connect with the Little Shen (spirit within the Heart), or to summon the Big Shen (universal spirit). Tan Xiang is nourishing for the blood which houses the emotions and memories, the aspect of the Shen Spirit that is carried in the blood as an extension of the heart. To the Chinese, the Heart, Mind, and Shen Spirit are inseparable. Tan Xiang benefits the Heart, blood, and spirit.

Within the body, Tan Xiang focuses on expanding the region of the chest where the heart and lungs reside. It opens the altar residing in the chest at Tan Zhong (CV17) to help with letting go of attachments. In the brain, its aroma stimulates the pineal gland and the release of endorphins to relieve pain, calm the mind, and deepen the breath.

Of these two Sandalwood species *Santalum album* is the one commonly used in Chinese herbal medicine. In most ways, the essential oils of the two species have similar attributes, however in comparison, the flowers of the *S. album* are red, giving it relatively more of an affinity to the Heart and indeed *S. album* contains the highest heartwood oil content out of all species of Sandalwood. *S. lanceolatum*'s white flowers give it a relatively greater affinity to the Lung.

Aroma: *Santalum album*: Exotic, sweet, creamy smooth and warm spice.
Santalum lanceolatum: Woody, earthy with soft honey spice and floral tones.

Note: Base.

Part of Plant: Wood.

Extraction Method: Steam distillation.

Color: Amber.

Growing Region: *S. album*: Northwest Australia (sustainably grown).
S. lanceolatum: Northern Queensland, Australia (sustainably grown).

Major Chemical Components:* Sesquiterpenoids, sequiterpenic alcohols (> 90%): santalol, lanceol, nuciferol, farnesol, bergamotol, bisabolol, nerloidol, curcumene, bisabolene, santalene, sinensal.

* *The two species also differ somewhat in their percentage of particular sesquiterpenes found in both.* S. album *contains a greater percentage of types of* santolol *while* S. lanceolatum *contains more of the lanceol, farnesol, and nuciferol.*

CM Category: Regulating Qi.

Nature and Taste: Acrid, aromatic, bitter, slightly cool.

Affinities: Spleen, Stomach, Lung. As essential oil, also Pericardium, Kidney.

Average Dilution: 8-10%.

Pharmacological Actions: Anti-inflammatory, COX-2 inhibitor, analgesic, sedative, antidepressant, anxiolytic, antimicrobial, and bacteriostatic, respiratory, mucolytic.

Actions and Indications:

- Releases the Qi of the chest and eases diaphragmatic, epigastric, and abdominal constriction and pain to treat cough, dyspnea, nausea, heartburn, or hiccups.
- Breaks up mucus and phlegm.
- Relieves chest oppression, angina, and shortness of breath.
- Moves blood, calms the Heart, opens the Pericardium, and treats PTSD.
- Grounds and calms anxiety, depression, restlessness, panic attacks, nightmares, and hypertension.
- Relieves physical or emotional Heart pains.
- Nourishes the Heart blood and benefits the Kidneys.
- Relieves menopausal symptoms, insomnia, and fatigue.
- Considered an aphrodisiac and benefits gonadal hormones for fertility.
- Drains damp congestion in the lower burner.
- Treats hot Bi syndrome with red, swollen, painful joints or atrophy.
- Increases white blood cell production.
- Benefits the adrenal glands for recovery from adrenal exhaustion.

CM Concepts, Channel Systems, and Patterns:

- Calm the Shen.
- Affinity with CV17/Tan Zhong.
- Descend Heart blood to the Kidneys
- Balance the Fire Water relationship

Application and Blends:

To move the blood, calm the Heart, and open the Pericardium, or calm the Spirit for anxiety, depression, restlessness, panic attacks, insomnia, or PTSD, inhale the aroma neat with deep breaths. Wear as perfume and place on acupoints of Heart, Pericardium, or Yin Wei Mai/Yin Link Vessel such as P6, KI9, SP15. For heart pain combine with Jiang Xiang (*Dalbergia*).

- For relaxation and calming, add 10-15 drops of Sandalwood to 1/3 cup of pink Himalayan salt in the bath water.
- As an anointment or incense to summon the Shen Spirit or invoke a dream state, diffuse and place neat on Yin Tang (Third Eye).
- To release the chest and ease diaphragmatic, epigastric, and abdominal constriction and pain, blend Tan Xiang 40% with 10% Qing Pi (Green Tangerine Peel) or Zhi Ke (*Citrus aurantium*), 25% Hou Po (Magnolia Bark) and 25% Mu Xiang (Saussurea) or Xiang Fu (*Cyperus*) as a 4-6% dilution in black cumin seed oil to gently spread over the affected area and apply to acupoints such as TE6, BL17, ST21, ST25, CV17, CV12, and CV6.
- To increase white blood cells, blend Tan Xiang with Chuan Xiong (*Ligusticum wallichii*), Huang Qi (*Astragalus*) and a small percentage of An Shu Ye (Eucalyptus) as a top note.
- Dilute 10% in black cumin seed oil and massage onto the chest around the region of CV17 and the thymus gland.

Wu Wei Zi 五味子

SCHISANDRA FRUIT

Schisandra Fruite chinensis Fructus

The Chinese name Wu Wei Zi translates to "Five Flavor Seed" (the Chinese character for Wei 味 in the name means both flavor and aroma). The flavors and aromas of the essential oil extracted from the seed embody the qualities of the five elements: the fruit skin is sweet, the fleshy part is sour, the seed core is bitter and pungent, and all parts have a salty taste. Inhalation of its subtle, balanced aroma seems to spread moisture to all of the senses.

In its essential oil form, this is one of the rare substances that consolidates Jing Essence. It nourishes the Yin aspect of all five Yin Organs: Kidney, Heart, Liver, Spleen, and Lung. While Wu Wei Zi nourishes the body's Yin essences and fluids, it is also an astringent which can bind fluids to prevent their loss as in the case of excessive sweating, urination, or bleeding. Wu Wei Zi essential oil has beneficial effects for both body and mind. According to modern research it is known to be adaptogenic. This adaptogenic quality helps one to adapt to both physical and emotional stressors. It quiets the Heart, benefits the brain and senses, relaxes nerves, aids concentration and memory.

Aroma: Subtle, fruity, lightly tart.

Note: Base.

Part of Plant: Seed.

Extraction Method: CO2 extraction.

Color: Golden yellow.

Growing Region: Heilongjiang and Ji Lin Province, China. Harvested September—October.

Major Chemical Components: Bioactive lignans: schisandrin [33], schisandrol. Sesquiterpenoids: ylangene, himachalene, bergomatene. Phytosterol: B-sistosterol, daucosterol. Ester: 5-dimethyl citrate.

CM Category: Stabilizing and Binding.

Nature and Taste: Sour and warm.

Affinities: Heart, Kidney, Lung.

Average Dilution: 15-20%. Gentle, may be applied neat.

Pharmacological Actions: Astringent, adaptogenic, CNS stimulant, cognitive, hepatoprotective, immunomodulatory, metabolic, antibiotic, cardiotonic, vasodilating.

ACTIONS AND INDICATIONS:

- Benefits Jing Essence, Qi, and Yin.
- Generates fluids and clears heat.
- Astringes leakages: stops sweating, nocturnal emissions, frequent urination, bleeding, deficiency diarrhea, and runny nose.
- Stabilizes the Zhi Will. Anchors the Lung Qi to the Kidneys to treat wheezing, cough, dyspnea, and asthma. Its stabilizing, grounding effect brings down blood pressure.
- Restorative, aids recovery from Lau syndrome, "burn out," depression, exhaustion, weakness, chronic cough, spontaneous sweating, or difficulty gaining or losing weight.
- Benefits the endocrine system by balancing progesterone.
- Aids recovery from adrenal exhaustion, low thyroid, and gonadal function.
- Regulates blood sugar and diabetes.
- Eases menopause symptoms: hot flashes, night sweats, insomnia, anxiety, palpitations, and fatigue.
- Consolidates to maintain latency. Slows disease progression and astringes to hold cancer treatments longer in the body.

CM CONCEPTS, CHANNEL SYSTEMS, AND PATTERNS:

- Consolidate the Root as part of Divergent Meridian treatment strategy.
- Maintain latency.
- Bind leakage.
- Aid Kidneys to grasp Lung Qi.

APPLICATION AND BLENDS:

As a restorative and adaptogen, to benefit Jing Essence, Qi, blood and Yin, take by internal ingestion. Wu Wei Zi 30% with essential oils of Huang Qi (*Astragalus*) 15%, Gou Qi Zi (Goji Berry) 40%, and Ren Shen (Ginseng) 15%, as a 2% dilution in Ling Zhi (Ganoderma) spore oil. 1/3 tsp twice per day.

To benefit the brain and senses, relax the nerves, and aid concentration and memory, blend equal parts Wu Wei Zi with Shi Chang Pu (Acorus), Bai Zi Ren (Biota Seed), and Chuan Xiong (*Ligusticum wallichii*). Dilute 4% in walnut or sesame oil. Deeply inhale the aroma or diffuse into the air. May be placed on acupoints of the GB, BL, and GV channels on the head region such as GB20, BL10, GV20, and on Jing Well points to open the sensory orifices. Topical application on points three days on, three days off. Hydrosols of Yuan Zhi

(*Polygala tenuifolia*) and Bai Ren Shen (Ginseng) are also recommended as a refreshing spray on the face and head or in the mouth.

- To aid the Kidney's function to anchor the Lung's Qi in the case of wheezing, cough, dyspnea, or asthma when there is underlying deficiency, blend Wu Wei Zi 25% with Yun Shan (Black Spruce) 40%, Bai Zi Ren (Biota Seed) 25%, and Chen Pi (Aged Tangerine Peel) 10%; diffuse into the air neat and place on acupoints as a 10% dilution in Zi Su Zi (cold-pressed Perilla Seed) or sesame seed carrier oils. Apply on Mu Accumulation and Shu Transport points of Lung and Kidney: LU1, BL13, GB25, BL23, as well as their Yuan Source points: LU9, KI3. A few drops may also be spread over the chest.
- To descend high blood pressure, rub a drop of Wu Wei Zi, neat, on the soles of the feet.
- Take by internal ingestion to bind leakages such as sweating, nocturnal emissions, frequent urination, bleeding disorders, or deficiency diarrhea. Place on Xi Cleft points of affected channels. Take internally as well, to maintain latency in order to slow metastatic cancer and as an astringent to hold cancer treatments longer in the body.
- Three drops three times per day neat for acute, emergency situations or diluted 15% in pomegranate seed oil or Ling Zhi spore oil 1/3 tsp two to three times per day for longer term use.
- To stop runny nose with clear, watery discharge, place neat on acupoints GB15 or BL3.
- Include Wu Wei Zi in essential oil blends to benefit the endocrine system along with other supportive oils according to the particular case. A few specific examples are: Adrenal and Thyroid: Song Zhen (Pine) or Yun Shan (Black Spruce); Thyroid: Ho Luo Bo Zi (Carrot Seed); Gonadal: Mei Gui Hua (Damascus Rose), Mo Li Hua (Jasmine), or Hu Lu Ba (Fenugreek); Pituitary: Ai Ye (*Artemisia argyi*) or Bi Cheng Qie (Litsea); Pineal: Bai Zi Ren (Biota Seed) or Tan Xiang (Sandalwood).

Wu Zhu Yu 吴茱萸

EVODIA FRUIT

Evodiae rutaecarpa Fructus

ALTHOUGH WU ZHU YU, as a Chinese medicine herb, is considered to be acrid and hot, as an essential oil it is warming and quite soothing. Its aroma is strikingly similar to that of marijuana resin and, interestingly, the two share similar properties. Both calm the nervous system and relieve pain. Another area where the two share beneficial effects is the stomach. Wu Zhu Yu, like cannabis, stops nausea and recovers lost appetite and taste for food which is helpful during chemotherapy treatment or debilitating illness. In large doses though, either as essential oils or plant material, if ingested (or smoked), both of them can cause psychedelic effects on the brain. Inhalation of the essential oil's aroma is perfectly safe and quite enough to be highly effective.

Aroma: Strong, herbaceous, earthy, and sweet with a hint of tart citrus. Distinctly reminiscent of fresh cannabis.

Note: Middle.

Part of Plant: Fruit.

Extraction Method: CO2 extraction.

Color: Dark olive green.

Growing Region: Guilin, China. Harvested before the fruit turns red in June to July, in the morning on a sunny day.

Major Chemical Components: Monoterpenes: evodene, myrcene, thujene, limonene, ocimene [34]. Sesquiterpenes: trans-caryophyllene, elemene. Triterpenoid (furanolactone): evodin/limonin.

CM Category: Warming the Interior and Expelling Cold.

Nature and Taste: Acrid, bitter, hot.

Affinities: Liver, Spleen, Stomach.

Average Dilution: 4-6%.

Cautions and Contraindications: Large doses of *Fructus Evodia* by internal consumption have a stimulatory effect on the central nervous system and can lead to visual disturbances and hallucinations.

Pharmacological Actions: Antifungal, antimicrobial, antiviral, anti-inflammatory, antioxidant, antacid, nervine, analgesic, CNS stimulant, psychedelic.

Actions and Indications:

- Strongly warms the middle and lower burners.
- Settles rebellious Stomach Qi downward to treat acid regurgitation, epigastric pain, nausea, and vomiting.
- Prevents and treats stomach ulcers, reduces gastric acid secretions.
- Regulates Liver Qi to calm strong emotion affecting the Stomach.
- Resolves Liver and Stomach Qi accumulation in the throat, such as goiter or Plum Pit Qi (a feeling of something stuck in the throat).
- Warms and resolves stagnation and cold in the Liver channel causing cold bulging disorders, hernia, and abdominal masses.
- Descends excessive fire rising to the head to treat hypertension, headaches, and oral ulcers.
- Use in gynecology: warms lower burner coldness causing menstrual irregularity, pain, and infertility.
- Calms the nerves and eases pain.
- Eliminates fungal infections, ringworms, candida, athlete's foot.

CM Concepts, Channel Systems, and Patterns:

- Warm coldness of Chong/Thoroughfare Vessel and Ren/Conception Vessel.
- Treat Jue Yin stage headaches.
- Harmonize Liver overacting on the Stomach.
- Lead fire downward.

Application and Blends:

To warm and resolve cold stagnation in the Liver channel causing bulging disorders, hernias, or abdominal masses, apply a castor oil pack over the affected area with essential oils of Xiao Hui Xiang (Fennel) 40%, Hu Lu Ba (Fenugreek) 40%, and Wu Zhu Yu (Evodia) 20% as a 4% dilution in castor oil. Soak a flannel cloth in the oil and compress with heat for twenty minutes, twice per day, three days on, and three days off for one month.

To regulate Liver overacting on the Stomach resulting in rebellious Stomach Qi with acid regurgitation, vomiting, stomach ulcers, hyperacidity, and pain, blend Wu Zhu Yu 35% with Zhi Ke (*Citrus aurantium*) 30% and Mu Xiang (Saussurea) 35% as a 4% dilution with black cumin seed oil as the carrier. Apply over the right ribs, upper stomach and esophageal area, three days on and three days off. May be taken by mouth for occasional, acute symptoms, 3 drops in yogurt, kefir, honey water or soy milk.

- In gynecology, when lower burner cold causes menstrual irregularity, pain, or infertility due to cold blockage of Chong and Ren Mai (Thoroughfare and Conception Vessels), Wu Zhu Yu can be part of an essential oil blend for topical application as a warm compress over the lower abdominal region with Ai Ye (*Artemisia argyi*) 40%, Dang Gui (*Angelica sinensis*) 40%, Rou Gui (Cinnamon Bark) 5%, and Wu Zhu Yu 15%. For infertility, add Mei Gui Hua (Damascus Rose). For menstrual irregularity, add Xiang Fu (*Cyperus*) 20% and reduce Ai Ye and Dang Gui to 30% each. To move the blood and Qi for cramping and pain add Chuan Xiong (*Ligusticum wallichii*) 30% and remove Ai Ye.
- Dilute 4-6% in safflower oil for blood stasis, in olive oil for blood deficiency, in sesame oil for issues of Jing Essence. Application of the blend directly on acupoints such as KI2 and SP8 may be included. Once or twice per day, three days on and three days off.
- To treat ringworms and other fungal skin infections, make a wash or spray with 2 tbsp apple cider vinegar in 1 quart of water. 2% dilution with Wu Zhu Yu alone or together with Zhang Nao (White Camphor) or Long Nao (*Borneolum*).
- For goiter, add 15 drops of Wu Zhu Yu to 3 tbsp of sea salt in 1 cup of water. Soak a cheesecloth in the dilution, apply on the throat and on the bottom of the feet (KI1). Retain for twenty minutes once per day for a total of four days. Long term use may raise the blood pressure.

NOTES:

Xi Xin 細辛

WILD GINGER

Asari Herba, Asarum

Inhalation of Xi Xin essential oil's powerfully pungent aroma immediately rises upward opening the nasal passages and clearing the mind and senses. On the skin or mucus membranes the oil feels hot and numbing, but when diluted it is warming and pain relieving. Xi Xin can be utilized either to warm the exterior of the body in order to release wind-cold that results in a common cold, or to warm more deeply, relieving cold and damp that has penetrated into the joints or channels causing pain and lack of mobility. Long-standing cold conditions can eventually cause stagnation of the fluids in the body resulting in phlegm that accumulates until it becomes a mass. Xi Xin's strong, dispersing warmth is able to break up this type of accumulation.

The *Shen Nong Ben Cao Jing/Divine Farmer's Materia Medica Classic* identifies Xi Xin as a superior grade herb and describes that, "It mainly treats cough and counterflow, headache and shaking brain, hypertonicity of the hundred joints, wind damp impediment, pain and dead muscles. It brightens the eyes and disinhibits the nine orifices."

Aroma: Sharp, earthy, musty, with a powerful, pungent overtone.

Note: Top/Middle.

Part of Plant: Leaf and twig.

Extraction Method: CO2 extraction.

Color: Pale greenish tan.

Growing Region: Northeastern China, eastern provinces of Fujian and Zhejiang.

Major Chemical Components: Phenols (phenylpropanoid): methyl eugenol [35], safrole, asaricin. Monoterpene: eucarvone.

CM Category: Exterior Releasing and Interior Warming.

Nature and Taste: Acrid, warm.

Affinities: Lung, Heart, Kidney.

Average Dilution: 2-3%. External use only. Strongly pungent.

Pharmacological Actions: Anesthetic, analgesic, antioxidant, respiratory stimulant, decongestant, mucolytic, antiviral.

Actions and Indications:

- Warms the Lung and stimulates the respiratory system to treat colds, nasal discharge, and cough with clear thin sputum.

- Provides a local anesthetic effect for headaches or toothaches.
- Penetrates to the bones, relieves cold-damp induced Bi syndrome, joint pain and stiffness.
- Resolves chronic damp lower limb swelling with numbness, weakness, and pain.
- Unblocks the sensory orifices, clears the nasal passages, brightens the eyes, improves mental clarity, and restores loss of consciousness.
- Breaks up mucus and phlegm accumulation, masses, fibroids, and cysts. Clears the lymphatic system.

CM Concepts, Channel Systems, and Patterns:

- Expel wind-cold.
- Open the sensory portals.
- Warm the interior.
- Treat cold-damp leg Qi.

Application and Blends:

- To clear the nasal passages, add 3-5 drops to 1 pint of steaming hot water and inhale the steam with eyes closed.
- Add to blends for wind-cold type common cold with chills, runny nose with clear nasal discharge, and cough with thin sputum. For this purpose, combine Xi Xin with other essential oils such as Zi Su Ye (Perilla Leaf), Jing Jie (*Schizonepeta*), and An Shu Ye (Eucalyptus) as a 4% dilution in Zi Su Zi (Perilla Seed) or almond cold-pressed carrier oil. Apply the blend to areas of the upper back and occipital region that affect the lungs and where points that expel wind are located, such as around BL11, BL12, Bl13, and GB20. May apply with cupping if desired. For runny nose apply on acupoint BL3.
- To open or unblock the sensory orifices, increase awareness, brighten the eyes and perception, or restore consciousness, place directly, undiluted, on Jing Well points with a pointed stone, glass, porcelain, or wooden tool and inhale as a smelling salt.
- As a local anesthetic:
  For toothache, apply a 1% dilution of Xi Xin in sesame oil on bit of cotton or swab soaked with the blend directly on the affected tooth.
  For headache, dilute 2 to 3% in safflower oil, apply to the area of pain and on associated channel points.
- For cold-damp Bi syndrome joint pain, make a liniment of 2 to 3% Xi Xin diluted in ethyl alcohol and rub into the joints.
- To resolve chronic damp Leg Qi, lower limb edema, numbness, weakness and pain combine Xi Xin 10% with Yi Yi Ren (Coix Seed) essential oil 90% as liniment in a 10% dilution using ethyl alcohol as the carrier. Apply on the affected areas twice per day, three days on, three days off.

XIANG FU 香附

NUTGRASS RHIZOME, *CYPERUS*

Cyperi rotundus Rhizoma

THE AROMA OF XIANG FU ESSENTIAL OIL embodies the Qi rectifying qualities of the Wood element. Consequently, it is one of the most important tools for treating depression. It deeply relaxes body and mind while freeing impediments to change. It resolves attachment, addictions, neediness, accumulation of excess weight, and eating disorders. With its affinity to the San Jiao (Triple Energizer), its actions course throughout the body.

In traditional Chinese medicine, Xiang Fu is said to be able to free the Qi aspect of the 12 primary channels (those named after their respective organs) and the 8 Vessels (meaning the 8 Extraordinary Vessels). The Qi moves the blood and so it is also called "an immortal herb for women" in its role of correcting all types of menstrual irregularities and easing premenstrual syndrome. As an essential oil, it nourishes the blood as well. According to some modern research, Xiang Fu is said to break down hormones and therefore may be contraindicated during pregnancy. On the other hand, one of its benefits in this regard is to treat polycystic ovarian syndrome.

Xiang Fu essential oil has a major effect on regulating circadian rhythm, which means it is helpful for jet lag or sleep disorders.

Aroma: Woody, piercing, pungent.

Note: Middle.

Part of Plant: Rhizome.

Extraction Method: CO2 extraction.

Color: Dark brown.

Growing Region: Zhejiang and Shandong Provinces of China.
Where it grows wild, it is considered an invasive weed.

Major Chemical Components: Sesquiterpenoids: a-cyperolone, B-selinene, cyperine, patchoulenone. Sesquiterpenic ketol: sugeonol. Monoterpenes: pinene, camphene, limonene. Monoterpene ether oxide: 1-8 cineole.

CM Category: Regulating, Rectifying Qi.

Nature and Taste: Acrid, bitter, sweet, neutral.

Affinities: Liver, San Jiao, Gallbladder.

Average Dilution: 3-4%.

Pharmacological Actions: Anti-inflammatory, antipyretic, analgesic, sedative, antidepressant, uterine relaxant, cardiovascular relaxant, antibiotic.
In Ayurvedic medicine, valued as antioxidant.

ACTIONS AND INDICATIONS:

- Cooling and clearing.
- Releases Qi stagnation, clears heat and inflammation.
- Frees and calms the spirit.
- Relieves pain.
- Opens the chest, diaphragm, and Liver Qi constraint for pent up emotion, insomnia, sleep apnea, asthmatic breathing, or phlegm stagnation.
- Releases anger, resentment, frustration, depression.
- Harmonizes the Liver and Stomach with emotional indigestion causing nausea, vomiting, and discomfort.
- Moves the Qi within the blood, regulates and promotes menses, eases menstrual pain.
- Treats PCOS (polycystic ovarian syndrome).
- Reduces excess cholesterol and hormones.

CM CONCEPTS, CHANNEL SYSTEMS, AND PATTERNS:

- Drain the Dai Mai/Belt Vessel.
- Reduce Yin Stasis.
- Open Yang Qiao Mai/Yang Heel Vessel.
- Harmonize Liver overacting on Stomach.

APPLICATION AND BLENDS:

To free the Qi of the chest for pent up emotion, or respiratory constraint, blend Xiang Fu 30% with Tan Xiang (Sandalwood) 50% and Qing Pi (Green Tangerine Peel) 20%. Dilute 4-6% in almond oil. Topically apply over chest and diaphragm region and directly on acupoints such as PC6, SP21, GB26, and LR13. Deeply inhale the aroma.

For insomnia and to reset the circadian rhythm, combine with Xun Yi Cao (Lavender) and Bai Zi Ren (Biota Seed). Diffuse in the sleeping room, with 10-15 drops of combined essential oils in the diffuser. Apply on the Four Gates, bilateral LI4 and LR3 and on Yin Tang.

To regulate menstruation and resolve premenstrual syndrome, Xiang Fu essential oil's dual attributes of nourishing and moving the blood, along with regulating the Qi, make it a harmonious match with Dang Gui (*Angelica sinensis*). These two essential oils may be used as the foundation of blends for this purpose, combining them with other essential oils according to the individual presentation.

- To release depression, create an aromatic blend for inhalation combining Xiang Fu with a floral aroma such as Mei Gui Hua (Rose), Qi Li Xiang (Orange Jessamine), or Zhi Zi Hua (Gardenia Flower) and Bo He (Peppermint) as a top note oil. Use neat as direct inhalation, diffused into the air and applied on acupoints according to the individual case; for example: HT5, LR5, PC6.
- To resolve attachment, neediness, accumulation of excess weight, or eating disorders, create an aromatic blend with other essential oils that have an affinity with the Spleen and Gallbladder and that transform dampness and turbidity such as: Huo Xiang (Patchouli), Su He Xiang (Styrax), Cang Zhu (Atractylodes), Bai Yu Lan Ye (Magnolia Leaf), and Fo Shou (Buddha's Hand). Apply on acupoints of the Gallbladder, San Jiao, channels and Dai Mai/Belt Vessel such as GB41, GB26, TE10, UB20, SP3, three days on and three days off.
- Yin stasis, and the accumulation of turbid Yin fluids can cause swellings, cysts, nodules, or masses. To reduce Yin stasis and regulate water by supporting the San Jiao's Yang Qi, and to free the Qi of Kidney and Bladder to move the water, Xiang Fu may be combined with Ze Xie (Alisma) and a small percentage of Ding Xiang (Clove) applied directly on UB40, UB39, and KI10 three days on and three days off.

NOTES:

XIAO HUI XIANG 小茴香

FENNEL SEED

Foeniculi vulgare Fructus

FENNEL IS A TRADITIONAL KITCHEN SPICE POPULAR in the cuisine of many cultures, not only for its flavor, but also for its beneficial effects on appetite and digestion. As an essential oil, its aroma alone can stimulate these benefits. Additionally, the oil is edible. Ingestion of a few drops can quickly settle upset stomach. Xiao Hui Xiang brings its warming energy all the way from the upper burner where it helps the lungs, to the middle burner's stomach and spleen, continuing downward to keep the intestines moving. Also, in the lower burner, it warms up coldness in the Liver channel which can result in bulging or pain, as with a hernia for example. Xiao Hui Xiang also warms and strengthens the kidneys and the adrenal glands which are located atop the kidneys. Its essential oil helps to reduce cortisol, the stress hormone which is excreted by the adrenals as a fight or flight response to trauma or perceived fearful, dangerous situations. Overall, its stimulating warmth increases one's appetite for life, motivation, and will power.

Aroma: Herbaceous, sweet, pleasantly fresh, spicy and lightly camphorous.

Note: Middle.

Part of Plant: Seed.

Extraction Method: CO2 extraction or distillation.

Color: Light amber-brown.

Growing Region: Inner Mongolia. Harvested May – June and September – October.

Major Chemical Components: Phenolic ethers 50-90%: trans-anethole [36], methyl chavicol. Monoterpenoid and ketone: fenchone (< 5%). Diterpenes.

CM Category: Warming the Interior and Expelling Cold.

Nature and Taste: Acrid, sweet, warm.

Affinities: Liver, Kidney, Spleen, Stomach.

Average Dilution: 4-6%.

Cautions and Contraindications: Naturally estrogenic, contraindicated during pregnancy, or with estrogen receptive tumors, cancers.

Pharmacological Actions: Antibacterial, antifungal, antiviral, antiseptic, antiparasitic, insecticide, stomachic, analgesic, antispasmodic, estrogenic, cholagogue, diuretic, emmenagogue.

Actions and Indications:

- Warms cold stagnation in Liver channel to treat lower abdominal or genital area pain and swelling, hernia, or amenorrhea.
- Warms the abdomen and back.
- Promotes digestion, relieves stomach and abdominal pain and digestive disharmonies.
- Induces peristaltic activity and increases the appetite.
- Promotes the discharge of bile.
- Benefits and warms the upper burner to treat bronchitis, cough, wheezing, and to expectorate phlegm.
- Brings energy from the upper burner downward to move the bowels and promotes urination.
- Stimulates delayed menstruation, promotes labor and delivery, repositions the fetus for the birthing process, and promotes lactation.
- Strengthens the Kidney Yang, regulates cortisol, adrenaline, and repairs the adrenals.
- Simulates Yang to nourish Yin.
- Anchors Yang and treats hyperthyroid.
- Regulates fluid metabolism, edema, and cellulite.
- Treats gout.
- Benefits wound healing.
- Disinfects dog bites, snake bites, spider, and insect bites.
- Kills worms.
- Neutralizes alcohol and aids alcoholism recovery.

CM Concepts, Channel Systems, and Patterns:

- Warm and tonify Kidney Yang.
- Anchor the Yang.
- Harmonize the Stomach, Spleen and Liver.
- Disperse lower burner cold bulging disorders

Application and Blends:

- To reposition baby for birthing process, apply Xiao Hui Xiang neat on acupoint BL67 in place of moxa cones.
- To promote labor, apply directly on acupoints LI4, SP6, and GB21 with or without needling.

- To promote lactation, dilute 4% in olive oil and apply on acupoints such as SI1, ST18, CV17, PC6, ST36, BL17, GB21.
- To move the digestive Qi by inducing peristaltic activity, dilute to 4% with black cumin seed carrier oil and apply over the abdomen or on acupoint ST25. Three days on, three days off. May use as a single oil or combine with Zhi Ke (*Citrus aurantium*).
- To relieve acute stomach and abdominal pain due to Stomach Qi stagnation and/or cold, 3 drops of Xiao Hui Xiang on the tongue, emulsified with 1 tsp of honey, yogurt, or black cumin seed carrier oil, settles the stomach and eases pain. For more cold, add 1 drop of Gan Jiang (Dry Ginger) and prepare as a warm drink made with 1/2 cup honey water.
- To promote wound healing after surgery, to protect and generate new tissue, make a poultice with Ru Xiang (CO2 extracted *Boswellia carterii* Frankincense) 50%, Mo Yao (CO2 extracted Myrrh) 30%, and Xiao Hui Xiang 20%. The sticky quality of the CO2 extracted Frankincense and Myrrh essential oils binds the wound and the Fennel prevents infection.
- As an antiseptic, apply a poultice made with 20 drops Fennel essential oil and 1/2 cup green clay powder on dog bites to prevent infection and tetany, or on snake bites, spider, and insect bites.
- For inguinal hernia and bulging disorders of the lower abdomen related to cold in the Liver channel, apply a warm compress of essential oils: Xiao Hui Xiang 40%, Hu Lu Ba (Fenugreek) 40%, and Wu Zhu Yu (Evodia) 20% as a 4% dilution in castor oil. Soak a flannel cloth in the oil and compress with heat for twenty minutes, twice per day, three days on, and three days off for one month as one course of treatment.
- As an aid to alcoholism recovery, create an aromatic blend using Xiao Hui Xiang with other essential oils such as Chai Hu (Bupleurum), Xiang Fu (*Cyperus*), Xun Yi Cao (Lavender), and Bo He (Peppermint) to inhale directly from the bottle as needed or diffuse into the air. Xiao Hui Xiang may be ingested as a 3% dilution in an edible carrier oil, 3 drops three times per day for three days to neutralize alcohol during the beginning stage of withdrawal.
- Add Xiao Hui Xiang to aromatic blends for PTSD to calm the fight or flight response, to reduce fear and promote feelings of hope, strengthen will power, and restore self-love, dignity, and appetite for life. The blend may be used as inhalation, diffused, or in the bath and applied on UB23, UB52, GV4, PC6, and points of the Yin Wei Mai/Yin Link Vessel.

Xing Ren 杏仁 / Bei Xing Ren 北杏仁
Ku Xing Ren 苦杏仁

BITTER ALMOND, APRICOT KERNEL

Pruni armeniacae amarum Semen

Xing Ren essential oil has the strong, delicious aroma of almond extract. It is highly concentrated and a little goes a long way. Its nature is descending and lubricating, which makes it helpful to thin out and expel thick phlegm congested in the lungs and to deepen the breath, especially when diffused together with other aromatic essential oils that open the lungs. *Pruni armeniacae amarum Semen* is referred to as Apricot Kernel as well as Bitter Almond. The oil from the interior of the pit is slightly toxic. Its use in cancer treatment is based on the Chinese medicine strategy called "toxin against toxin," which describes the principle behind many chemotherapy drugs. Because Xing Ren's main affinity is to the Lungs and since the Lungs open to the skin, this essential oil, diluted and applied topically, is a useful ingredient in blends to treat cancerous skin conditions.

Aroma: Nutty, almond extract.

Note: Middle/Base.

Part of Plant: Kernel.

Extraction Method: CO2 extraction.

Color: Light amber.

Growing Region: Northwestern China.

Major Chemical Components: Aldehyde: benzaldehyde [37] (~90%), mandelonitrile* (~5%) and benzoic acid (~4%). Monoterpene alcohol: linalool, 4-terpinenol, a-terpineol.

Average Dilution: 1-2%. External use only or under doctor's guidance.

CM Category: Relieving Coughing and Wheezing.

Nature and Taste: Bitter, slightly warm, slightly toxic.

Affinities: Lung, Large Intestine.

Pharmacological Actions: Antitussive, anti-asthmatic, mucolytic, antimicrobial, antioxidant, anticarcinogenic.

* *Mandelonitrile is a common structural component of both laetrile and amygdalin used in experimental cancer treatments that are not approved in the U.S. partly because mandelonitrile contains trace amounts of cyanide.*

Actions and Indications:

- Benefits respiratory function, stops coughing, dyspnea, wheezing.
- Lubricates and decongests the lungs.
- Moves the Lung Qi downward to the large intestine, promotes peristalsis and lubricates the intestines.
- Arrests free radicals, supports apoptosis (cancer cell death), prevents cellular damage. Has strong antimicrobial activity.

Application and Blends:

- To benefit respiration in cases of coughing, dyspnea, wheezing, Xing Ren works best diffused into the air with Song Zhen (Pine Needle) essential oil. Add 3 drops of Xing Ren and 9 drops of Song Zhen (Pine Needle) in a diffuser. If there is more phlegm congestion add An Shu Ye (Eucalyptus) and Zi Su Ye (Perilla Leaf). A combination of these essential oils along with Bo He (Peppermint) can also be diluted to 4% in Zi Su Zi (Perilla Seed) cold-pressed carrier oil and prepared as a topical application over the chest and upper back as well as applied to acupoints of the Lung channel.
- Add 1-2 drops of Xing Ren to 1 oz of topical applications for skin or other cancers. Other essential oils to consider in a blend for this purpose are: She Chuang Zi (Cnidium Fruit), E Zhu (*Curcuma zedoaria*), Ru Xiang (*Boswellia carterii*), and Ye Ju Hua (Wild Chrysanthemum). Dilute the blend to 3% in calophyllum (tamanu oil). Apply 1-3 drops directly on the lesion or affected region. Avoid sun exposure, apply at night and cover during the day, three days on, three days off.

Xun Yi Cao 薰衣草

LAVENDER

Lavendula augustifolia Flos

In Western aromatherapy, Lavender is often thought of for its calming effect. The same idea is shared in the context of Chinese medicine, where this lack of calm, in the case of Lavender, is mainly due to Liver Qi Stagnation. The role of the Liver is to provide the smooth flowing of the Qi and blood. It harmonizes the emotions and the relationships among the organs of the body. Lavender essential oil plays this role by harmonizing the oils in a blend. Emotions that injure the Liver are anger, resentment, and frustration, especially if unexpressed. When emotion affects the Liver Qi, smooth flow is lost, normal cycles are interrupted, tension, depression, irritability, and difficulty moving on ensue. The aroma of Lavender is helpful to soothe the emotions, relax the body, and restore the free flow of the Liver Qi. It reminds us that it's ok to slow down, take a breath and reflect.

Applied directly on the skin, Lavender is cooling and soothing. It works like magic to soothe and heal burns, insect bites, and sunburn. It restores normal circadian rhythm and cures jet lag. Diffused into the air or as a sachet, it acts to fumigate, to get rid of pestilence or negativity.

Aroma: Sweet, floral, slight spice.

Note: Middle/Top.

Part of Plant: Flower.

Extraction Method: Distillation.

Color: Clear to pale yellow.

Growing Region: Xinjiang Province, China. Harvested June to July on sunny, dry days.

Major Chemical Components: Esters (> 50%): linalyl acetate, lavender acetate. Monoterpene alcohols: linalool, geraniol, lavandulol, terpineol, borneol. Sesquiterpene: caryophyllene. Monoterpene: a-Pinene. Ketones (< 0.55%).

CM Category: Regulating Qi.

Nature and Taste: Cooling, sweet, spicy.

Affinities: Lung, Liver, Pericardium.

Average Dilution: 10-15%. May be applied neat.

Pharmacological Actions: Analgesic, nervine, antispasmodic, hypotensive, insect repellent.

ACTIONS AND INDICATIONS:

- Promotes the free movement of Liver and Lung Qi.
- Opens the chest and diaphragm.
- Eases nervous tension, headaches, muscle spasms and tightness, irritability, and hypertension.
- Relaxes tubular ring muscles, such as sphincter muscles of the digestive tract to relieve irritable bowel syndrome, gassiness after eating, bloating, and pain.
- Calms the Heart and Spirit, to treat palpitations, anxiety, insomnia, and restlessness.
- Breaks up old patterns, habits, or addictions.
- Clears heat.
- Boosts the immune system.
- Balances circadian rhythm and treats jet lag.
- Decreases cortisol levels and regulates GABA to relieve anxiety and depression.
- Stops itching and speeds healing of burns, insect bites, sunburn, and scars.

CM CONCEPTS, CHANNEL SYSTEMS, AND PATTERNS:

- Regulate Ying and Wei Qi as part of Divergent Meridian treatment strategy.
- Calm the Spirit.
- Release diaphragmatic constriction, Lung and Liver Qi.

APPLICATION AND BLENDS:

To free the Liver and Lung Qi, and open the chest and diaphragm, formulate an aromatic blend of Xun Yi Cao (Lavender) and Tan Xiang (Sandalwood) for direct deep inhalation or by diffusion. A few drops may be spread on the chest and ribs area or applied to acupoints such as CV17 (Influential point of Qi), BL17, along with the Mu and Shu points of Lung and Liver: BL13, LU1, BL18, and LR14.

To ease nervous tension causing headaches, muscular spasms or tightness, apply Lavender alone or with Chuan Xiong (*Ligusticum wallichii*) in equal parts. For one-time use, may be applied neat with massage on the affected areas and along the Yang Sinew Meridians or add 10 to 15 drops to the bath with Epsom salt. Dilute to 10% in black cumin seed carrier oil for repeated applications.

To calm the Heart and Spirit, palpitations, anxiety, insomnia, restlessness, create an aromatic blend with Bai Zi Ren (Biota Seed) for deep inhalation. For insomnia, diffuse in the sleeping room. Apply on acupoints such as PC6, HT7, and the Mu Accumulation point of the Heart, CV14, three days on and three days off, or as needed for relief.

- To bring down high blood pressure, combine Lavender with Jiang Xiang (*Dalbergia*) and Wu Wei Zi (*Schisandra Fruit*). Deeply inhale the aroma or diffuse and apply on the bottom of the feet. Note that in higher percentages and with repeated use, Lavender can be stimulating, causing the opposite effect. Be sure to use the three days on, three days off application method and rotate blend ingredients periodically.
- To assist in breaking up stuck psychological patterns or addictions, blend Lavender 40% with Chai Hu (Bupleurum) 20% and Huo Xiang (Patchouli) 40%. Dilute to 15% in olive or safflower oil for deep inhalation. May also apply on acupoints appropriate to the particular case, three days on and three days off.

NOTES:

YE JU HUA AND YE JU HUA ABSOLUTE 野菊花

WILD CHRYSANTHEMUM and SHEN NONG JU

Chrysanthemi/Dendranthema indicum Flos

YE JU HUA IS THE BRASH, WILD COUSIN of Ju Hua (Chrysanthemum). Both flowers share some characteristics. For example, both are hardy and grow abundantly all year round. Their essential oils clear heat and inflammation, regulate Qi, break up swellings and accumulations. Both treat skin and eye conditions and lower blood pressure. However, the aroma and actions of Wild Chrysanthemum are fiercer and sharper, strongly detoxifying and disinfecting. It can clear intense heat conditions that are referred to as fire toxins. It treats chronic inflammatory or cancerous conditions. It cuts through stubborn conditions that have become latent or difficult to change. As a floral essential oil, these qualities apply to entrenched mental emotional conditions as well. Wild Chrysanthemum extracted by CO2 and the solvent-extracted absolute have similar therapeutic functions; however, the absolute is considered to be more of a base note with a thicker consistency and a longer lasting aroma. There are numerous varieties of Wild Chrysanthemum. The variety called Shen Nong Ju is named after the original Divine Farmer of the *Shen Nong Ben Cao Jing*. It grows wild in the Shen Nong Jia Nature Preserve, a UNESCO World Heritage site.

Aroma: Clean, sharp, acrid, floral.

Note: CO2 – Middle. Absolute – Middle/Base.

Color: CO2 – Yellow green. Absolute – Opaque dark green.

Growing Region: Ye Ju Hua – Guilin, China. Shen Nong Ju – Shen Nong Jia Forestry District, Hubei Province, China. Harvested September – November. Flowers are dried prior to extraction.

Part of Plant: Flower.

Extraction Method: CO2 extraction. Absolute – Solvent extraction using edible hexane.*

Average Dilution: 3-4%. External use. Contains ketone components not recommended for internal ingestion.

Major Chemical Components: Monoterpene alcohols: borneol, terpineol. Monoterpene ether oxide: 1-8 cineole (eucalyptol). Sesquiterpenes: zingeberene, caryophyllene. Sesquiterpene alcohol: bisabolol. Ester: bornyl acetate. Monoterpene ketones: camphor (~6%), thujone (~3%).

CM Category: Heat Clearing and Toxin Eliminating.

* *Although the hexane solvent used is considered edible, absolutes are not recommended for internal consumption.*

Nature and Taste: Bitter, acrid, cool.

Affinities: Lung, Liver.

Pharmacological Actions: antimicrobial, anti-inflammatory, antipyretic, antihypertensive.

Actions and Indications:

- Strongly clears heat and toxins.
- Use in dermatology: clears fire toxins from skin, treats basal cell carcinoma, eczema, psoriasis, psoriatic arthritis, carbuncle, furuncle, sores and various skin problems with redness and inflammation.
- Lightens dark pigmentation such as moles or age spots.
- Clears heat and inflammation from eyes: stye, swollen eyelids, redness, infections.
- Resolves latency in certain eye diseases such as glaucoma or eye tumors.
- Cools and disinfects sore throat.
- Lowers blood pressure and relieves migraine headache due to Liver fire or excessive Liver Yang.

Application and Blends:

- As a topical application for skin inflammations such as eczema, psoriasis, or psoriatic arthritis, use alone or add other essential oils such as Lian Qiao (Forsythia) or Jin Yin Hua (Honeysuckle) to further clear heat. Combine Ye Ju Hua with Bai Zhi (*Angelica dahurica*) to draw out pustular swellings or abscesses. In both cases add a citrus peel top note oil such as Qing Pi (Green Tangerine Peel) to direct the blend outward. Dilute to 3% in a carrier oil such as calophyllum (tamanu), almond, or coconut oil. Three days on, three days off. If there is pus or abscess, make a paste with grapeseed oil to dry up, and green clay powder to draw out. Apply the paste directly on the lesions.

- For skin cancers, combine Ye Ju Hua with She Chuang Zi (Cnidium Fruit), E Zhu (*Curcuma zedoaria*), and 1 drop of Xing Ren (*Prunus armeniaca*). Dilute to 3% in calophyllum (tamanu) oil. Apply directly on the lesion. Avoid sun exposure, apply at night and cover during the day, three days on, three days off.

- To treat inflammation, redness, and swelling of the eyes, combine Ye Ju Hua 40% with Bo He (Peppermint) 10% and Man Jing Zi (Vitex Seed) 50%. Make a 1-2% dilution in almond, coconut or hazelnut oil. Apply as a compress over the affected eye. Be sure to wring the compress out completely, close the eyes and do not let the oil drip into the eye.

- To cool sore throat, dilute two drops of Ye Ju Hua in 1/2 cup of warm salt water and gargle.

YI YI REN 薏苡仁

JOB'S TEARS, COIX SEED

Coicis lacryma-jobi Semen

YI YI REN ESSENTIAL OIL is very gentle and not irritating to the skin or mucus membranes. It may be applied neat for short-term or diluted for longer term use. Although aromatically this oil is somewhat unremarkable, certain effects of the essential oil itself are quite potent. For one, its prominent triterpene content provides aspirin-like anti-inflammatory pain relief when used topically. Another very interesting fact is that Coix Seed has a long history as an anticancer agent in China, and an extract of the oil has been developed into an injectable product for this purpose. It is also an excellent ingredient in skin care due to its soothing, non-irritating nature and ability to draw out.

Aroma: Mild, nutty.

Note: Base.

Part of Plant: Seed.

Extraction Method: CO2 extraction.

Color: Pale tan.

Growing Region: Fujian, Hebei, and Liaoning Provinces of China.

Major Chemical Components: Phytosterols: beta-sitosterol, stigmasterol. Triterpenoid saponin: coixenolide. Triterpenes. Phenol: coixol. Aldehyde: nonalactone. Fatty acids: hexanoic acid, nonanoic acid, octanoic (caprilic) acid, dilinoleic acid-triolein, palmic acid-dilinolein.

CM Category: Draining Dampness and Regulating Water.

Nature and Taste: Sweet and bland.

Affinities: Spleen, Stomach, Lung, Kidney.

Average Dilution: 15-20%. Very gentle, may be applied neat and ingested.

Pharmacological Actions: Steroidal, cortico-steroid regulating, anti-inflammatory, analgesic, COX-2 regulating, anticancer [38], antitumor, antiproliferative, chemoprotective, immune enhancing.

ACTIONS AND INDICATIONS:

- Regulates water metabolism.
- Draws out dampness from bones, sinews, and muscles to resolve swelling, pain, spasms, hypertonicity, arthritis, rheumatism.
- Balances adrenal glands to relieve stress, pain, and increases joint mobility in chronic damp cases with numbness, atrophy, and weakness.

- Expels pus, clears acne, and resolves abscesses.
- Supports cancer treatment and reduces tumor growth and cell proliferation.

CM Concepts, Channel Systems, and Patterns:

- Leach out dampness.
- Regulate water.

Application and Blends:

- As a topical application for skin conditions to expel pus, clear acne, and resolve abscesses, make a plaster using green clay powder to draw out and dry up. Combine the essential oils of Yi Yi Ren and Bai Zhi (*Angelica Dahurica*) as a 10% dilution with grapeseed oil and mix with the green clay powder to a paste-like consistency. Apply directly on the lesions.
- To support cancer therapy, Yi Yi Ren essential oil may be ingested daily, 3 drops with 1/3 tsp Ling Zhi (Ganoderma) spore oil, three times per day.
- To leach out dampness in chronic Bi syndrome, Leg Qi, with swelling and numbness or pain, combine Yi Yi Ren with Cang Zhu (Atractylodes), Song Zhen (Pine) or Yun Shan (Black Spruce) and Jing Jie (*Schizonepeta*) in a 10% dilution using witch hazel and safflower oil together as the carrier with Yi Yi Ren as the primary essential oil ingredient (60% of the blend). Apply to the affected areas twice per day, three days on, three days off.
- In the case of atrophy and weakness resulting from chronic damp conditions like rheumatism and arthralgia, combine Yi Yi Ren with equal parts Du Huo (*Angelica pubescentis)*, Dang Gui (*Angelica sinensis*), and Chuan Xiong (*Ligusticum wallichii*) as a 10% dilution in safflower oil and apply to the affected areas twice per day, three days on, and three days off.

Yin Chen Hao 茵陳

REDSTEM WORMWOOD

Artemisiae scopariae Herba, Artemisia capillaris

Yin Chen Hao's fresh, sharp aroma is cooling and clarifying. This essential oil is a powerful, broad-spectrum antibiotic, strongly antiviral and antifungal. It is also good at breaking up accumulations and fats. Its main activities are focused on the Liver and Gallbladder where it clears up congestion and inflammation. In Chinese medicine, Yin Chen Hao is a famous herb for treating jaundice. It benefits the skin by clearing up sores and infections.

Aroma: Fresh, herbaceous, sharp, bitter.

Note: Middle.

Part of Plant: Leaf and twig.

Extraction Method: CO2 extraction.

Color: Golden yellow.

Growing Region: Native mainly to semi-arid, low elevation areas of southern China.

Major Chemical Components: Monoterpenes: pinene, cymene, myrcene, limonene, terpinene, ocimene. Monoterpene ether oxide: 1-8 cineole (eucalyptol). Monoterpene ketones: thujone, carvone, camphor. Monoterpene alcohol: thujyl alcohol. Monoterpene aldehyde: citronellol. Sesquiterpenes: germacrene, caryophyllene, santalene.

CM Category: Draining Dampness and Heat.

Nature and Taste: Bitter, slightly cold.

Affinities: Liver, Gallbladder, Spleen, Stomach.

Average Dilution: 2-4%. Topical application only.

Cautions and Contraindications: Contraindicated for children and cats.

Pharmacological Actions: Antibiotic, antiviral, antifungal, anti-inflammatory, antipyretic, antihypertensive, antilipidemic, detergent, mucolytic, hepatoprotective.

Actions and Indications:

- Resolves conditions of dampness and heat.
- Benefits the Liver and Gallbladder: regenerates liver cells, regulates bile production, clears inflammation, eliminates stones, treats cholestasis, cirrhosis, hepatitis and jaundice.

- Use in dermatology: urticaria, eczema, rashes, sores, viral, bacterial and fungal infections of the skin.
- Reduces fever, blood pressure, and cholesterol.
- Breaks up belly fat.
- Eliminates infections and clears toxins.

CM Concepts, Channel Systems, and Patterns:

- Clear the Dai Mai/Belt Vessel.
- Clear damp-heat.

Application and Blends:

- For Liver/Gallbladder diseases, combine Yin Chen Hao 35% with essential oils of Zhi Zi (Gardenia Fruit) 35%, and Qing Pi (Green Tangerine Peel) 30% as a 4-6% dilution in castor oil and apply as a compress over the Liver/Gallbladder area of the right ribs twice per day for three days, then take three days off and repeat the cycle for one month as one course of treatment.

- As a hepatoprotective agent, to benefit the Liver and generate liver cells, combine Yin Chen Hao 20%, Ho Luo Bo Zi (Carrot Seed) 25%, Chai Hu (Bupleurum) 25%, Chuan Xiong (*Ligusticum wallichii*) 25%, and Bo He (Peppermint) 5%. Dilute 4-6% in olive oil. Apply on acupoints such as UB18, LR14, LR3, and LR8. Spread a few drops gently over the Liver area. Apply once or twice per day for three days, then take three days off and repeat the cycle for one to three months.

- In blends for skin problems expressing with heat, such as urticaria, eczema, rashes, herpes sores, or fungal infections, make a 3% dilution applied topically to the affected areas using calophyllum (tamanu) or grapeseed as the carrier oil. Other essential oils may be combined such as Ye Ju Hua (Wild Chrysanthemum), Lian Qiao (Forsythia), Long Nao (*Borneolum*), or Qing Hao (*Artemisia annua*).

YUN SHAN 雲杉

BLACK SPRUCE NEEDLE

Picea mariana

THE EVERGREEN AROMA OF BLACK SPRUCE is both calming and energizing. It aids recovery from the tired-wired state of adrenal exhaustion. It brings a sense of quietude. It also benefits the lungs and respiration by freeing and anchoring the breath while fighting respiratory infections. In that regard, diffusing into the air is a good way to use Yun Shan. While other types of Spruce essential oils elicit similar properties, the color black, associated with the Water element, gives this one a more direct effect on the kidneys and adrenals, the lower back and the joints. Emotionally, because of this essential oil's strong support of the Kidneys and Lung, it helps one to overcome fear and grief. Applied topically, it is useful to ease pain and inflammation of the joints, muscles, and tendons.

Aroma: Balsamic, sweet.

Note: Middle/Top.

Part of Plant: Needle.

Extraction Method: Distillation.

Color: Clear.

Growing Region: Northern North America, Canada.

Major Chemical Components: Ester: bornyl acetate. Monoterpenes: pinene, camphene, carene, myrcene, limonene, santene, phellandrene. Monoterpene alcohols: borneol, terpineol, 1,8-cineole, Sesquiterpene: cadinene

CM Category: Dispelling Wind-Damp and Relieving Pain.

Nature and Taste: Spicy, warming.

Affinities: Lung, Kidney.

Average Dilution: 6-10%.

Pharmacological Actions: Antimicrobial, antioxidant, analgesic, anti-inflammatory, respiratory, antitussive, mucolytic, hormone modulatory.

ACTIONS AND INDICATIONS:

- Benefits Lung, treats bronchitis, asthma, and cough. Breaks up mucus and phlegm.
- Anchors the Lung Qi downward to the Kidneys.
- Warms the Kidney Yang. Aids recovery from adrenal exhaustion and stimulates the adrenal cortex.

- Balances the hormonal system (pituitary-thyroid-adrenal-ovary).
- Enhances memory and concentration.
- Cortisone-like, eliminates pain and inflammation, joint pain, muscle stiffness, and spasms.

CM Concepts, Channel Systems, and Patterns:

- Aid Kidney to grasp Lung Qi.
- Tonify Kidney Yang.
- Dispel wind-cold-damp Bi Obstruction.
- Lung and Large Intestine meridians, deep-superficial-deep strategy. Apply to confluent points.

Application and Blends:

- Diffuse alone or with An Shu Ye (Eucalyptus) to open the lungs for acute respiratory infections, cough, phlegm, bronchitis, or asthma. 10-15 drops of combined oils in the diffuser, or directly inhale the steam from 3-5 drops placed in 1 pint of hot, steaming water.
- For chronic respiratory conditions with underlying deficiency and to aid the Kidneys' function of grasping the Lung Qi, combine Yun Shan 60% with Wu Wei Zi (*Schisandra Fruit*) 40% as a 4-6% dilution in a carrier oil such as Zi Su Zi (cold-pressed Perilla Seed) or sesame seed oil. Apply on acupoints of the Kidney channel on the chest that affect the Lung such as KI24 to KI27, on KI23 and on Yuan Source points of Lung and Kidney channels, LU9 and KI3. Apply three days on and three days off. Diffuse neat with 15-20 drops in a diffuser.
- To regulate adrenaline, repair the adrenals, and benefit the Kidney Yang, use together with Xiao Hui Xiang (Fennel), dilute 4-6% in sesame seed oil and gently spread a few drops across the kidney treatment area of the lower back from UB23 on one side to UB23 on the other, three days on and three days off.
- Add Yun Shan to liniments for wind-cold-damp Bi, joint pain, muscle stiffness, spasms, impaired mobility. Combine with essential oils such as Du Huo (*Angelica pubescentis*), Jing Jie (*Schizonepeta*), Gui Zhi/Gui Ye (Cinnamon Twig and Leaf), or Chuan Xiong (*Ligusticum wallichii*). Use ethyl alcohol as the carrier in a 4% dilution. Cinnamon should be no more than 2% of total essential oils in the blend because its spicy nature may irritate the skin. Apply to affected areas and related Sinew Meridians with massage or cupping if desired.

ZE XIE 澤瀉

WATER PLANTAIN, ALISMA

Alismatis plantago Rhizoma

ZE XIE ESSENTIAL OIL profoundly supports the Water element. Its aroma and material essence connect with this element to promote physical health as well as to cultivate qualities associated with the Water temperament. It is an ally to help with tapping into the Kidney's attribute of Zhi Will in order to strengthen one's foundation, resolve, and motivation, and to overcome fear. Ze Xie oil can be used in shamanic practices to drain the "swamp," draw closer to the water terrain, and delve into the mystery of the source of creation.

Physically, Ze Xie facilitates distribution of Kidney's Yin essences and essential Qi throughout the body under the direction of the San Jiao (Triple Energizer). It helps to regulate the body's pilot light, the Ming Men Life Gate fire. This means that Ze Xie assists in maintaining the balance of Yin and Yang, water and fire. When Yin fluids become stagnant and their circulation becomes impeded, Ze Xie helps to get rid of the accumulation of dampness that results, restoring the normal metabolism and distribution of essential fluids needed to nourish and moisten. When excessive Liver or Heart fire results from a lack of Yin, with flaring up of emotional disturbances, Ze Xie helps to clear the fire by freeing the water pathways.

The Shen Nong Ben Cao Jing/Divine Farmer's Materia Medica Classic identifies Ze Xie as a superior grade herb and says, "It disperses water, nourishes the five viscera, boosts the Qi...makes one strong...renders the face brilliant and enables one to walk over water." Walking over water in this case means mastery over the Water element, in all of its aspects.

Aroma: Sweet, musky, earthy.

Note: Base.

Part of Plant: Rhizome.

Extraction Method: CO2 extraction.

Color: Opaque dark brown/black with red and gold highlights.

Growing Region: Fujian Province, China.

Major Chemical Components:* Triterpenoids: alisol. Sesquiterpenoids: alismol, alismoxide, orientalol.

CM Category: Draining Dampness.

Nature and Taste: Sweet, bland, cold.

* *The chemical composition of* Ze Xie *essential oil is unusual, with a predominance of sesquiterpenoids and triterpenoids unique to* Alismatis plantago.

Affinities: Kidney, Bladder.

Average Dilution: 8-10%.

Pharmacological Actions: Diuretic, antihyperlipidemic, antihypertensive, anti-inflammatory, steroidal, hepatoprotective, analgesic, immunomodulatory, hormone modulatory.

Actions and Indications:

- Promotes urination, eliminates dampness and turbidity.
- Disperses stagnation in lower burner due to accumulation of dampness and heat causing urinary tract infection, painful or difficult urination, dribbling, edema, or diarrhea.
- Benefits the prostate gland.
- Removes accumulation of excess water weight.
- Treats dizziness and vertigo.
- Drains fire due to Kidney Yin deficiency.
- Drains Kidney fire causing semen leakage, premature ejaculation, and nocturnal emissions.
- Lowers blood pressure and cholesterol.

CM Concepts, Channel Systems, and Patterns:

- Leach out dampness.
- Balance ministerial fire.

Application and Blends:

- To clear dampness and heat affecting the urinary tract, combine equal parts Ze Xie with Nan Mu (Cedarwood), Cang Zhu (Atractylodes), Yi Yi Ren (Coix), and Zhi Zi (Gardenia Fruit). Apply on the Front Mu Accumulation and the Back Shu Transport points of the Bladder: CV3 and BL28 along with the lower He Sea point of the San Jiao (Triple Energizer) BL39.
- To balance fire and water when insufficient Kidney Yin and strong emotions such as anxiety or anger cause Heart or Liver fire to blaze up, create an aromatic blend of Ze Xie with Tan Xiang (Sandalwood), Zhi Zi (Gardenia Fruit), and Zhi Zi Hua (Gardenia Flower). Deeply inhale the aroma. May also apply on acupoints, for example: KI3 (Yuan Source point of Kidney) along with CV14 (Mu Accumulation point of Heart), CV15 (Source point of Yin) or LR14 (Mu Accumulation point of Liver).
- To connect with the Water element, anoint KI21 whose point name, You Men, means "Mystery Gate", with a drop of Ze Xie and deeply inhale the aroma with intention.

ZHANG NAO 樟腦

WHITE CAMPHOR

Cinnnamomom camphora

THE POWERFULLY SHARP AROMA OF WHITE CAMPHOR has the immediate effect of a smelling salt. It is one of the strongest of the essential oils that are said to open the sensory portals. This means that merely by smelling these oils, they can bring one back from a faint, shock, or altered mental state. This oil is also used topically, always diluted, in blends for traumatic injuries and pain. Zhang Nao effectively kills microbes, parasites, or fungal infections on the skin. Traditionally, White Camphor is used to prevent decay and drive away infestations.

Aroma: Strong, sharp, spicy.

Note: Top.

Part of Plant: Leaves, twigs, and sap.

Extraction Method: Distillation.

Color: Clear.

Growing Region: Hunan Province, China.

Major Chemical Components: Monoterpene ketone: camphor. Ester: methyl cinnamate. Monoterpenes: camphene, pinene, sabinene, cymene. Monoterpene ether oxide: 1-8 cineole (eucalyptol). Monoterpene alcohol: terpenin-4-ol.

CM Category: Substances for Topical Application.

Nature and Taste: Acrid, hot, toxic.

Affinities: Heart, Spleen, Lung.

Average Dilution: 1-2%. External, topical use only. For acute care, not for long-term use.

Cautions and Contraindications: Contraindicated for children and pregnant women.

Pharmacological Actions: Stimulant, antiparasitic, antifungal, antitoxin, antimicrobial, anti-epidemic, mucolytic.

ACTIONS AND INDICATIONS:

- Revives the senses for shock, seizure, delirium, loss of consciousness, or a severely depressive state.
- Enlivens insufficient Heart Qi with low blood pressure, weak limbs, palpitations, shortness of breath, and sweat upon exertion.

- Clears toxins and turbidity.
- Breaks up mucus, phlegm, and lymph congestion.
- Repels and kills insects.
- Kills parasites, scabies, ringworms, fungal infections, and itching skin sores.
- Stimulates circulation and relieves pain.

CM Concepts, Channel Systems, and Patterns:

- Open the Sensory Portals.
- Clear Toxin
- Open Yang Qiao Mai/Yang Heel Vessel.

Application and Blends:

- Inhale briefly, as a smelling salt for emergency medicine. Make a smelling salt by mixing 5 drops in 1/2oz of salt and keep in a closed container for ready use as needed. Not for long-term use.
- On acupuncture points to open the sensory portals and restore consciousness, place neat directly on the Jing Well points, LI20, GV20, and GV26.
- For wind stroke or epilepsy, place on GV15, GV24, GV25, and KI1.
- Used topically as a plaster or compress for traumatic injuries with pain, swelling, bruising, inflammation, blend with equal parts Yi Yi Ren (Coix), Ru Xiang (Frankincense), and Mo Yao (Myrrh). Make a 10% dilution in safflower oil with Zhang Nao being 1-2% of the total of essential oils in the blend.
- As a topical application for parasites, scabies, tinea, weeping, itching skin lesions, combine Zhang Nao with She Chuang Zi (Cnidium Fruit) essential oil in a 1-2% dilution. Use grapeseed oil as the carrier. Make a paste with green clay powder to draw out. For parasites, scabies, ringworms, and fungal infections, make a wash or spray with equal parts apple cider vinegar and water.
- For oral herpes, make a salve of equal parts Zhang Nao and Qing Hao (*Artemisia annua*) diluted to 1% in calophyllum (tamanu) oil. Apply directly on the lesion.
- Sprinkle Zhang Nao on salt and place into a cloth bag as a sachet to keep moths and insects away from stored clothing.

ZHI KE 枳壳

BITTER ORANGE FRUIT

Citrus aurantium, Aurantii Fructus

ZHI KE ESSENTIAL OIL IS A LIVELY, UPLIFTING TOP NOTE. Its effect gets stuck Qi moving. It especially works on the digestive tract to relieve intestinal sluggishness and discomfort, and on the chest to break up congestion in the lungs and free the breath. One of its qualities as a citrus top note is to cleanse and gently exfoliate the skin. This makes it a helpful and pleasantly aromatic addition to blends for beauty products or skin conditions. Many of Zhi Ke's effects can be explained by its dominant chemical component, limonene. Commonly found in citrus essential oils, this monoterpene is a high-spectrum antimicrobial agent. It has been found to neutralize gastric acid and support normal peristalsis. Limonene is also a natural solvent of cholesterol and has been used clinically to dissolve cholesterol containing gallstones.

Aroma: Sweet citrus with bright, tart notes.

Note: Top.

Part of Plant: Fruit and Peel.

Extraction Method: Distillation.

Color: Golden yellow.

Growing Region: Southern China, Sichuan, Jiangxi, Hunan, Jiangsu, Zhejiang Provinces.

Major Chemical Components: Monoterpenes: limonene, terpinene, pinene, ocimene. Ester: myrcenyl acetate. Monoterpene aldehyde: citral. Monoterpene alcohol: linalool. Coumarin [14].

CM Category: Regulating Qi.

Nature and Taste: Bitter, acrid, slightly cold.

Affinities: Spleen, Stomach, Large Intestine. As essential oil, also Lung.

Average Dilution: 4-6%.

Cautions and Contraindications: Photosensitive, caution on exposed skin.

Pharmacological Actions: Antimicrobial, digestive, antacid, antihyperlipidemic, smooth muscle stimulant, decongestant.

ACTIONS AND INDICATIONS:

- Activates Qi circulation and regulates digestion.
- Relieves distention and pressure in the abdomen.

- Supports descending of the digestive Qi and moves accumulation in the intestines.
- Promotes peristalsis.
- Neutralizes gastric acid, heartburn, and GERD.
- Expands the chest and unbinds the diaphragm.
- Stimulates bile, breaks up phlegm, cholesterol, and stones.
- Benefits the skin.

CM Concepts, Channel Systems, and Patterns:

- Regulate Qi as part of Divergent Meridian treatment strategy.

Application and Blends:

For excessive Stomach acidity due to Stomach fire, combine Zhi Ke with Zhi Zi (Gardenia Fruit) as a 3% dilution with black cumin seed oil as the carrier. Apply over the stomach area. This may be orally ingested, for short-term acute symptom relief, three drops as a dose in yogurt or honey water.

If indigestion is due to emotions such as anger or frustration, with Liver Wood overacting on the Stomach Earth causing Qi stagnation, pain, and nausea, create an aromatic blend of Zhi Ke with Mu Xiang (Saussurea) and Zhi Zi Hua (Gardenia Flower) as a 3% dilution in cumin seed oil and apply topically over the hypochondriac areas and on acupoints such as LR3 and PC6 along with direct inhalation of the aroma.

For nausea and vomiting:
If morning sickness, combine Zhi Ke with Zi Su Ye (Perilla Leaf). Inhale directly as needed.

If due to excessive cold diet affecting the stomach, combine Zhi Ke with Ding Xiang (Clove Bud) and Gan Jiang (Dry Ginger). Dilute 3% in black cumin seed oil and compress on the abdomen with gentle heat.

In both cases apply on acupoints such as P6, SP4, ST36, and CV12.

Add Zhi Ke as a top note to blends addressing respiratory infections with congestion and chest constraint to help regulate the Qi of the lungs and chest and to break up phlegm. Diffuse with An Shu Ye (Eucalyptus) and Song Zhen (Pine Needle) for cough and congestion, and to rid the air of pathogens. This blend may also be applied on the chest as a 4% dilution in almond oil.

For the skin, 1-2% Zhi Ke may be added to facial masks, scrubs, or creams. Apply at night to avoid reaction to sun exposure.

ZHI ZI 梔子

GARDENIA FRUIT

Gardeniae jasminoides Fructus

THE ESSENTIAL OIL, EXTRACTED FROM THE RED GARDENIA FRUIT, with its pink color and its aroma's bitter edge, aligns with the Fire element. Excessive heat or fire in the body can arise from internal or external factors. Internally, strong emotions like anger or anxiety can cause a flaring up of Liver or Heart fire which further disturbs the mind and results in physical symptoms as well. On the other hand, fire caused by external factors such as diet, excessive alcohol intake, or environmental toxins will not only cause physical symptoms but will disturb the mind and stir up strong emotions. Gardenia essential oil clears the fire and calms the emotions. Zhi Zi works throughout the San Jiao, thereby, reaching the entire body. The San Jiao mechanism is the means by which Yuan Source Qi is distributed to the internal organs and by which the movement of fire and water are regulated. When fire and water are unregulated, the normal functions of metabolism are disrupted, and conditions of damp-heat can arise causing illness. If damp-heat conditions are not resolved they can turn into fire toxins, a much more serious illness. Zhi Zi clears damp-heat and toxins from all three burners as well as fire toxins manifesting as skin conditions.

Aroma: Rich and herbaceous with a piercing bitter edge.

Note: Middle/Top.

Part of Plant: Fruit.

Extraction Method: CO2 extraction.

Color: Red orange.

Growing Region: Henan Province, China. A large evergreen shrub native to southern China with red fruit and fragrant white flowers.

Major Chemical Components: Monoterpenoids: gardenamide [39], jasminoside. Irodoid glycoside: geniposide. Fatty acids: linoleic acid, squalene, palmitic acid, n- hexadecanoic acid, myristic acid, and caproic acid. Phenols. Aldehydes. Esters. Alcohols.

CM Category: Clearing Heat and Purging Fire.

Nature and Taste: Bitter and cold.

Affinities: San Jiao, Heart, Lung, Liver, Stomach.

Average Dilution: 4-6%

Pharmacological Actions: Analgesic, antacid, antihypertensive, antihyperlipidemic, antipyretic, antibiotic, hepatoprotective, antidepressant, sedative, antioxidant.

Actions and Indications:

- Calms irritability, restlessness, sleep disorders, and short temper by sedating fire.
- Benefits the brain and nervous system.
- Clears fire toxin and damp-heat from all three burners.
- Cools heat in the blood to stop bleeding.
- Quells Stomach fire, decreases secretion of gastric acid and increases pH in the stomach to treat stomach pain, burning, hyperacidity.
- Lowers blood pressure and cholesterol.
- Breaks up belly fat.
- Clears congestion and inflammation, in liver and gallbladder, and resolves jaundice.
- Treats injuries with pain, inflammation, redness, swelling, bruising.

CM Concepts, Channel Systems, and Patterns:

- Clear damp-heat as part of Divergent Meridian treatment strategy.
- Open and clear the Dai Mai/Belt Vessel.
- Clear Liver and Gallbladder damp-heat.
- Benefit the Health Palace of the Nine Palaces.

Application and Blends:

- To cool and calm irritability, restlessness, and short temper with feelings of heat in the upper body due to Heart and Liver fire, create an aromatic blend of Zhi Zi with Zhi Zi Hua (Gardenia Flower), or another aromatic floral essential oil such as Xun Yi Cao (Lavender) or Mei Gui Hua (Rose). Add Bo He (Peppermint) as a top note to release the heat outward. Inhale directly or diffuse. May also apply to acupoints of the Pericardium and Liver channels that clear heat.
- To lower blood pressure, combine Zhi Zi with Jiang Xiang (*Dalbergia*). Inhale directly or diffuse and apply to the bottom of the feet, on and around KI1. Additionally, if elevated blood pressure causes symptoms such as headache with heat and bloodshot eyes, combine with Ju Hua (Chrysanthemum) and Bo He (Peppermint), inhale the aroma and dilute 4-6% to apply on the painful areas of the head.
- For excessive stomach acidity due to Stomach fire, blend with Zhi Ke (*Citrus aurantium*) essential oil as a 4% dilution with black cumin seed oil as the carrier. Apply a few drops gently spread over the upper abdominal and stomach area. May be ingested to relieve acute stomach and abdominal pain. Three drops on the tongue, emulsified with 1 tsp of honey, yogurt, or black cumin seed carrier oil, settles the stomach and eases discomfort.
- To break up belly fat and cellulite, combine Zhi Zi with Hu Lu Ba (Fenugreek) and Wu Wei Zi (*Schisandra Fruit*) essential oils diluted to 2% in cod liver or castor oil and vigorously rub over the waistline area, then compress with a hot washcloth.

ZHI ZI HUA 栀子花

GARDENIA FLOWER

Gardeniae jasminoides Flos

BOTH ZHI ZI, THE GARDENIA FRUIT, AND ZHI ZI HUA, THE GARDENIA FLOWER, travel throughout the San Jiao. As essential oils, they reach all three levels of Jing Essence, Qi, and Shen Spirit. While the flower and fruit share many attributes, by way of comparison, Zhi Zi, the red fruit of Gardenia, works more on the material aspects of the Qi, blood, and fluids: clearing heat, draining damp, clearing toxin, and quieting emotions that arise due to flaring fire, damp encumbrance, and blood stagnation. The beautiful, fragrant Gardenia flower works more on the immaterial level, cleansing and clearing away what has gotten in the way of emotional and spiritual transformation. Its aroma invites white light and is deeply calming and freeing. The pure white color of the blossom reflects its affinity with the Metal element and specifically with the Lungs, which deal with feelings of loss and the ability to let go. Zhi Zi Hua essential oil cools entrapped Lung heat, thereby releasing overwhelming grief and sorrow trapped deep inside out to the surface. Gardenia blooms in the spring, season of the Wood element, and so its fragrance is imbued with the blossoming of growth, renewal, and transcendence.

Aroma: Heady, sweet floral, fruity and gently spicy.

Note: Middle/Base.

Part of Plant: Flower.

Extraction Method: CO2 extraction.

Color: Golden amber.

Growing Region: Henan Province, China. A large evergreen shrub, native to southern China, with red fruit and fragrant white flowers.

Major Chemical Components: Sesquiterpenes: alpha-farnesene, trans-beta-ocimene, hexenyl tiglate. Monoterpene alcohol: linalool.

CM Category: Clearing Heat, Calming the Spirit.

Nature and Taste: Sweet, spicy, cool.

Affinities: San Jiao, Heart, Lung, Liver.

Average Dilution: 2-4%.

Pharmacological Actions: Sedative, anxiolytic antipyretic, antihypertensive, antimicrobial, antifungal, antioxidant.

Actions and Indications:

- Calms the spirit. Cools Liver and Heart fire.
- Lowers blood pressure.
- Calms irritability, anxiety, and insomnia.
- Clears Lung heat and frees the chest and diaphragm.

Application and Blends:

- To calm the spirit, the best use of Zhi Zi Hua is to inhale the aroma, neat, and wear as a perfume on the inner wrist.
- To subdue shock or fright, combine with Ju Hua (Chrysanthemum) and Zhi Ke (*Citrus aurantium*) neat for direct inhalation.
- Combine the fruit and flower of Gardenia together as an aromatic blend to treat both physical and emotional issues. For example, to work on resolving emotional and spiritual angst arising from the challenge of a serious illness. For topical application, dilute 4-6% in jojoba oil and gently spread over the physically affected area with intention. Deeply inhale the aroma.
- To clear Lung heat, free the chest and diaphragm, or to treat depression, create an aromatic blend of Zhi Zi Hua, Tan Xiang (Sandalwood), Xiang Fu (*Cyperus*), and Qing Pi (Green Tangerine Peel). Inhale the aroma and dilute 4% in almond oil to spread a few drops over the chest and diaphragm.
- Anoint Zhi Zi Hua on Bai Hui (GV20) and Yin Tang (Third Eye) to invite white light during meditation. Apply neat. Diffuse to bring light into the meditation space.

Zi Su Ye 紫蘇葉

PERILLA LEAF, SHISO

Perillae fructescens Folium

ZI SU YE ESSENTIAL OIL BENEFITS both the respiratory and digestive system. It is an effective preventative as well as curative for respiratory infections, "stomach bugs" like a digestive flu, and allergies. It decongests and clears inflammation of the nose, eyes, and ears. Zi Su Ye is best used, and highly effective, diffused into the air or applied topically. It is not recommended for internal ingestion due to its ketone chemical constituents which, on the other hand, are valuable for breaking up mucus and phlegm and killing germs.

Aroma: Herbaceous, apple fruity, and minty, with a gently bitter undertone.

Note: Middle.

Part of Plant: Leaf.

Extraction Method: CO2 extraction.

Color: Amber-olive.

Growing Region: Hubei Province, China. An invasive plant native to mountainous areas.

Major Chemical Components: Monoterpene aldehyde: perillaldehyde > 32%. Monoterpenes: limonene, pinene. Ketones: perilla ketone, elsholtzia ketone. Phenols (Phenylpropanoid): cis-asarone, eugenol.

CM Category: Releasing the Exterior.

Nature and Taste: Acrid, aromatic, slightly warm.

Affinities: Lung, Spleen.

Average Dilution: 4-6%.

Cautions and Contraindications: Ketone components, contraindicated for topical use or ingestion during pregnancy.

Pharmacological Actions: Digestive, anti-emetic, mucolytic, anti-inflammatory, immunomodulating (interferon), preventative, antiviral, anti-allergic, anti-asthmatic, analgesic, antimicrobial, antibacterial.

ACTIONS AND INDICATIONS:

- Harmonizes the digestion, stops nausea and vomiting, morning sickness, abdominal pain, and sluggish digestion.
- Expands the chest, dissolves phlegm, treats colds and upper respiratory infections, coughing, wheezing, asthma, and allergies.
- Supports Wei Protective Qi, boosts immunity, increases interferon.

- Preventative during cold and allergy season.
- Resolves children's cough and upper respiratory infections.
- Treats conjunctivitis (pink eye).
- Opens the senses, nose, ears.
- Benefits the eyes and declining vision.
- Detoxifies seafood poisoning and waterborne pathogens.
- Breaks up scars, fibrotic tissue, skin tags, and masses.
- Stimulates hair growth.
- Lowers cortisol levels.

Application and Blends:

- Diffuse into the air as a preventative during cold, flu, and allergy seasons. 10-15 drops of Zi Su Ye, neat, in the diffuser.
- To tonify the Qi and increase interferon in order to prevent and treat viruses, apply on ST36 and dilute 4% in almond oil for massaging into areas with more sweat glands such as the bottom of the feet and center of the chest.
- Very effective and safe diffused for children's cough/upper respiratory infections.
- For conjunctivitis, steam the eye area by placing 3-5 drops in a pint of hot water. Allow the steam to rise from the water to the eye area for 5 to 10 minutes, once or twice per day. If a stinging sensation occurs, increase distance from the water. Or apply a warm compress of Zi Su Ye and Ju Hua (Chrysanthemum) essential oils diluted to 2% in almond or other gentle carrier oil. Wring the cloth well. Do not allow the oil to drip into the eyes.
- For nausea, including morning sickness, inhale briefly directly from the bottle or inhale the steam by placing 3-5 drops in a pint of hot water.
- To break up scar tissue after surgery, especially concave scars, combine with resins such as Ru Xiang (Frankincense) and Mo Yao (Myrrh), apply a 4-6% dilution in calophyllum (tamanu) oil. May also be applied this way to break up fibrotic tissue such as warts or skin tags. For uterine fibroids, combine Zi Su Ye with E Zhu (*Curcuma zedoaria*) and Qing Pi (Green Tangerine Peel), use a higher concentration 6-8% dilution and compress over the affected area once per day three days on and three days off.
- To stimulate hair growth, add Zi Su Ye, Ce Bai Ye (Biota Leaf), Bai Zi Ren (Biota Seed), and Rosemary. 50 total drops of essential oil to 4 oz of shampoo.
- Zi Su Ye may be applied neat or diluted on acupuncture points such as on the Stomach channel for digestive issues, Lung channel for respiratory, Jing Well points and GV20 to open the senses.

Zi Su Zi 紫蘇子

PERILLA SEED

Perillae fructescens Fructus

ZI SU ZI ESSENTIAL OIL very specifically benefits the Metal element and its organs, the Lung and Large Intestine. Its function in Chinese medicine is to stop coughing and wheezing by dissolving phlegm and directing the Lung Qi downward. It is widely used in traditional herbal formulas for asthmatic and cough conditions of various types. The lubricating nature of the oil loosens and breaks up congestion so that it can more easily be expelled. Upon inhalation, the gentle, complex aroma of Zi Su Zi essential oil leads its energy downward from the nose into the chest where it opens the breath and then continues downward into the lower abdomen. Combining Perilla Seed with An Shu Ye (Eucalyptus) or Song Zhen (Pine) will add a more aromatic and stimulating lung opening effect for diffusers or chest rubs.

Working on the emotional level, blending together the attributes of both the seed (Zi Su Zi) and the leaf (Zi Su Ye) essential oils of the Perilla plant broaden and deepen their effect. Both affect the Metal element to deal with issues of loss, grief, guilt, and judgment. Perilla Leaf's combined Earth and Metal affinities are harmonizing. It transforms damp, ingrained thought patterns regarding family and relationships, while Perilla Seed gently softens what is stuck and congested. Together they make it possible to breathe freely, to take in and digest what is going on in our lives, and to exhale and eliminate what is holding us back.

Aroma: Herbaceous, sweet, lightly pungent overtone and mildly bitter undertone.

Note: Base.

Part of Plant: Seed.

Extraction Method: CO2 extraction.

Color: Golden yellow.

Growing Region: Hubei Province, China. Harvested in October. An invasive plant native to mountainous areas.

Major Chemical Components: Monoterpene aldehyde: perillaldehyde. Sesquiterpenes: caryophyllene, farnesene. Phenol (phenylpropanoid): eugenol. Fatty acids: Palmitic acid,* oleolic acid, linoleic acid. Monoterpene ketone: perilla ketone.

* *Palmitic acid, a saturated long chain fatty acid, is a major constituent of Zi Su Zi essential oil. It is the most common saturated fatty acid found in animals, plants and microorganisms. It is found throughout human tissue, and in all parts of human cells as well as in body fluids such as sweat and cerebral spinal fluid. In the lungs, palmitic acid exhibits efficient surfactant activity. Pulmonary surfactant is essential for breathing. It reduces surface tension at the air/liquid interface of the alveoli. Insufficiency causes respiratory distress.*

CM Category: Transforming Phlegm and Stopping Cough.

Nature and Taste: Acrid, aromatic, warm, moistening.

Affinities: Lung, Large Intestine.

Average Dilution: 10-15%. Gentle and nonirritating to average skin.

Pharmacological Actions: Antitussive, anti-asthmatic, mucolytic, expectorant, antibacterial.

Actions and Indications:

- Stops cough and calms wheezing, directs the Lung Qi downward and dissolves phlegm.
- Moistens dryness inhibiting the free movement and descension of the Lung and Large Intestine Qi.
- Warms the lungs to resolve cold phlegm obstruction. Relieves shortness of breath and chest discomfort.

CM Concepts, Channel Systems, and Patterns:

- Redirect rebellious Lung Qi.
- Moisten the intestines and unblock the stool.

Application and Blends:

- For cold phlegm obstructing the lungs, diffuse and inhale the steam from Zi Su Zi with essential oils of An Shu Ye (Eucalyptus) and Gui Zhi/Gui Ye (Cinnamon Twig and Leaf).
- To stop coughing, wheezing, and asthmatic conditions, blend Zi Su Zi Si 30% with Xing Ren (*Prunus armeniaca*) 10%, Hou Po (Magnolia Bark) 20%, and Song Zhen (Pine) 40% as a 4-6% dilution in almond or Zi Su Zi (Perilla Seed) cold-pressed carrier oil. Apply on the chest and diffuse the essential oils neat in a diffuser.
- To work with issues of grief and guilt, create an aromatic blend with the seed and leaf oils of Perilla (Zi Su Zi and Zi Su Ye) together with the bark and leaf oils of Magnolia (Hou Po and Bai Yu Lan Ye). Inhale the aroma, wear as perfume, or in the bath. Apply on the Yuan Source and Luo Connecting points of the Lung and Spleen channels: LU9, LU7, SP3, SP4.

Hydrosols & Hydrolats

Hydrosols

One of the main methods of extracting essential oils from plants is steam distillation. During this process two products are created: essential oil and hydrosol. Essential oils are extractions of the oils and oil-soluble compounds contained in the plant. Hydrosols contain the water-soluble compounds present in the plant which are created as a result of steam and condensation produced during the distillation process. Plants contain more water than oil, and so the amount of hydrosol produced during distillation far exceeds that of essential oil. Hydrosols embody medicinal and energetic properties of the plants; however, they are much less concentrated than their essential oil counterparts and very gentle on the skin. The aroma of hydrosol is lighter and more subtle compared to the aroma exuded by essential oil.

Hydrolats

A hydrolat contains both hydrosol and a small amount of essential oil, which can be collected during the process of separating the essential oil from the hydrosol. Hydrolats are used similarly to hydrosols, but the presence of essential oil tends to potentiate the medicinal qualities and aroma.

Hydrosols and hydrolats are commonly used in beauty and skin care and can also be used as an aromatherapy spray to affect mental emotional states and to benefit and awaken the senses. They can be spritzed on the face, head, body, or into the air to affect the environment. Hydrosols and hydrolats are also safe for internal ingestion due to their gentle, dilute nature.

Hydrosols, Hydrolats, and Skin Care

Many hydrosols and hydrolats, like normal healthy skin, tend to have a mildly acidic pH. Maintaining normal pH balance is essential to support the skin's natural protective barrier, called the acidic mantle, its moisture retention, and healthy bacterial flora. When the skin becomes too alkaline, it loses the integrity of the acidic mantle and is prone to develop conditions such as acne, rosacea, rashes, fungal or yeast infections. Products with lower pH, meaning more acidic, are anti-inflammatory. In the language of Chinese medicine, this means that they help to clear heat and toxin.

For Mental Emotional Balance

Peacefulness and quietude are Yin states. Yin nourishing substances tend to be moistening and neutral or cooling. The mildly acidic pH of hydrosols and hydrolats means that many of them are calming for anxiety, insomnia, post-trauma, mood disorders, and depending on the additional actions of the particular herb, they are useful for various types of mental illness or neurological disorders.

Bai Li Xiang / Thyme Hydrosol

Thymus mongolicus Herba

Aroma: Herbaceous spice. pH: 6.3

Thyme is a low bushy plant with various species that are found all over the world. It is well known for its effects as a digestive as well as a strong antiseptic. The hydrosol maintains the plant's greenish color and distinctive aroma. It can be quite concentrated and viscous. Thyme hydrosol can be sprayed to refresh, protect, and sanitize. This species of Thyme has been shown to have antifungal properties and can be used topically to help control fungal infections of the skin such as athlete's foot.

Bai Ren Shen/ White Ginseng Root Hydrosol

Panax Ginseng Radix

Aroma: Light, earthy. pH: 6.0

White Ginseng hydrosol is energizing and stimulating. It invigorates the body and awakens the senses. Relative to Red Ginseng, which is very warm natured, White Ginseng is slightly cool in nature; this hydrosol can enliven the body and spirit without adding additional heat into the body.

Ginseng is a highly regarded herbal medicinal, and in addition to having a tonifying effect on all of the organs, it benefits the immune system and is one of the few herbs that can boost the Yuan Source Qi.

Mei Gui Hua/ Damascus Rose Hydrosol

Rosa damascena Flos

Aroma: Light, true rose floral. pH: 4.0 - 4.4

Damascus Rose nourishes the Yin and Jin Ye body fluids, including hormonal secretions, and is a wonderful herbal ally for moistening and restoring aging skin. It calms the spirit and relaxes the blood pressure and heart rate. The aroma of Rose inspires feelings of nourishment, beauty, love, and transcendence.

Damascus Rose hydrosol is balancing and gentle and can be used for all skin types including sensitive skin. Due to its gently astringent nature, it can be used alone as a facial toner. It is anti-inflammatory, antiseptic, and can be applied to calm irritated skin or acne.

Rose hydrosol has a relaxing and moving effect on the bladder and lower intestine. It can be used as an enema, abdominal massage, or sitz bath to produce a gentle laxative effect for children and the elderly. Ingested, Rose hydrosol is diuretic, to move the urine when it is inhibited, for example, in the case of prostatitis.

HUANG QIN/ SKULLCAP HYDROSOL

Scutellaria baicalensis Radix

Aroma: Light earthy, woody, bitter. pH 5.8

Commonly known as Skullcap, Huang Qin hydrosol is produced from the golden yellow colored root of the *Scutellaria baicalensis* plant. It has a subtle woody, bitter aroma and taste. In traditional Chinese medicine, the root is used to clear damp-heat conditions. This hydrosol, with a pH slightly more alkaline than normal skin, is balancing for oily skin. It helps to even the skin tone and assist in lightening dark pigmentation. Plus, considering Huang Qin's attributes as an herbal medicine, it may be applied for purulent, damp skin conditions and infections. It can also be used as a mouthwash for sores, or gargle for sore throat.

LAN LIAN HUA / BLUE LOTUS HYDROSOL

Nymphaea tetragona Flos

Aroma: Light sweet floral. Ph 6.6

The blue water lily, called blue lotus, is a perennial aquatic plant that has been revered in Asian culture for centuries for its spiritual and medicinal benefits. Its extensive underground root system aids its environment in water purification and can absorb heavy metals and filter microorganisms. Its cooling and purifying nature can be used to calm emotional disturbances such as anxiety, restlessness, depression, and short temper. This plant can be used in skin care to retain moisture in the skin due to its astringent nature and can also be used topically to reduce inflammation of skin legions, rashes, and allergic reactions or bacterial infections. This wondrous plant also contains compounds that have been shown to maintain healthy cells within the hair, skin, and nails.

Ma Chi Xian / Purselane Hydrolat

Portulaca oleracea Herba

Aroma: Light, herbaceous. pH: 7.0

Ma Chi Xian hydrolat can be used topically for damp-heat fire toxin type skin problems with redness, swelling, and oozing such as poison ivy, carbuncles, and sores. It can also be used as an antidote for pain and swelling from insect stings or spider bites. It has strong antibacterial and antimicrobial properties.

The Chinese herb Ma Chi Xian is contraindicated for internal ingestion during pregnancy.

Ru Xiang / Sacred Frankincense Hydrosol

Boswellia sacra, Olibanum

Aroma: Resinous, balsamic. pH 5.0

Sacred Frankincense is so named because of its traditional use as incense or anointment in sacred ceremonies. The resin of the Boswellia tree is well known for its capacity to promote the healing of wounds to both body and spirit. The hydrolat embodies its resinous intensity.

It can be poured directly into the bath or applied topically onto areas of injury for pain, bruising, swelling, or to hasten healing response and stimulate tissue generation.

A spritz on the face stirs the Qi and blood and swirls in the head, initiating a shift in consciousness or an opening for transport to other realms. Be sure to ground yourself.

Shi Che Ju / Blue Cornflower Hydrolat

Centaurea cyanus Flos

Aroma: Light sweet floral with mild tart spice. pH: 3.5-4.0

The bright blue color of this flower illustrates its affinity with the Liver and by extension its relationship to the eyes. Shi Che Ju hydrolat can be used to brighten and benefit the eyes for cases of eye strain, puffy eyes, or inflammation, conjunctivitis, or blepharitis. It can be sprayed on the skin to clear heat, and reduce swelling, sores, abscesses, itching, and inflammation. It helps to repair wounds, prevent infection, break up scars and fibrotic tissue. Its aroma releases pent up emotion. It is cooling, calming, and freeing.

For skin care, Cornflower hydrosol is astringent. It brings and retains moisture and helps to reduce wrinkles.

YUAN ZHI / POLYGALA HYDROSOL

Polygala tenuifolia Radix

Aroma: Herbaceous, earthy. pH: 5.5

Yuan Zhi's traditional usage in Chinese medicine is to calm the spirit and nourish the Heart. It quiets the mind and emotions and treats depression, anxiety, insomnia, palpitations, and restlessness. Its special function to clear phlegm enveloping the orifices of the Heart and obstructing the senses makes it a commonly used herb to relieve mental and emotional disorientation, quell seizures, and to aid mental clarity and memory. Yuan Zhi strengthens the Will (Zhi 志) and opens the sensory orifices including the eyes, fostering the ability to see by literally benefiting the vision, and figuratively, to see the world differently and have the will power to change.

It can also be applied for topical use to reduce abscess and swelling.

ZHI ZI HUA / GARDENIA FLOWER HYDROSOL

Gardeniae jasminoides Flos

Aroma: Light sweet floral. pH: 4.5

The fruit of the Gardenia flower is used in Chinese medicine for clearing heat in the body. Heat tends to rise to the head and upper body, giving rise to mental emotional symptoms. The descending nature of this herb will guide the heat downward. In addition, its cooling nature counterbalances accumulated heat in the body. As a fully blossomed flower, the mental, emotional, and spiritual attributes of Gardenia are enhanced. Zhi Zi Hua hydrosol is calming for mood disorders such as anxiety, depression, restlessness, short temper, and irritability. It is especially helpful for sleep disorders and trouble falling asleep. The aroma of this hydrosol is spiritually uplifting.

On the skin, it reduces swelling and inflammation, and can be applied topically to heal wounds and reduce acne, eczema, boils, and rashes.

Gardenia is antibacterial, antibiotic, analgesic, antihypertensive, antihyperlipidemic, anti-inflammatory.

Endnotes

(See Bibliography for citations)

1. **Cineole/Eucalyptol** – An Shu (*Eucalyptus*), a monoterpene ether oxide, is known to be mucolytic, bronchodilating, anti-inflammatory, to reduce exacerbation rates in COPD patients, and to ameliorate symptoms in patients suffering from asthma and rhinosinusitis.

   Juergens, U R. "Anti-inflammatory properties of the monoterpene 1.8-cineole: current evidence for co-medication in inflammatory airway diseases." *Drug research,* Vol. 64,12 (2014): 638-46. doi:10.1055/s-0034-1372609.

2. **Linalool** – Bai Yu Lan Ye (*Magnolia denudate*), Mo Li Hua (*Jasminum sambac*) a monoterpene alcohol found in many essential oils, especially florals, is shown to have sedative and protective effects on the central nervous system. It is anti-inflammatory, antihyperalgesic, and antinociceptive.

   Batista, Patricia Aparecida et al. "The antinociceptive effect of (-)-linalool in models of chronic inflammatory and neuropathic hypersensitivity in mice." *The journal of pain,* Vol. 11,11 (2010): 1222-9. doi:10.1016/j.jpain.2010.02.022.

3. **Cedrol** – Bai Zi Ren (*Biota orientalis Seed*), Ce Bai Ye (*Biota Orientalis Leaf*) a sesquiterpene alcohol has been shown to exert astringent, antiseptic, anti- inflammatory, antispasmodic, sedative, tonic, insecticidal, and antifungal activities. *Platycladus orientalis* Leaf is traditionally known to potentiate hair growth promotion. In the current work, cedrol as a major constituent from *P. orientalis* was evaluated for its potential on hair growth in vivo. Results indicated that cedrol significantly promoted hair growth in a dose-dependent manner. Further observation of the hair follicle demonstrated that cedrol exerted a remarkable effect on the hair follicle length. These findings suggested that cedrol may be the main active ingredient of *P. orientalis* and have the potential of becoming a new hair growth promoter.

   Zhang, Yan et al. "Hair growth promoting activity of cedrol isolated from the leaves of Platycladus orientalis." *Biomedicine & pharmacotherapy = Biomedecine & pharmacotherapie,* Vol. 83 (2016): 641-647. doi:10.1016/j.biopha.2016.07.022.

   Kagawa, Daiji et al. "The sedative effects and mechanism of action of cedrol inhalation with behavioral pharmacological evaluation." *Planta medica,* Vol. 69,7 (2003): 637-41. doi:10.1055/s-2003-41114.

Umeno, Katsumi et al. "Effects of direct cedrol inhalation into the lower airway on autonomic nervous activity in totally laryngectomized subjects." *British journal of clinical pharmacology,* Vol. 65,2 (2008): 188-96. doi:10.1111/j.1365-2125.2007.02992.x.

4. **Cuparene** – Bai Zi Ren (*Biota orientalis*) Though the medicinal properties of cuparene have not been explored as broadly as those of other conifer terpenes, cuparene has been documented as being beneficial in the fight against blood cancer and for treating inflammation and bacterial infections.

   Eybna Technologies. "Cuparene Profile: Sesquiterpenes."

5. **Bi Cheng Qie/Shan Ji Jiao** (*Litsea cubeba*) Beside *Litsea cubeba's* traditional medicinal uses its essential oil has protective action against several bacteria and cytoxicity. It possesses antioxidant and antiparasitic properties and has been shown to prevent several cancers.

   Kamle, Madhu et al. "Ethnopharmacological Properties and Medicinal Uses of *Litsea cubeba*." *Plants (Basel, Switzerland),* Vol. 8,6 150. 1 Jun. 2019, doi:10.3390/plants8060150.

6. **Atractylone** – Cang Zhu (*Atractylodis lancea Rhizoma*) shows beneficial effects on allergic inflammatory diseases. It has antimicrobial anti-inflammatory and anti-ulcer activities.

   Jun, Xie et al. "Pharmacological effects of medicinal components of *Atractylodes lancea* (Thunb.) DC." *Chinese Medicine,* Vol. 30, 59 (2018). doi: 10.1186/s13020-018-0216-7.

7. **Saikosaponins** – Chai Hu (*Bupleurum chinensis Radix*) are the main active compounds in Radix Bupleuri. They have been shown to possess many beneficial pharmacological effects including neuroregulation, sedation, anticonvulsant, antipyretic, antiviral, antitumor, pro-immune, anti-inflammation, antioxidant, and hepatoprotective.

   Yuan, Bochuan et al. "A systematic review of the active saikosaponins and extracts isolated from Radix Bupleuri and their applications." *Pharmaceutical biology,* Vol. 55,1 (2017): 620-635.doi:10.1080/13880209.2016.1262433.

8. **Ligustilide** – Chuan Xiong (*Ligusticum wallichii*), Dang Gui (*Angelica sinensis*) a phthalide, is a major component in both Dang Gui (*Angelica sinensis*) and Chuan Xiong (*Ligusticum wallichii*) which relaxes smooth muscle, and is responsible,

specifically, for antispasmodic effect on uterine muscle. A recent study found that ligustilide could improve cognitive dysfunction and brain damage which fits particularly well with Chuan Xiong's attribute in Chinese medicine to benefit the head and brain.

Tang, Yuping et al. "Identification and comparative quantification of bio-active phthalides in essential oils from si-wu-tang, fo-shou-san, radix angelica and rhizoma chuanxiong." *Molecules (Basel, Switzerland),* Vol. 15,1 341-51. 15 Jan. 2010, doi: 10.3390/molecules15010341.

9. **Eugenol** – Ding Xiang (*Caryophylli aromaticus Flos, Eugenia caryophyllata)* Clove oil contains over 80% eugenol. Eugenol is thought to have anti-aging properties because it is shown to protect against DNA damage by free radicals and to benefit the immune system by boosting white blood cells. It has been the focus of a great deal of research. Its powerful antioxidant and anti-inflammatory properties have been shown to be effective anticarcinogenic agents. As one example, a series of test tube and animal experiments identifies eugenol's effectiveness in slowing the growth of colon and lung cancer tumors by initiating apoptosis (cancer cell death). See: XI XIN (Asarum) for more about eugenol.

   Liu, Haizhou et al. "Clove extract inhibits tumor growth and promotes cell cycle arrest and apoptosis." Oncology Research, Vol.21 5(2014): 247 - 59 . doi: 10.3727/096504014X13946388748910.

   Hussain, Arif et al. "Eugenol enhances the chemotherapeutic potential of gemcitabine and induces anticarcinogenic and anti-inflammatory activity in human cervical cancer cells." Cancer Biotherapy & Radiopharmaceuticals, Vol. 26,5 (2011): 519-27. doi: 10.1089/cbr.2010.0925.

   Wikipedia. "Bcl-2."

   Dwivedi, Vinay et al. "Comparative anticancer potential of clove (*Syzygium aromaticum*) – an Indian spice – against cancer cell lines of various anatomical origin." Asian Pacific journal of cancer prevention: APJCP, Vol. 12,8 (2011): 1989-93.

   Sarmistha Banerjee et al. "Clove (*Syzygium aromaticum L.*), a potential chemopreventive agent for lung cancer." Carcinogenesis, Volume 27, Issue 8, August 2006, Pages 1645–1654. https://doi.org/10.1093/carcin/bgi372.

10. **Angelol** – Du Huo (*Angelica pubescentis Radix)* Research into *Angelica pubescentis* has shown its benefits to the brain and central nervous system with improvement of memory, cognition, vascular dementia, and Alzheimer's. These effects are largely due to certain phenols including angelol and osthole (See: SHE CHUANG ZI for more about osthole).

Yaqi, Lu et al. "Traditional Chinese Medicine of *Angelicae Pubescentis Radix*: A Review of Phytochemistry, Pharmacology and Pharmacokinetics." *Frontiers in Pharmacology.* March 2020. https://doi.org/10.3389/fphar.2020.00335.

11. **Sesquiterpenes** – E Zhu (*Curcumae zedoaria Rhizoma*) in E Zhu have been the focus of a great deal of research regarding various anticancer properties. As an example, one particular study found them to be cytotoxic against human gastric cancer AGS cells.

    Lee, Tae Kyoung et al. "Sesquiterpenes from Curcuma zedoaria rhizomes and their cytotoxicity against human gastric cancer AGS cells." *Bioorganic chemistry* Vol. 87 (2019): 117-122. doi:10.1016/j.bioorg.2019.03.015

12. **Germacrone** – E Zhu (*Curcumae zedoaria Rhizoma*) in various studies is shown to inhibit proliferation of breast cancer cell lines by inducing cell cycle arrest and promoting apoptosis. Germacrone has also been shown to have strong antiviral properties.

    Ye, Lianbao et al. "Novel anti-cancer agents based on germacrone: design, synthesis, biological activity, docking studies and MD simulations." *RSC Advances* Issue 7 (2017): 3760-3767. doi: 10.1039/c6ra26944c.

13. **Limonene** – Fo Shou (*Citri sarcodactylis Swingle Fructus*) a monoterpene commonly found in citrus essential oils, is a high- spectrum antimicrobial agent. It has been found to neutralize gastric acid and support normal peristalsis. Limonene is a natural solvent of cholesterol and has been used clinically to dissolve cholesterol containing gallstones.

    Sun, Jidong. "D-Limonene: safety and clinical applications." *Alternative medicine review: a journal of clinical therapeutic,* Vol. 12,3 (2007): 259-64.

14. **Coumarin** – Fo Shou (*Citri sarcodactylis Swingle Fructus*) a benzenoid lactone found in many plants, is a prominent component of Cassia as well as many citrus fruits and their peels. It has been widely studied for its pharmacological and medical benefits. Findings include: anti-infectious, anticoagulant, anti-inflammatory, anticancer, antitumor, and side effects of radiation therapy. It is also known for its lipid lowering activity and is a potent antioxidant. Coumarins are used as an immunostimulatory drug for the treatment of chronic infections. Due to its hormonal sensitivity and immune modulating effects, coumarin has been found to be useful in prostate cancer. Some types of coumarins tend to be reactive to sun exposure.

Rohini, K. and P.S. Srikumar. "Therapeutic Role of Coumarins and Coumarin-Related Compounds." Journal of Thermodynamics and Catalysis, 2014. 5:2.

Das, A. et al. "Phenolic Compounds as Functional Ingredients in Beverages." The Science of Beverages, 2019, Vol. 14. Pages 285-323.

15. **Gingerol** – Gan Jiang (*Zingiberis officinalis Rhizoma*) the main bioactive chemical component of Ginger, has been extensively studied. Ginger is one of highest antioxidant essential oils and gingerol has been found to reduce oxidative stress, including age-related oxidative stress markers, and to elongate shortened telomeres believed to be an indicator of anti-aging activity.

    Bode, AM, and Z. Dong. "The Amazing and Mighty Ginger." Benzie IFF and S. Wachtel- Galor, editors. *Herbal Medicine: Biomolecular and Clinical Aspects.* 2nd edition. *CRC Press/Taylor & Francis,* 2011. Chapter 7. Available from: https://www.ncbi.nlm.nih.gov/ books/NBK92775/.

16. **Benzyl benzoate** – Gui Zhi/Gui Ye (*Cinnamomi cassia Ramulus et Folium*) is lethal to the mite that causes scabies. It is one of the older preparations used to treat scabies. It is also used to treat lice infestation of the head and body. It fell out of favor as a first-choice treatment due to its irritant properties.

    Bachewar, Narendra P et al. "Comparison of safety, efficacy, and cost effectiveness of benzyl benzoate, permethrin, and ivermectin in patients of scabies." *Indian Journal of Pharmacology,* Vol. 41,1 (2009): 9-14. doi:10.4103/0253-7613.48882.

    Buffet, M, and N Dupin. "Current treatments for scabies." *Fundamental & clinical pharmacology,* Vol. 17,2 (2003): 217-25. doi:10.1046/j.1472-8206.2003.00173.x.

17. **Honokiol** – Huo Po (*Magnolia officinalis Cortex*) has been the subject of much pharmacological research including its positive effect on insomnia and anxiety due to its benzodiazepene-like activity as a GABA agonist. It has also shown anti-inflammatory, antioxidant, antibacterial and anticancer benefits. Healing effect on gastric ulcers and relaxation of the digestive tract were also noted results of studies.

    Alexeev, Mikhail et al. "The natural products magnolol and honokiol are positive allosteric modulators of both synaptic and extra-synaptic GABAA receptors." *Neuropharmacology* Vol. 62, 8 (2012): 2507-2514. doi: 10.1016/j.neuropharm.2012.03.002.

18. **Trigonelline** – Hu Lu Ba (*Trigonellae foenum-gracum Semen*) is a plant hormone that has regulatory functions which help with survival and growth of plants. It was first isolated from Fenugreek Seeds (Trigonellae) and is found in significant

quantity in Fenugreek (and coffee beans). It is a methylation product of niacin. It has been shown to have hypoglycemic, neuroprotective, anti-invasive, estrogenic, and antibacterial activities.

Ramesh, C. Garg. "Fenugreek: Multiple Health Benefits." *Nutraceuticlas: Efficacy, Safety and Toxicity*, 2016, Pages 599-617.

Arauz, J et al. "Coffee and the Liver." Muriel, Pablo, editor. *Liver Pathophysiology*. Elsevier Inc, 2017.

19. **Lupenone triterpene** – Huang Qi (*Astragali membranaceus Radix*) pharmacological screening revealed various pharmacological activities including anti-inflammatory, antivirus, antidiabetic, anticancer, and improving of Chagas disease without major toxicity.

Xu, Feng et al. "Beneficial health effects of lupenone triterpene: A review." *Biomedicine & pharmacotherapy = Biomedecine & pharmacotherapie,* Vol. 103 (2018): 198-203. doi: 10.1016/j.biopha.2018.04.019.

20. **Nepetalactone** – Jing Jie (*Schizonepeta tenuifolia Herba*) is related to catnip. Both herbs arouse the Yin and cats are Yin natured animals. The nepetalactone in the essential oil of these plants binds to the olfactory receptors of cats, affecting their brains like a pheromone, resulting in a temporary euphoria.

Brunning, Andy. "The Chemical Behind Catnip's Effect on Cats." Compound Interest. 2014.

21. **Terpinen-4-ol** – Long Nao (*Dryoblanops aromatica, Borneolum*) also found as the main component in Melaleuca (Tea Tree) essential oil, is known for its antifungal activity against a variety of fungal infections including candida. It is also an antibacterial and antiviral agent and clears heat and inflammation.

Brilhante, Raimunda Sâmia Nogueira et al. "Terpinen-4-ol, tyrosol, and β-lapachone as potential antifungals against dimorphic fungi." Brazilian journal of microbiology: [publication of the Brazilian Society for Microbiology] vol. 47,4 (2016): 917-924. doi: 10.1016/j.bjm.2016.07.015

Mondello, F., De Bernardis, F., Girolamo, A. *et al.* "*In vivo* activity of terpinen-4-ol, the main bioactive component of *Melaleuca alternifolia* Cheel (tea tree) oil against azole- susceptible and -resistant human pathogenic *Candida* species." *BMC Infectious Diseases* **6,** 158 (2006). doi: 10.1186/1471-2334-6-158.

22. **Sesquiterpenoid** – Mo Yao (*Commiphorae myrrahae Resina*) substances found in resinous trees such as Myrrh, Frankincense, and Sandalwood have psycho-neuro-

logical activity. For example, those in Myrrh have been shown to bind with opioid receptors in the brain.

Xu, Jing et al. "Four new sesquiterpenes from *Commiphora myrrha* and their neuroprotective effects." *Fitoterapia.* Vol. 83,4 (2012): 801-5. doi:10.1016/j.fitote.2012.03.016.

Xu, Jing et al. "Sesquiterpenoids from the resinous exudates of *Commiphora myrrha* and their neuroprotective effects." *Planta medica.* Vol. 77,18 (2011): 2023-8. doi: 10.1055/s-0031-1280087.

23. Costunolide – Mu Xiang (*Aucklandiae lappa Radix*) is a bioactive sesquiterpene lactone with diverse therapeutic potential. It possesses anti-inflammatory, antioxidative, anti-allergic, bone remodeling, neuroprotective, hair growth promoting, anticancer, and antidiabetic effects. For example, several studies have demonstrated its potential in improving bone health for osteoporosis. Another study demonstrated the mechanisms by which costunolide shows potential in the management of Parkinson's and other neurodegerative diseases, largely by mediating oxidative neuronal cell death.

Kim, Dae Yong, and Bu Young Choi. "Costunolide-A Bioactive Sesquiterpene Lactone with Diverse Therapeutic Potential." *International journal of molecular sciences,* Vol. 20,12 2926. 14 Jun. 2019, doi:10.3390/ijms20122926.

24. **Artemisinin** – Qing Hao (*Artemisiae annuae Herba*) Research into the unique sesquiterpene lactone, artemisinin, discovered in *Artemisiae annuae* led to the 2015 Nobel Prize for Medicine being awarded to Dr. Yuyou Tu for the discovery of an effective antimalarial drug.

Kim, Wan-Su. "Anti-inflammatory, Antioxidant and Antimicrobial Effects of Artemisinin Extracts from *Artemisia annua L.*" *Korean J Physiol Pharmacol,* 2015 Jan;19(1):21-27. https://doi.org/10.4196/kjpp.2015.19.1.21.

25. Herniarin – Qing Hua Jiao (*Zanthoxyli schinifolium Pericardium*) also found in Barley, is shown be antitumor and cytotoxic to breast cancer and to enhance the effect of cisplatin in vitro.

Mousavi, Seyed Hadi et al. "Comparative analysis of the cytotoxic effect of 7- prenyloxycoumarin compounds and herniarin on MCF-7 cell line." *Avicenna journal of phytomedicine,* Vol. 5,6 (2015): 520-30.

26. **Myristicin** – Rou Dou Kou (*Myristicae fragrans Semen*) is a strong hallucinogen. It is an anticholinergic and is the traditional precursor to the psychedelic and empathogenic drug MDMA. Caution with internal ingestion: only in very small doses and for short time.

    Holstege, Christopher P. "Nutmeg." Encyclopedia of Toxicology (2005): 276–277. doi: 10.1016/b0-12-369400-0/00700-6

27. **Elemicin** – Rou Dou Kou (*Myristicae fragrans Semen*) also an anticholinergic, and the traditional precursor in synthesizing the alkaloid mescalin, contributes to this psychedelic effect.

    Holstege, Christopher P. "Nutmeg." Encyclopedia of Toxicology (2005): 276–277. doi: 10.1016/b0-12-369400-0/00700-6

28. **Cinnamaldehyde** – Rou Gui (*Cinnamomi cassis Cortex*) is widely used in agriculture as a nontoxic way to prevent and treat funguses that threaten crops. Additionally, it is an effective insecticide including against mosquitoes, mosquito larvae, and repels animals that threaten crops.

    Rao, Pasupuleti Visweswara, and Siew Hua Gan. "Cinnamon: a multifaceted medicinal plant." *Evidence-based complementary and alternative medicine: eCAM*, Vol. 2014 (2014): 642942. doi:10.1155/2014/642942.

29. **Boswellic acids** – Ru Xiang (*Olibanum Gummi, Boswellia carterii*) have been shown to possess anticancer activities through their cytostatic and apoptotic effects in multiple human cancer cell lines including meningioma, leukemia, hepatoma, melanoma, fibrosarcoma, and colon cancer cells. One particular study showed that whole Frankincense essential oil is able to distinguish between bladder cancer cells and healthy urothelial cells in culture, suppress cell survival and induce apoptosis in cultured bladder cancer cells.

    Frank, M.B., Yang, Q., Osban, J. *et al.* "Frankincense oil derived from *Boswellia carteri* induces tumor cell specific cytotoxicity." *BMC Complement Altern Med* 9, 6 (2009). https://doi.org/10.1186/1472-6882-9-6.

    Schnaubelt, Kurt. *The Healing Intelligence of Essential Oils, The Science of Advanced Aromatherapy*. Healing Arts Press, 2011, pg.158.

30. **11 keto-B-boswellic acid** – Ru Xiang (*Olibanum Gummi, Boswellia carterii*) the most potent anti-inflammatory component of the Frankincense resin, selectively blocks leukotriene biosynthesis providing protective effects on ulcerative colitis.

Frank, M.B., Yang, Q., Osban, J. *et al.* "Frankincense oil derived from *Boswellia carteri* induces tumor cell specific cytotoxicity." *BMC Complement Altern Med* 9, 6 (2009). https://doi.org/10.1186/1472-6882-9-6.

Schnaubelt, Kurt. *The Healing Intelligence of Essential Oils, The Science of Advanced Aromatherapy.* Healing Arts Press, 2011, pg.158.

31. **Osthole** – She Chuang Zi (*Cnidii monnieri Fructus*) the main component of Cnidium, has been the subject of a great deal of research. It is responsible for many of this essential oil's beneficial effects, including pro- libido effects, and the inhibition of histamine dependent itching. Osthole suppresses inflammatory responses and has been used in treatments for inflammation, osteoporosis, and tumors for many years. It has been the subject of numerous recent research studies that have found that Osthole inhibits alcohol or dietary fat induced fatty liver disease and is a good candidate in treatment of liver cancer because of its unique chemical structure. Osthole has been found to be as effective as 17 beta-estradiol in suppressing bone loss and benefiting those with osteoporosis. It lowers blood pressure, inhibits platelet aggregation, and inhibits smooth muscle contraction. It has also been found to be neuroprotective, analgesic, and to reduce lipid accumulation. Studies show that osthole alone exhibits antitumor activity against HER2 positive gastric cancer cells and breast cancer cells.

Zhang, Zhong-Rong. "Osthole: A Review on Its Bioactivities, Pharmacological Properties, and Potential as Alternative Medicine." *Hindawi* (2015). doi: 10.1155/2015/919616.

Dau, Thuy Duong et al. "Effects of *Cnidium monnieri* (L.) Cuss. fruit extract on sexual behaviors in male rats." *Clinical Phytoscience* 6, 80 (2020). doi: 10.1186/s40816-020-00227-3.

32. **Asarone** – Shi Chang Pu (*Acori tatarinowii Rhizoma)* is one of the most widely researched phytochemicals and possesses a wide range of pharmacological activities including antidepressant, anti-anxiety, anti- Alzheimer's, anti-Parkinson's, antiepileptic, anticancer, antihyperlipidemic, antithrombotic, anticholestasis, and radioprotective activities. It is important to note that toxicology studies find that oral ingestion of asarone, in high concentrations, can cause hepatomas.

Han, Ping et al. "Antidepressant-like effects of essential oil and asarone, a major essential oil component from the rhizome of Acorus tatarinowii." Pharmaceutical biology vol. 51,5 (2013): 589-94. doi:10.3109/13880209.2012.751616

Chellian, Ranjithkumar et al. "Pharmacology and toxicology of α- and β-Asarone: A review of preclinical evidence." Phytomedicine : international journal of phytotherapy and phytopharmacology vol. 32 (2017): 41-58. doi:10.1016/j.phymed.2017.04.003

33. Schisandrin – Wu Wei Zi (*Schisandrae Chinensis Fructus*) a main component of Schisandra, is classified as a lignin which is a polyphenolic compound. It has been shown to ameliorate memory impairment, at least in part, due to its antioxidant and free radical scavenging activity. Its low molecular mass and high lipid solubility allow it to pass through the blood brain barrier.

Hu, Di et al. "Schizandrin, an Antioxidant Lignan from Schisandra chinensis, Ameliorates Aβ1–42-Induced Memory Impairment in Mice." *Oxidative Medicine and Cellular Longevity*, Vol. 12 (2012). doi: 10.1155/2012/721721.

34. Ocimene – Wu Zhu Yu (*Evodiae rutecarpa Fructus*) also a prominent cannabis terpene, is responsible for several of the medicinal effects of both plants as well as for the characteristic aroma that they share. In nature, this terpene protects against harmful agents. It has anti-inflammatory, antifungal, antiviral, and antibacterial properties. As an antifungal agent it is used to prevent and treat mycoses such as athlete's foot, candidiasis, and ringworm.

Neoflora. "What is Ocimene and What Does this Terpene Do?" *CBD 101*. neoflora.co/ ocimene/. Accessed 10 June 2021.

35. Methyl Eugenol – Xi Xin (*Asari Herba, Asarum*) a major component of Xi Xin (Asarum) as well as Ding Xiang (Clove), is a powerful antioxidant. It is thought to be anti-aging because it is shown to protect against DNA damage by free radicals. This includes preventing free radicals from attacking lipids embedded in cell walls while increasing antioxidant enzymes. The anticancer action of eugenol is seen in its influence on a certain family of regulator proteins responsible for cancer cell death and apoptosis. This effect was found to be the case in studies of prostate, esophageal, breast and other cancer cells. Eugenol was also noted to decrease the spread of cervical tumors and early stage lung cancer. It is also antiviral. See DING XIANG (Clove) for more on eugenol.

Liu, Haizhou et al. "Clove extract inhibits tumor growth and promotes cell cycle arrest and apoptosis." *Oncology research*, Vol. 21, 5 (2014) : 247 - 59 . doi: 10.3727/096504014X13946388748910.

Hussain, Arif et al. "Eugenol enhances the chemotherapeutic potential of gemcitabine and induces anticarcinogenic and anti-inflammatory activity in human cervical cancer cells." *Cancer biotherapy & radiopharmaceuticals*, Vol. 26,5 (2011): 519-27. doi: 10.1089/cbr.2010.0925.

Wikipedia. "Bcl-2."

Dwivedi, Vinay et al. "Comparative anticancer potential of clove (*Syzygium aromaticum*) – an Indian spice – against cancer cell lines of various anatomical origin." *Asian Pacific journal of cancer prevention*: APJCP, Vol. 12,8 (2011): 1989-93.

Sarmistha Banerjee et al. "Clove (Syzygium aromaticum L.), a potential chemopreventive agent for lung cancer." *Carcinogenesis*, Volume 27, Issue 8, August 2006, Pages 1645–1654. https://doi.org/10.1093/carcin/bgi372

36. Anethole – Xiao Hui Xiang (*Foeniculi vulgare Fructus*) contributes a large component to the flavor and aroma of Fennel. It has potent antimicrobial activity against bacteria, yeasts, and fungi, is an insecticide, and is estrogenic.

Akhbari, Maryam et al. "Analysis and evaluation of the antimicrobial and anticancer activities of the essential oil isolated from Foeniculum vulgare from Hamedan, Iran." Natural product research vol. 33,11 (2019): 1629-1632. doi: 10.1080/14786419.2017.1423310

Mazaheri, Safoora et al. "Effects of Fennel Essential Oil on Cisplatin-induced Nephrotoxicity in Ovariectomized Rats." Toxicology international vol. 20,2 (2013): 138-45. doi:10.4103/0971-6580.117256

37. Benzylaldehyde – Xing Ren (*Pruni armeniacae amarum Semen*)is the simplest aromatic aldehyde constituent of almonds and many fruits and is abundant in *Prunus armeniaca*. The anticancer effect of benzylaldehyde was first reported in 1980 and multi-institutional clinical trials were performed at the time in Japan. These trials attested to the therapy's safety. More recently the mechanism effect was verified and benzyladehyde is now considered a new class of anticancer agent for pancreatic and small cell lung cancer.

Saitoh, Jun and Hideyuki Saya. "Abstract 4758: Benzaldehyde suppresses multiple signal pathways in cancer cells by regulating 14-3-3ζ-mediated protein-protein interactions." *Cancer Res*, July 15, 2016 (76) (14 Supplement) 4758; doi: 10.1158/1538-7445.AM2016-4758.

38. Yi Yi Ren *(Coicis lacryma-jobi Semen)* Coix seed oil is well known to possess diverse antitumor activities and has been widely applied to treat multiple primary malignant tumors. It has shown various exceptional properties in enhancing the immunocompetence and effect of natural killer cells on tumor cells and helping to prevent the decrease of white cells during chemotherapy.

Qu, Ding et al. "Triterpene-loaded microemulsion using Coix lacryma-jobi seed extract as oil phase for enhanced antitumor efficacy: preparation and in vivo evaluation." *International Journal of Nanomedicine* vol. 9 (2014): 109-19. doi:10.2147/IJN.S54796

Zhu, Jiayi et al. "Formulation, Preparation and Evaluation of Nanostructured Lipid Carrier Containing Naringin and Coix Seed Oil for Anti-Tumor Application Based on "Unification of Medicines and Excipients"." Drug Design, Development and Therapy vol. 14 1481-1491. 16 Apr. 2020, doi:10.2147/DDDT.S236997

39. Gardenamide – Zhi Zi (*Gardeniae jasminoides Fructus*) has been studied and utilized for its neurotropic and neuroprotective actions and has been found to improve cognition in Alzheimer's disease.

Zhang, Zuzhi et al. "The synthesis and biological evaluation of novel gardenamide A derivatives as multifunctional neuroprotective agents." MedChemComm, Vol. 10,7 1180-1186. 24 May. 2019, doi:10.1039/c9md00211a.

Carta, Gianfranca et al. "Palmitic Acid: Physiological Role, Metabolism and Nutritional Implications." Frontiers in Physiology, Vol. 8 902. 8 Nov. 2017, doi:10.3389/fphys.2017.00902.

Appendices & Index

Books for Readers' Further Exploration

Acupuncture Points and Channels Location:

Ellis, Andrew, Nigel Wiseman, and Ken Boss. *Fundamentals of Chinese Acupuncture.* Ken Boss. Paradigm Publications, 1991.

Deadman, Peter, and Mazin Al-Khafaji, with Kevin Baker. *A Manual of Acupuncture.* Journal of Chinese Medicine Publications, 1998.

Aromatherapy:

Yuen, Jeffrey C. *Materia Medica of Essential Oils.* Lotus Center for Integrative Medicine, 2000.

Schnaubelt, Kurt. *Advanced Aromatherapy.* Healing Arts Press, 1998.

Schnaubelt, Kurt. *Healing Intelligence of Essential Oils.* Healing Arts Press, 2011.

Chinese Herbs:

Chen, John K., and Tina Chen. *Chinese Medical Herbology and Pharmacology.* Art of Medicine Press, Inc., 2004.

Bensky, Ben, Steven Clavey, and Erich Stoeger. *Chinese Herbal Materia Medica* 3rd edition. Eastland Press, Inc., 2004.

Classical Chinese Philosophy and Philosophy of Chinese Medicine:

For translations and commentary on classical texts, including organ systems, five elements and philosophy, see the many works of Elisabeth Rochat de la Valleé published by Monkey Press and Station Hill Press.

Eight Extraordinary Vessels:

Chace, Charles, and Miki Shima. *An Exposition on the Eight Extraordinary Vessels: Acupuncture, Alchemy, and Herbal Medicine.* Eastland Press, 2010.

Farrell, Yvonne R. *Psycho-Emotional Pain and the Eight Extraordinary Vessels.* Singing Dragon, 2016.

Stones:

Franks, Leslie J. *Stone Medicine: A Chinese Medical Guide to Healing with Gems and Stones.* Inner Traditions/Bear, 2016.

REFERENCE BOOKS

Yuen, Jeffrey C. *Materia Medica of Essential Oils.* Lotus Center for Integrative Medicine, 2000.

Schnaubelt, Kurt. *Advanced Aromatherapy.* Healing Arts Press, 1998.

Schnaubelt, Kurt. *Healing Intelligence of Essential Oils.* Healing Arts Press, 2011.

Rochat de la Vallée, Elisabeth. *Wu Xing: The Five Elements In Chinese Classical Texts.* Monkey Press, 2012.

Divine Farmer's Materia Medica: A Translation of the Shen Nong Ben Cao Jing. Translated by Yang Shou-Zhong. Blue Poppy Press, 1998.

Chen, John K., and Tina Chen. *Chinese Medical Herbology and Pharmacology.* Art of Medicine Press, Inc, 2004.

Bensky, Ben, Steven Clavey, and Erich Stoeger. *Chinese Herbal Materia Medica,* 3rd edition. Eastland Press, Inc, 2004.

Ellis, Andrew, Nigel Wiseman, and Ken Boss. *Fundamentals of Chinese Acupuncture.* Paradigm Publications, 1991.

Deadman, Peter, and Mazin Al-Khafaji, with Kevin Baker. *A Manual of Acupuncture.* Journal of Chinese Medicine Publications, 1998.

Chinese Pinyin Name Cross Reference

Mandarin Pinyin	Chinese	Common Name	Pharmaceutical Botanical	Pg.
Ai Ye	艾葉	Mugwort Leaf	*Artemisiae argyi Folium*	65
An Shu Ye	桉 樹 葉	Eucalyptus Leaf	*Eucalyptus globulus, Eucalyptus radiata Folium*	67
Bai Dou Kou	白豆蔻	Round Cardamom	*Amomi rotundus Fructus*	69
Bai Ju Hua	白菊花	White Chrysanthemum	*Chrysanthemi morifolium Flos*	71
Bai Li Xiang	百里香	Thyme Leaf	*Thymus mongolicus Herba*	231
Bai Yu Lan Ye	百玉蘭葉	Magnolia Leaf	*Magnoliae denudata Folium*	76
Bai Zhi	白芷	Angelica Dahurica Root	*Angelicae dahuricae Radix*	78
Bai Zi Ren	柏子仁	Biota Seed, Arborvitae	*Platycladi orientalis Semen*	80
Bi Cheng Qie	華澄茄	Litsea Fruit	*Litseae cubeba Fructus*	82
Bo He	薄荷	Peppermint Leaf	*Menthae haplocalyx Herba*	85
Cang Zhu	蒼術	Atracylodes Root	*Atractylodis lancea Rhizoma*	87
Ce Bai Ye	側柏葉	Biota Leaf, Arborvitae	*Platycladi orientalis Cacumen*	90
Chai Hu	柴胡	Bupleurum Root	*Bupleuri chinensis Radix*	92
Chen Pi	陳皮	Aged Tangerine Peel	*Citri reticulatae Pericarpium*	95
Chuan Xiong	川芎	Sichuan Lovage Root	*Ligustici wallichii Rhizoma*	97
Dang Gui	當歸	Angelica sinensis Root	*Angelicae sinenis Radix*	100
Ding Xiang	丁香	Clove Bud	*Caryophylli aromaticus Flos*	103
Du Huo	獨活	Angelica Pubescentis Root	*Angelicae pubescentis Radix*	106
E Zhu	莪術	Curcuma Rhizome	*Curcumae zedoaria Rhizoma*	108
Fo Shou	佛手	Buddha's Hand Fruit, Finger Citron	*Citri sarcodactylis Fructus*	110
Gan Jiang	乾姜	Dried Ginger Root	*Zingiberis officinale Rhizoma*	112
Gou Qi Zi	枸杞子	Goji Berry	*Lycii barbarum Fructus*	114
Gui Zhi / Gui Ye	桂枝	Cinnamon Twig and Leaf	*Cinnamomi cassia Ramulus et Folium*	116
Hou Po	厚朴朴	Magnolia Bark	*Magnoliae officinalis Cortex*	119
Hu Lu Ba	葫蘆巴	Fenugreek Seed	*Trigonellae foenum-gracum Semen*	121
Hu Luo Bo Zi	胡蘿蔔子	Carrot Seed	*Daucus carota Semen*	124
Hu Po	琥珀	Amber	*Succinum*	126
Huang Qi	黄芪	Astralagalus, Milk Vetch Root	*Astragali membranaceus Radix*	128
Huang Qin	黄芩	Baical Skullcap Root	*Scutellaria baicalensis Radix*	233
Huo Xiang	藿香	Patchouli	*Pogostemonis cablin Herba*	130
Jiang Xiang	降香	Rosewood	*Dalbergiae odoriferae Lignum*	132
Jin Yin Hua	金銀花	Honeysuckle	*Lonicerae japonica Flos*	134
Jing Jie	荊芥	Nepeta	*Schizonepetae tenufolia Herba*	137
Ju Hua	菊花	Chrysanthemum	*Chrysanthemi morifolium Flos*	71
Lan Lian Hua	藍蓮花	Blue Lotus	*Nymphaea tetragona Flos*	233
Lian Qiao	連翹	Forsythia Fruit	*Forsythiae suspensa Fructus*	139
Long Nao	龍腦	Dragon Brain, Borneol	*Dryoblanops aromatica, Borneolum*	141

Mandarin Pinyin	Chinese	Common Name	Latin Pharmaceutical Botanical	Pg.
Ma Chi Xian	马齿苋	Purslane	*Portulaca oleracea Herba*	233
Man Jing Zi	蔓荆子	Vitex, Chastetree Berry	*Viticis agnus castus Fructus*	143
Mei Gui Hua	玫瑰花	Damascus Rose	*Rosa damacena Flos*	145
Mo Li Hua	茉莉花	Jasmine Flower	*Jasminum sambac Flos*	148
Mo Yao	沒藥	Myrrh	*Commiphorae myrrhae Resina*	151
Mu Xiang	木香	Saussurea, Costus Root	*Aucklandiae lappa Radix*	153
Nan Mu	楠木	Southern Chinese Cedarwood	*Cupressus funebris Lignum*	155
Qi Li Xiang	七里香	Orange Jessamine Flower	*Murraya paniculata Flos*	157
Qing Hao	青蒿	Sweet Wormwood	*Artemisiae annuae Herba*	159
Qing Hua Jiao	青花椒	Green Sichuan Pepper	*Zanthoxyli schinifolium Pericarpium*	161
Qing Pi	青皮	Green Mandarin Tangerine Peel	*Citri reticulatae viride Pericarpium*	163
Ren Shen	人參	Ginseng Root	*Panax ginseng Radix*	165
Rou Dou Kou	肉豆蔻	Nutmeg	*Myristicae fragrans Semen*	167
Rou Gui	肉桂	Cinnamon Bark	*Cinnamomi cassia Cortex*	169
Ru Xiang	乳香	Frankincense	*Boswellia carterii*	172
Ru Xiang	乳香	Sacred Frankincense, White Omani Frankincense	*Boswellia sacra*	175
She Chuang Zi	蛇床子	Cnidium Fruit	*Cnidium monnieri Fructus*	177
Shi Chang Pu	石菖蒲	Acorus, Sweet Flag Root	*Acori tatarinowii Rhizoma*	180
Shi Che Ju	矢车菊	Blue Cornflower	*Centaurea cyanus Flos*	233
Song Zhen	松針	Pine Needle	*Pinus tabuliformis*	182
Su He Xiang	蘇合香	Styrax	*Liquidamber orientalis*	184
Tan Xiang	檀香	Sandalwood	*Santali album/lanceolatum Lignum*	186
Wu Wei Zi	五味子	Schisandra Fruit Fruit	*Schisandra Fruite chinensis Fructus*	189
Wu Zhu Yu	吳茱萸	Evodia Fruit	*Evodiae rutaecarpa Fructus*	192
Xi Xin	細辛	Asarum, Wild Ginger	*Asari Herba*	195
Xiang Fu	香附	Nutgrass Rhizome, Cyperus	*Cyperi rotundus Rhizoma*	197
Xiao Hui Xiang	小茴香	Fennel Seed	*Foeniculi vulgare Fructus*	200
Xing Ren	苦杏仁	Bitter Almond, Apricot Kernel	*Pruni armeniacae Semen*	203
Xun Yi Cao	薰衣草	Lavender	*Lavendula augustifolia Flos*	205
Ye Ju Hua	野菊花	Wild Chrysanthemum	*Dendranthema indicum Flos*	208
Yi Yi Ren	薏苡仁	Coix Seed, Job's Tears	*Coicis lacryma-jobi Semen*	210
Yin Chen Hao	茵陳	Redstem Wormwood	*Artemisiae scopariae Herba*	212
Yuan Zhi	远志	Polygala Root	*Polygala tenuifolia Radix*	234
Yun Shan	雲杉	Black Spruce Needle	*Picea mariana*	214
Ze Xie	澤瀉	Water Plantain, Alisma	*Alismatis plantago Rhizoma*	216
Zhang Nao	樟腦	White Camphor	*Cinnamomom camphora*	218
Zhi Ke	枳壳	Bitter Orange Fruit	*Citrus aurantium Fructus*	220
Zhi Zi	梔子	Gardenia Fruit	*Gardeniae jasminoides Fructus*	222
Zhi Zi Hua	梔子花	Gardenia Flower	*Gardeniae jasminoides Flos*	224
Zi Su Ye	紫蘇葉	Perilla Leaf	*Perillae fructescens Folium*	226
Zi Su Zi	紫蘇子	Perilla Seed	*Perillae fructescens Fructus*	228

Latin Pharmaceutical / Botanical Cross Reference

Latin Pharmaceutical Botanical	Mandarin Pinyin	Chinese	Common Name	Pg.
Acori tatarinowii Rhizoma	Shi Chang Pu	石菖蒲	*Acorus, Sweet Flag Root*	180
Alismatis plantago Rhizoma	Ze Xie	澤瀉	*Water Plantain, Alisma*	216
Amomi rotundus Fructus	Bai Dou Kou	白豆蔻	*Round Cardamom*	69
Angelicae dahuricae Radix	Bai Zhi	白芷	*Angelica Dahurica Root*	78
Angelicae pubescentis Radix	Du Huo	獨活	*Angelica Pubescentis Root*	106
Angelicae sinenis Radix	Dang Gui	當歸	*Angelica Sinensis Root*	100
Artemisiae annuae Herba	Qing Hao	青蒿	*Sweet Wormwood*	159
Artemisiae argyi Folium	Ai Ye	艾葉	*Mugwort Leaf*	65
Artemisiae scopariae Herba	Yin Chen Hao	茵陳	*Redstem Wormwood*	212
Asari Herba	Xi Xin	細辛	*Asarum, Wild Ginger*	195
Astragali membranaceus Radix	Huang Qi	黃芪	*Astralagus, Milk Vetch Root*	128
Atractylodis lancea Rhizoma	Cang Zhu	蒼術	*Atracylodes Root*	87
Aucklandiae lappa Radix	Mu Xiang	木香	*Saussurea, Costus Root*	153
Boswellia carterii	Ru Xiang	乳香	*Frankincense*	172
Boswellia sacra	Ru Xiang	乳香	*"Sacred Frankincense, White Omani Frankincense"*	175
Bupleuri chinensis Radix	Chai Hu	柴胡	*Bupleurum Root*	92
Caryophylli aromaticus Flos	Ding Xiang	丁香	*Clove Bud*	103
Cupressus funebris Lignum	Nan Mu	楠木	*Southern Chinese Cedarwood*	155
Centaurea cynus Flos	Shi Che Ju	矢车菊	*Blue Cornflower*	233
Chrysanthemi morifolium Flos	Ju Hua, Bai Ju Hua	菊花, 白菊花	*White Chrysanthemum*	71
Dendranthema indicum Flos	Ye Ju Hua	野菊花	*Wild Chrysanthemum*	208
Cinnamomom camphora	Zhang Nao	樟腦	*White Camphor*	218
Citri reticulatae Pericarpium	Chen Pi	陳皮	*Aged Tangerine Peel*	95
Citri reticulatae viride Pericarpium	Qing Pi	青皮	*Green Mandarin Tangerine Peel*	163
Citri sarcodactylis Fructus	Fo Shou	佛手	*Buddha's Hand Fruit, Finger Citron*	110
Citri aurantium Fructus	Zhi Ke	枳壳	*Bitter Orange Fruit*	220
Cnidium monnieri Fructus	She Chuang Zi	蛇床子	*Cnidium Fruit*	177
Coicis lacryma-jobi Semen	Yi Yi Ren	薏苡仁	*Coix Seed, Job's Tears*	210
Commiphorae myrrhae Resina	Mo Yao	沒藥	*Myrrh*	151
Cinnamomi cassia Cortex	Rou Gui	肉桂	*Cinnamon Bark*	169
Cinnamomi cassia Ramulus et Folium	Gui Zhi / Gui Ye	桂枝	*Cinnamon Twig & Leaf*	116
Curcumae zedoaria Rhizoma	E Zhu	莪術	*Curcuma Rhizome*	108
Cyperi rotundus Rhizoma	Xiang Fu	香附	*Nutgrass Rhizome, Cyperus*	197
Dalbergiae odoriferae Lignum	Jiang Xiang	降香	*Rosewood*	132
Daucus carota Semen	Hu Luo Bo Zi	胡蘿蔔子	*Carrot Seed*	124
Dendrathema indicicum Flos	Ye Ju Hua	野菊花	*Wild Chrysanthemum*	208

Latin Pharmaceutical Botanical	Mandarin Pinyin	Chinese	Common Name	Pg.
Dryoblanops aromatica, Borneolum	Long Nao	龍腦	*Dragon Brain, Borneol*	141
Eucalyptus globulus/ radiata Folium	An Shu Ye	桉 樹 葉	*Eucalyptus Leaf*	67
Evodiae rutecarpa Fructus	Wu Zhu Yu	吳茱萸	*Evodia Fruit*	192
Foeniculi vulgare Fructus	Xiao Hui Xiang	小茴香	*Fennel Seed*	200
Forsythiae suspensa Fructus	Lian Qiao	連翹	*Forsythia Fruit*	139
Gardeniae jasminoides Flos	Zhi Zi Hua	梔子花	*Gardenia Flower*	224
Gardeniae jasminoides Fructus	Zhi Zi	梔子	*Gardenia Fruit*	222
Jasminum sambac Flos	Mo Li Hua	茉莉花	*Jasmine Flower*	148
Lavendula augustifolia Flos	Xun Yi Cao	薰衣草	*Lavender*	205
Ligustici wallichii Rhizoma	Chuan Xiong	川芎	*Sichuan Lovage Root*	97
Liquidamber orientalis	Su He Xiang	蘇合香	*Styrax*	185
Litseae cubeba Fructus	Bi Cheng Qie	蓽澄茄	*Litsea Fruit*	82
Lonicerae japonica Flos	Jin Yin Hua	金銀花	*Honeysuckle*	134
Lycii barbarum Fructus	Gou Qi Zi	枸杞子	*Goji Berry*	114
Magnoliae denudata Folium	Bai Yu Lan Ye	玉蘭葉	*Magnolia Leaf*	76
Magnoliae officinalis Cortex	Hou Po	厚朴朴	*Magnolia Bark*	119
Menthae haplocalyx Herba	Bo He	薄荷	*Peppermint Leaf*	85
Murraya paniculata Flos	Qi Li Xiang	七里香	*Orange Jessamine Flower*	157
Myristicae fragrans Semen	Rou Dou Kou	肉豆蔻	*Nutmeg*	167
Nyphaea tetragona Flos	Lan Lian Hua	藍蓮花	*Blue Lotus*	233
Panax ginseng Radix	Ren Shen	人參	*White Ginseng Root*	165
Perillae fructescens Folium	Zi Su Ye	紫蘇葉	*Perilla Leaf*	226
Perillae fructescens Fructus	Zi Su Zi	紫蘇子	*Perilla Seed*	228
Picea mariana	Yun Shan	雲杉	*Black Spruce Needle*	214
Pinus tabuliformis	Song Zhen	松針	*Pine Needle*	182
Platycladi orientalis Cacumen	Ce Bai Ye	側柏葉	*Biota Leaf, Arborvitae*	90
Platycladi orientalis Semen	Bai Zi Ren	柏子仁	*Biota Seed, Arborvitae*	80
Pogostemonis cablin Herba	Huo Xiang	藿香	*Patchouli*	130
Polygala tenuifolia Radix	Yuan Zhi	远志	*Polygala Root*	234
Portulaca oleracea Herba	Ma Chi Xian	马齿苋	*Purslane*	233
Pruni Armeniacae Semen	Xing Ren	苦杏仁	*Bitter Almond, Apricot Kernel*	203
Rosa damacena Flos	Mei Gui Hua	玫瑰	*Damascus Rose*	145
Santali album/lanceolatum Lignum	Tan Xiang	檀香	*Sandalwood*	186
Schisandrae chinensis Fructus	Wu Wei Zi	五味子	*Schisandra Fruit*	189
Schizonepetae tenufolia Herba	Jing Jie	荊芥	*Nepeta*	137
Scutellaria baicalensis Radix	Huang Qin	黄芩	*Baical Skullcap Root*	233
Succinum	Hu Po	琥珀	*Amber*	126
Thymus mongolicus Herba	Bai Li Xiang	百里香	*Thyme Leaf*	321
Trigonellae foenum-gracum Semen	Hu Lu Ba	葫蘆巴	*Fenugreek Seed*	121
Viticis agnus castus Fructus	Man Jing Zi	蔓荆子	*Vitex, Chastetree Berry*	143
Zanthoxyli schinifolium Pericarpium	Qing Hua Jiao	青花椒	*Green Sichuan Pepper*	161
Zingiberis officinale Rhizoma	Gan Jiang	乾姜	*Dried Ginger Root*	112

English Common Name Cross Reference

Common Name	Mandarin Pinyin	Chinese	Latin Pharmaceutical Botanical	Pg.
Acorus, Sweet Flag Root	Shi Chang Pu	石菖蒲	*Acori tatarinowii Rhizoma*	180
Amber	Hu Po	琥珀	*Succinum*	126
Angelica Dahurica Root	Bai Zhi	白芷	*Angelicae dahuricae Radix*	78
Angelica Pubescentis Root	Du Huo	獨活	*Angelicae pubescentis Radix*	106
Angelica Sinensis Root	Dang Gui	當歸	*Angelicae sinenis Radix*	100
Astralagus, Milk Vetch Root	Huang Qi	黄芪	*Astragali membranaceus Radix*	128
Atracylodes Root	Cang Zhu	蒼術	*Atractylodis lancea Rhizoma*	87
Biota Leaf, Arborvitae	Ce Bai Ye	側柏葉	*Platycladi orientalis Cacumen*	90
Biota Seed, Arborvitae	Bai Zi Ren	柏子仁	*Platycladi orientalis Semen*	80
Bitter Almond, Apricot Kernel	Xing Ren	苦杏仁	*Pruni Armeniacae Semen*	203
Bitter Orange Fruit	Zhi Ke	枳壳	*Citri aurantii Fructus*	220
Blue Cornflower	Shi Che Ju	矢车菊	*Centaurea cynus Flos*	233
Blue Lotus	Lan Lian Hua	蓝莲花	*Nyphaea tetragona Flos*	233
Borneol, Dragon Brain	Long Nao	龍腦	*Dryoblanops aromatica, Borneolum*	141
Buddha's Hand Fruit, Finger Citron	Fo Shou	佛手	*Citri sarcodactylis Fructus*	110
Bupleurum Root	Chai Hu	柴胡	*Bupleuri chinensis Radix*	92
Cardamom, Round	Bai Dou Kou	白豆蔻	*Amomi rotundus Fructus*	69
Carrot Seed	Hu Luo Bo Zi	胡蘿蔔子	*Daucus carota Semen*	124
Cedarwood, Southern Chinese	Nan Mu	楠木	*Cupressus funebris Lignum*	155
Chrysanthemum, White	Ju Hua, Bai Ju Hua	菊花, 白菊花	*Chrysanthemi morifolium Flos*	71
Chrysanthemum, Wild	Ye Ju Hua	野菊花	*Dendranthema indicum Flos*	208
Cinnamon Bark	Rou Gui	肉桂	*Cinnamomi cassia Cortex*	160
Cinnamon Twig and Leaf	Gui Zhi / Gui Ye	桂枝	*Cinnamomi cassia Ramulus et Folium*	116
Clove Bud	Ding Xiang	丁香	*Caryophylli aromaticus Flos*	103
Cnidium Fruit	She Chuang Zi	蛇床子	*Cnidium monnieri Fructus*	177
Coix Seed, Job's Tears	Yi Yi Ren	薏苡仁	*Coicis lacryma-jobi Semen*	210
Curcuma Rhizome	E Zhu	莪術	*Curcumae zedoaria Rhizoma*	108
Eucalyptus Leaf	An Shu Ye	桉 樹 葉	*Eucalyptus globulus, Eucalyptus radiata Folium*	67
Evodia Fruit	Wu Zhu Yu	吳茱萸	*Evodiae rutecarpa Fructus*	192
Fennel Seed	Xiao Hui Xiang	小茴香	*Foeniculi vulgare Fructus*	200
Fenugreek Seed	Hu Lu Ba	葫蘆巴	*Trigonellae foenum-gracum Semen*	121
Forsythia Fruit	Lian Qiao	連翹	*Forsythiae suspensa Fructus*	139
Frankincense	Ru Xiang	乳香	*Boswellia carterii*	172
Frankincense, Sacred	Ru Xiang	乳香	*Boswellia sacra*	175
Gardenia Flower	Zhi Zi Hua	梔子花	*Gardeniae jasminoides Flos*	224
Gardenia Fruit	Zhi Zi	梔子	*Gardeniae jasminoides Fructus*	222
Ginger Root, Dry	Gan Jiang	乾姜	*Zingiberis officinale Rhizoma*	112

Common Name	Mandarin Pinyin	Chinese	Latin Pharmaceutical Botanical	Pg.
Ginseng Root	Ren Shen	人參	*Panax ginseng Radix*	165
Goji Berry	Gou Qi Zi	枸杞子	*Lycii barbarum Fructus*	114
Green Sichuan Pepper	Qing Hua Jiao	青花椒	*Zanthoxyli schinifolium Pericarpium*	161
Honeysuckle	Jin Yin Hua	金銀花	*Lonicerae japonica Flos*	134
Jasmine Flower	Mo Li Hua	茉莉花	*Jasminum sambac Flos*	148
Lavender	Xun Yi Cao	薰衣草	*Lavendula augustifolia Flos*	205
Litsea Fruit	Bi Cheng Qie	華澄茄	*Litseae cubeba Fructus*	82
Lovage Root	Chuan Xiong	川芎	*Ligustici wallichii Rhizoma*	97
Magnolia Bark	Hou Po	厚朴朴	*Magnoliae officinalis Cortex*	119
Magnolia Leaf	Bai Yu Lan Ye	玉蘭葉	*Magnoliae denudata Folium*	76
Mugwort Leaf	Ai Ye	艾葉	*Artemisiae argyi Folium*	65
Myrrh	Mo Yao	沒藥	*Commiphorae myrrhae Resina*	151
Nepeta	Jing Jie	荊芥	*Schizonepetae tenufolia Herba*	137
Nutgrass Rhizome, Cyperus	Xiang Fu	香附	*Cyperi rotundus Rhizoma*	197
Nutmeg	Rou Dou Kou	肉豆蔻	*Myristicae fragrans Semen*	167
Orange Jessamine Flower	Qi Li Xiang	七里香	*Murraya paniculata Flos*	157
Patchouli	Huo Xiang	藿香	*Pogostemonis cablin Herba*	130
Peppermint Leaf	Bo He	薄荷	*Menthae haplocalyx Herba*	85
Perilla Leaf	Zi Su Ye	紫蘇葉	*Perillae fructescens Folium*	226
Perilla Seed	Zi Su Zi	紫蘇子	*Perillae fructescens Fructus*	228
Pine Needle	Song Zhen	松針	*Pinus tabuliformis*	182
Polygala Root	Yuan Zhi	远志	*Polygala tenuifolia Radix*	234
Purslane	Ma Chi Xian	马齿苋	*Portulaca oleracea Herba*	233
Rose, Damascus	Mei Gui Hua	玫瑰	*Rosa damacena Flos*	145
Rosewood	Jiang Xiang	降香	*Dalbergiae Odoriferae Lignum*	132
Sandalwood	Tan Xiang	檀香	*Santali album/lanceolatum Lignum*	186
Saussurea, Costus Root	Mu Xiang	木香	*Aucklandiae lappa Radix*	153
Schisandra Fruit	Wu Wei Zi	五味子	*Schisandrae chinensis Fructus*	189
Skullcap Root	Huang Qin	黄芩	*Scutellaria baicalensis Radix*	233
Spruce Needle, Black	Yun Shan	雲杉	*Picea mariana*	214
Styrax	Su He Xiang	蘇合香	*Liquidamber orientalis*	184
Tangerine Peel, Aged	Chen Pi	陳皮	*Citri reticulatae Pericarpium*	95
Tangerine Peel, Green Mandarin	Qing Pi	青皮	*Citri reticulatae viride Pericarpium*	163
Thyme Leaf	Bai Li Xiang	百里香	*Thymus mongolicus Herba*	231
Vitex, Chastetree Berry	Man Jing Zi	蔓荊子	*Viticis agnus castus Fructus*	143
Water Plantain, Alisma	Ze Xie	澤瀉	*Alismatis plantago Rhizoma*	216
White Camphor	Zhang Nao	樟腦	*Cinnamomom camphora*	218
Wild Ginger, Asarum	Xi Xin	細辛	*Asari Herba*	195
Wormwood, Redstem	Yin Chen Hao	茵陳	*Artemisiae scopariae Herba*	212
Wormwood, Sweet	Qing Hao	青蒿	*Artemisiae annuae Herba*	159

Pharmacological Actions

This index lists known and studied pharmacological actions which appear in the pharmacological actions section of the materia medica entry for each oil.

Pharmaceutical Action	Pinyin	Common Name
Adaptogenic	Bai Zi Ren	Biota Seed
	E Zhu	Curcuma zedoaria Rhizome
	Gou Qi Zi	Goji Berry
	Huang Qi	Astragalus Root
	Ren Shen	White Ginseng
	Wu Wei Zi	Schisandra Fruit
Analgesic	Ai Ye	Mugwort
	Bai Yu Lan Ye	Magnolia Leaf
	Bai Zhi	Angelica dahurica Root
	Bi Cheng Qie	Litsea Fruit
	Bo He	Peppermint
	Chai Hu	Bupleurum Root
	Chuan Xiong	Sichuan Lovage Root
	Dang Gui	Angelica sinensis Root
	Ding Xiang	Clove
	Du Huo	Angelica pubescentis Root
	Gan Jiang	Dry Ginger
	Gui Zhi/Gui Ye	Cinnamon Twig and Leaf
	Hu Lu Ba	Fenugreek Seed
	Hu Po	Amber
	Jiang Xiang	Rosewood
	Lian Qiao	Forsythia
	Long Nao	Borneol
	Man Jing Zi	Vitex
	Mo Li Hua	Jasmine
	Mo Yao	Myrhh
	Nan Mu	Southern Chinese Cedarwood
	Qi Li Xiang	Orange Jessamine
	Qing Hua Jiao	Green Sichuan Pepper
	Rou Dou Kou	Nutmeg
	Ru Xiang	Frankincense
	She Chuang Zi	Cnidium Fruit
	Song Zhen	Pine Needle
	Su He Xiang	Styrax
	Tang Xiang	Sandalwood
	Wu Zhu Yu	Evodia Fruit
	Xi Xin	Asarum

Pharmaceutical Action	Pinyin	Common Name
	Xiang Fu	Cyperus
	Xiao Hui Xiang	Fennel Seed
	Xun Yi Cao	Lavender
	Yi Yi Ren	Coix Seed
	Yun Shan	Black Spruce Needle
	Ze Xie	Alisma
	Zhi Zi	Gardenia Fruit
	Zi Su Ye	Perilla Leaf
Anesthetic	Qing Hua Jiao	Green Sichuan Pepper
	Xi Xin	Asarum
Anodyne	Bai Zhi	Angelica dahurica Root
Antacid	Fo Shou	Buddha's Hand Fruit
	Wu Zhu Yu	Evodia Fruit
	Zhi Ke	Bitter Orange Fruit
	Zhi Zi	Gardenia Fruit
Anti-aging	Ding Xiang	Clove
	Gan Jiang	Dry Ginger
	Gou Qi Zi	Goji Berry
	Ren Shen	White Ginseng
Anti-allergic	Bai Yu Lan Ye	Magnolia Leaf
	Cang Zhu	Atroctlyodes Rhizome
	Zi Su Ye	Perilla Leaf
Anti-Alzheimers	Shi Chang Pu	Acorus
Anti-arrythmia	Dang Gui	Angelica sinensis Root
Anti-asthmatic	Ai Ye	Mugwort
	Bi Cheng Qie	Litsea Fruit
	Chen Pi	Aged Tangerine Peel
	Xing Ren	Apricot Kernel
	Zi Su Ye	Perilla Leaf
	Zi Su Zi	Perilla Seed
Anti-epidemic	Zhang Nao	White Camphor
Anti-epileptic	Su He Xiang	Styrax
Anti-infectious	Ding Xiang	Clove
	Gui Zhi/Gui Ye	Cinnamon Twig and Leaf
	Huo Xiang	Patchouli
	Rou Gui	Cinnamon Bark
Anti-inflammatory	An Shu Ye	Eucalyptus Leaf
	Bai Yu Lan Ye	Magnolia Leaf
	Bai Zhi	Angelica dahurica Root
	Bi Cheng Qie	Litsea Fruit

Pharmaceutical Action	Pinyin	Common Name
	Bo He	Peppermint
	Cang Zhu	Atroctlyodes Rhizome
	Ce Bai Ye	Biota Leaf
	Chai Hu	Bupleurum Root
	Dang Gui	Angelica sinensis Root
	Ding Xiang	Clove
	Du Huo	Angelica pubescentis Root
	Gan Jiang	Dry Ginger
	Gui Zhi/Gui Ye	Cinnamon Twig and Leaf
	Hu Luo Bo Zi	Carrot Seed
	Huang Qi	Astragalus Root
	Huo Xiang	Patchouli
	Jiang Xiang	Rosewood
	Jin Yin Hua	Honeysuckle
	Ju Hua	Chrysanthemum
	Long Nao	Borneol
	Man Jing Zi	Vitex
	Mo Li Hua	Jasmine
	Mo Yao	Myrhh
	Mu Xiang	Saussurea
	Nan Mu	Southern Chinese Cedarwood
	Qi Li Xiang	Orange Jessamine
	Rou Dou Kou	Nutmeg
	Rou Gui	Cinnamon Bark
	Ru Xiang	Frankincense
	She Chuang Zi	Cnidium Fruit
	Tan Xiang	Sandalwood
	Wu Zhu Yu	Evodia Fruit
	Xiang Fu	Cyperus
	Ye Ju Hua	Wild Chrysanthemum
	Yi Yi Ren	Coix Seed
	Yin Chen Hao	Redstem Wormwood
	Yun Shan	Black Spruce Needle
	Ze Xie	Alisma
	Zi Su Ye	Perilla Leaf
Antibacterial	An Shu Ye	Eucalyptus Leaf
	Bai Dou Kou	Round Cardamom
	Bi Cheng Qie	Litsea Fruit
	Ce Bai Ye	Biota Leaf
	Chen Pi	Aged Tangerine Peel

Pharmaceutical Action	Pinyin	Common Name
	Hu Lu Ba	Fenugreek Seed
	Huo Xiang	Patchouli
	Ju Hua	Chrysanthemum
	Lian Qiao	Forsythia
	Long Nao	Borneol
	Nan Mu	Southern Chinese Cedarwood
	Qing Hao	Sweet Wormwood
	Song Zhen	Pine Needle
	Xiao Hui Xiang	Fennel Seed
	Zi Su Ye	Perilla Leaf
	Zi Su Zi	Perilla Seed
Antibiotic	Ai Ye	Mugwort
	Bai Zhi	Angelica dahurica Root
	Cang Zhu	Atroctlyodes Rhizome
	Chai Hu	Bupleurum Root
	Chai Hu	Bupleurum Root
	Dang Gui	Angelica sinensis Root
	Du Huo	Angelica pubescentis Root
	Hou Po	Magnolia Bark
	Jing Jie	Schizonepeta
	Man Jing Zi	Vitex
	Mu Xiang	Saussurea
	Qing Hua Jiao	Green Sichuan Pepper
	Rou Dou Kou	Nutmeg
	Wu Wei Zi	Schisandra Fruit
	Xiang Fu	Cyperus
	Yin Chen Hao	Redstem Wormwood
	Zhi Zi	Gardenia Fruit
Anticancer	Bi Cheng Qie	Litsea Fruit
	Ding Xiang	Clove
	E Zhu	Curcuma zedoaria Rhizome
	Huang Qi	Astragalus Root
	Jin Yin Hua	Honeysuckle
	Rou Gui	Cinnamon Bark
	Ru Xiang (B. carterii)	Frankincense
	She Chuang Zi	Cnidium Fruit
	Xing Ren	Apricot Kernel
Anti-angiogenesis	Chuan Xiong	Sichuan Lovage Root
Chemopreventative	Ru Xiang (B. sacra)	Frankincense
Chemoprotective, Antiproliferative	Yi Yi Ren	Coix Seed

Pharmaceutical Action	Pinyin	Common Name
Anticoagulant	Chuan Xiong	Sichuan Lovage Root
	E Zhu	Curcuma zedoaria Rhizome
	Hou Po	Magnolia Bark
	Ru Xiang	Frankincense
Anticonvulsant	Shi Chang Pu	Acorus
	Su He Xiang	Styrax
Antidepressant	Hou Po	Magnolia Bark
	Mei Gui Hua	Rose
	Mu Xiang	Saussurea
	Shi Chang Pu	Acorus
	Tan Xiang	Sandalwood
	Xiang Fu	Cyperus
	Jiang Xiang	Rosewood
	Zhi Zi Hua	Gardenia Flower
Antidiabetic	Cang Zhu	Atroctlyodes Rhizome
	Fo Shou	Buddha's Hand Fruit
	Gou Qi Zi	Goji Berry
	Hu Lu Ba	Fenugreek Seed
	Huang Qi	Astragalus Root
	Ren Shen	White Ginseng
	Rou Gui	Cinnamon Bark
Antidiabetic (Insulin regulating)	Bai Zi Ren	Biota Seed
	Ce Bai Ye	Biota Leaf
Antidysenteric	Bi Cheng Qie	Litsea Fruit
Antiemetic	Bai Dou Kou	Round Cardamom
	Gan Jiang	Dry Ginger
	Zi Su Ye	Perilla Leaf
Antifibrotic	Ru Xiang	Frankincense
Antifungal	An Shu Ye	Eucalyptus Leaf
	Bai Yu Lan Ye	Magnolia Leaf
	Bai Zhi	Angelica dahurica Root
	Bi Cheng Qie	Litsea Fruit
	Ce Bai Ye	Biota Leaf
	Ding Xiang	Clove
	Hou Po	Magnolia Bark
	Hu Lu Ba	Fenugreek Seed
	Hu Luo Bo Zi	Carrot Seed
	Huo Xiang	Patchouli
	Long Nao	Borneol
	Mo Yao	Myrhh

Pharmaceutical Action	Pinyin	Common Name
	Mu Xiang	Saussurea
	Nan Mu	Southern Chinese Cedarwood
	Rou Dou Kou	Nutmeg
	Rou Gui	Cinnamon Bark
	She Chuang Zi	Cnidium Fruit
	Song Zhen	Pine Needle
	Su He Xiang	Styrax
	Wu Zhu Yu	Evodia Fruit
	Xiao Hui Xiang	Fennel Seed
	Yin Chen Hao	Redstem Wormwood
	Zhang Nao	White Camphor
	Zhi Zi Hua	Gardenia Flower
Antiglaucoma	Gou Qi Zi	Goji Berry
Antihistamine	Chen Pi	Aged Tangerine Peel
	Long Nao	Borneol
Antihyperalgesic	Mo Li Hua	Jasmine
Antihyperlipidemic	Mo Yao	Myrhh
	Rou Gui	Cinnamon Bark
	Yin Chen Hao	Redstem Wormwood
	Ze Xie	Alisma
	Zhi Ke	Bitter Orange Fruit
	Zhi Zi	Gardenia Fruit
Antihypertensive	Hou Po	Magnolia Bark
	Ju Hua	Chrysanthemum
	Ye Ju Hua	Wild Chrysanthemum
	Yin Chen Hao	Redstem Wormwood
	Ze Xie	Alisma
	Zhi Zi	Gardenia Fruit
	Zhi Zi Hua	Gardenia Flower
Antimalarial	Qing Hao	Sweet Wormwood
Antimicrobial	An Shu Ye	Eucalyptus Leaf
	Bai Zhi	Angelica dahurica Root
	Bi Cheng Qie	Litsea Fruit
	Chen Pi	Aged Tangerine Peel
	E Zhu	Curcuma zedoaria Rhizome
	Fo Shou	Buddha's Hand Fruit
Antimicrobial (and Antipathogenic)	Jin Yin Hua	Honeysuckle
	Man Jing Zi	Vitex
	Mo Li Hua	Jasmine

Pharmaceutical Action	Pinyin	Common Name
	Qing Pi	Green Mandarin Tangerine Peel
	Rou Gui	Cinnamon Bark
	Tan Xiang	Sandalwood
	Wu Zhu Yu	Evodia Fruit
	Xing Ren	Apricot Kernel
	Ye Ju Hua	Wild Chrysanthemum
	Yun Shan	Black Spruce Needle
	Zhang Nao	White Camphor
	Zhi Ke	Bitter Orange Fruit
	Zhi Zi Hua	Gardenia Flower
	Zi Su Ye	Perilla Leaf
Antinociceptive	Bai Yu Lan Ye	Magnolia Leaf
	Mo Li Hua	Jasmine
	Qi Li Xiang	Orange Jessamine
	Ru Xiang	Frankincense
Antioxidant	Bai Zi Ren	Biota Seed
	Bi Cheng Qie	Litsea Fruit
	Ce Bai Ye	Biota Leaf
	Chen Pi	Aged Tangerine Peel
	Ding Xiang	Clove
	Gan Jiang	Dry Ginger
	Gou Qi Zi	Goji Berry
	Hu Luo Bo Zi	Carrot Seed
	Mu Xiang	Saussurea
	Qi Li Xiang	Orange Jessamine
	Ren Shen	White Ginseng
	Rou Dou Kou	Nutmeg
	Rou Gui	Cinnamon Bark
	Wu Zhu Yu	Evodia Fruit
	Xi Xin	Asarum
	Xing Ren	Apricot Kernel
	Yun Shan	Black Spruce Needle
	Zhi Zi	Gardenia Fruit
	Zhi Zi Hua	Gardenia Flower
Antiparasitic	Bi Cheng Qie	Litsea Fruit
	Cang Zhu	Atroctlyodes Rhizome
	Ding Xiang	Clove
	Qing Hao	Sweet Wormwood
	Qing Hua Jiao	Green Sichuan Pepper
	Rou Dou Kou	Nutmeg

Pharmaceutical Action	Pinyin	Common Name
	Su He Xiang	Styrax
	Xiao Hui Xiang	Fennel Seed
	Zhang Nao	White Camphor
Antiplatelet	Hou Po	Magnolia Bark
	Chuan Xiong	Sichuan Lovage Root
	Dang Gui	Angelica sinensis Root
	E Zhu	Curcuma zedoaria Rhizome
	Jiang Xiang	Rosewood
	Su He Xiang	Styrax
Antipruritic	Bo He	Peppermint
	Jing Jie	Schizonepeta
	She Chuang Zi	Cnidium Fruit
Antipyretic	An Shu Ye	Eucalyptus Leaf
	Bai Zhi	Angelica dahurica Root
	Bo He	Peppermint
	Ce Bai Ye	Biota Leaf
	Chai Hu	Bupleurum Root
	Jin Yin Hua	Honeysuckle
	Jing Jie	Schizonepeta
	Ju Hua	Chrysanthemum
	Lian Qiao	Forsythia
	Man Jing Zi	Vitex
	Qing Hao	Sweet Wormwood
	Xiang Fu	Cyperus
	Ye Ju Hua	Wild Chrysanthemum
	Yin Chen Hao	Redstem Wormwood
	Zhi Zi	Gardenia Fruit
	Zhi Zi Hua	Gardenia Flower
Antiseizure	Long Nao	Borneol
	Shi Chang Pu	Acorus
	Su He Xiang	Styrax
Antiseptic	Bai Zhi	Angelica dahurica Root
	Bi Cheng Qie	Litsea Fruit
	Bo He	Peppermint
	Ju Hua	Chrysanthemum
	Qing Pi	Green Mandarin Tangerine Peel
	Xiao Hui Xiang	Fennel Seed
Antispasmodic	Bai Dou Kou	Round Cardamom
	Bai Zhi	Angelica dahurica Root
	Bi Cheng Qie	Litsea Fruit

Pharmaceutical Action	Pinyin	Common Name
	Bo He	Peppermint
	Cang Zhu	Atroctlyodes Rhizome
	Chuan Xiong	Sichuan Lovage Root
	Dang Gui	Angelica sinensis Root
	Ding Xiang	Clove
	Du Huo	Angelica pubescentis Root
	Jing Jie	Schizonepeta
	Nan Mu	Southern Chinese Cedarwood
	Ru Xiang	Frankincense
	Xiao Hui Xiang	Fennel Seed
	Xun Yi Cao	Lavender
Antitoxin	Zhang Nao	White Camphor
Antitumor	Ce Bai Ye	Biota Leaf
	E Zhu	Curcuma zedoaria Rhizome
	Ru Xiang	Frankincense
	She Chuang Zi	Cnidium Fruit
	Yi Yi Ren	Coix Seed
Antitussive	Ai Ye	Mugwort
	An Shu Ye	Eucalyptus Leaf
	Bai Zi Ren	Biota Seed
	Chen Pi	Aged Tangerine Peel
	Gou Qi Zi	Goji Berry
	Hou Po	Magnolia Bark
	Jiang Xiang	Rosewood
	Song Zhen	Pine Needle
	Xing Ren	Apricot Kernel
	Yun Shan	Black Spruce Needle
	Zi Su Ye	Perilla Leaf
	Zi Su Zi	Perilla Seed
Antiulcer	Cang Zhu	Atroctlyodes Rhizome
	Mu Xiang	Saussurea
	Ren Shen	White Ginseng
	Ru Xiang	Frankincense
Antiviral	Bai Dou Kou	Round Cardamom
	Cang Zhu	Atroctlyodes Rhizome
	Chai Hu	Bupleurum Root
	Chen Pi	Aged Tangerine Peel
	Ding Xiang	Clove
	Hu Luo Bo Zi	Carrot Seed
	Huang Qi	Astragalus Root

Pharmaceutical Action	Pinyin	Common Name
	Huo Xiang	Patchouli
	Lian Qiao	Forsythia
	Long Nao	Borneol
	Mo Yao	Myrhh
	Nan Mu	Southern Chinese Cedarwood
	Qing Hao	Sweet Wormwood
	Song Zhen	Pine Needle
	Wu Zhu Yu	Evodia Fruit
	Xi Xin	Asarum
	Xiao Hui Xiang	Fennel Seed
	Yin Chen Hao	Redstem Wormwood
	Zi Su Ye	Perilla Leaf
Anxiolytic	Bai Zi Ren	Biota Seed
	Gou Qi Zi	Goji Berry
	Jiang Xiang	Rosewood
	Jin Yin Hua	Honeysuckle
	Mei Gui Hua	Rose
	Mo Li Hua	Jasmine
	Mu Xiang	Saussurea
	Tan Xiang	Sandalwood
	Zhi Zi Hua	Gardenia Flower
Astringent	Ce Bai Ye	Biota Leaf
	Fo Shou	Buddha's Hand Fruit
	Qing Pi	Green Mandarin Tangerine Peel
	Rou Dou Kou	Nutmeg
	Wu Wei Zi	Schisandra Fruit
Bacteriostatic	Tan Xiang	Sandalwood
Cardiotonic	Wu Wei Zi	Schisandra Fruit
	Ren Shen	Panax Ginseng
Cardiovascular relaxant	Xiang Fu	Cyperus
Cardiovascular tonic	Rou Gui	Cinnamon Bark
Carminative	Bai Zhi	Angelica dahurica Root
	Bi Cheng Qie	Litsea Fruit
	Bo He	Peppermint
	Ding Xiang	Clove
	Gan Jiang	Dry Ginger
Cholagogue	Chai Hu	Bupleurum Root
	Mu Xiang	Saussurea
	Xiao Hui Xiang	Fennel Seed
Circulatory	Chuan Xiong	Sichuan Lovage Root
	Dang Gui	Angelica sinensis Root

Pharmaceutical Action	Pinyin	Common Name
	Du Huo	Angelica pubescentis Root
	Gui Zhi/Gui Ye	Cinnamon Twig and Leaf
	Hu Po	Amber
CNS modulatory	Hu Po	Amber
	Mei Gui Hua	Rose
	Shi Chang Pu	Acorus
	Wu Wei Zi	Schisandra Fruit
	Wu Zhu Yu	Evodia Fruit
CNS protective	Mo Li Hua	Jasmine
Cognitive	Ling Zhi	Reishi
	Ren Shen	White Ginseng
	Shi Chang Pu	Acorus
	Wu Wei Zi	Schisandra Fruit
COX-2 inhibitor	Gui Zhi/Gui Ye	Cinnamon Twig and Leaf
	Tan Xiang	Sandalwood
COX-2 regulating	Yi Yi Ren	Coix Seed
Decongestant	An Shu Ye	Eucalyptus Leaf
	Bai Dou Kou	Round Cardamom
	Bai Yu Lan Ye	Magnolia Leaf
	Song Zhen	Pine Needle
	Xi Xin	Asarum
	Zhi Ke	Bitter Orange Fruit
Diaphoretic	Bai Zhi	Angelica dahurica Root
	Bo He	Peppermint
	Jing Jie	Schizonepeta
Digestive	Bai Dou Kou	Round Cardamom
	Fo Shou	Buddha's Hand Fruit
	Huo Xiang	Patchouli
	Zhi Ke	Bitter Orange Fruit
	Zi Su Ye	Perilla Leaf
Disinfectant	Du Huo	Angelica pubescentis Root
	Song Zhen	Pine Needle
Diuretic	An Shu Ye	Eucalyptus Leaf
	Bai Zhi	Angelica dahurica Root
	Bi Cheng Qie	Litsea Fruit
	Cang Zhu	Atroctlyodes Rhizome
	Hu Lu Ba	Fenugreek Seed
	Hu Po	Amber
	Xiao Hui Xiang	Fennel Seed
	Ze Xie	Alisma

Pharmaceutical Action	Pinyin	Common Name
Emmenagogue	Gui Zhi/Gui Ye	Cinnamon Twig and Leaf
	Hu Lu Ba	Fenugreek Seed
	Hu Po	Amber
	Xiao Hui Xiang	Fennel Seed
Estrogenic	Hu Lu Ba	Fenugreek Seed
	Xiao Hui Xiang	Fennel Seed
Expectorant	Ai Ye	Mugwort
	Bi Cheng Qie	Litsea Fruit
	Gan Jiang	Dry Ginger
	Gou Qi Zi	Goji Berry
	Mo Yao	Myrhh
	Qing Hao	Sweet Wormwood
	Qing Pi	Green Mandarin Tangerine Peel
	Zi Su Zi	Perilla Seed
Galactagogue	Hu Lu Ba	Fenugreek Seed
	Mo Li Hua	Jasmine
Gastrointestinal relaxant	Cang Zhu	Atroctlyodes Rhizome
	Hou Po	Magnolia Bark
Gastrointestinal stimulant	Ai Ye	Mugwort
Hematopoietic	Chuan Xiong	Sichuan Lovage Root
	Mei Gui Hua	Rose
Hematopoietic (Red and white blood cells)	Gou Qi Zi	Goji Berry
Hemostatic	Ai Ye	Mugwort
	Bai Zi Ren	Biota Seed
	Ce Bai Ye	Biota Leaf
	Jiang Xiang	Rosewood
	Bai Zi Ren	Biota Seed
	Ce Bai Ye	Biota Leaf
	Hu Luo Bo Zi	Carrot Seed
Hepatoprotective	Chai Hu	Bupleurum Root
	Dang Gui	Angelica sinensis Root
	Hu Luo Bo Zi	Carrot Seed
	Wu Wei Zi	Schisandra Fruit
	Yin Chen Hao	Redstem Wormwood
	Ze Xie	Alisma
	Zhi Zi	Gardenia Fruit
Hepatoregenerative	Bo He	Peppermint
Hormone modulatory	Ai Ye	Mugwort

Pharmaceutical Action	Pinyin	Common Name
	Man Jing Zi	Vitex
	Mei Gui Hua	Rose
	Mo Li Hua	Jasmine
	Mo Yao	Myrhh
	Yun Shan	Black Spruce Needle
	Ze Xie	Alisma
Hydrating	Gou Qi Zi	Goji Berry
	Mei Gui Hua	Rose
	Mo Li Hua	Jasmine
	Qing Hao	Sweet Wormwood
Hypoglycemic	Hu Lu Ba	Fenugreek Seed
Hypotensive	Jiang Xiang	Rosewood
	Nan Mu	Southern Chinese Cedarwood
	Ren Shen	White Ginseng
	Xun Yi Cao	Lavender
Immunomodulatory	Chai Hu	Bupleurum Root
	Gou Qi Zi	Goji Berry
	She Chuang Zi	Cnidium Fruit
	Wu Wei Zi	Schisandra Fruit
	Ze Xie	Alisma
	Zi Su Ye	Perilla Leaf
Immunostimulant	Dang Gui	Angelica sinensis Root
	Ding Xiang	Clove
	Huang Qi	Astragalus Root
	Qi Li Xiang	Orange Jessamine
	Ren Shen	White Ginseng
	Ru Xiang	Frankincense
	Yi Yi Ren	Coix Seed
Insect repellant	Nan Mu	Southern Chinese Cedarwood
	Xun Yi Cao	Lavender
	Ai Ye	Mugwort
	Bi Cheng Qie	Litsea Fruit
Insecticide	Bi Cheng Qie	Litsea Fruit
	Long Nao	Borneol
	Qing Hao	Sweet Wormwood
	Xiao Hui Xiang	Fennel Seed
Metabolic	Gou Qi Zi	Goji Berry
	Huang Qi	Astragalus Root
	Wu Wei Zi	Schisandra Fruit

Pharmaceutical Action	Pinyin	Common Name
Mucolytic	An Shu Ye	Eucalyptus Leaf
	Bai Yu Lan Ye	Magnolia Leaf
	Chen Pi	Aged Tangerine Peel
	Fo Shou	Buddha's Hand Fruit
	Gan Jiang	Dry Ginger
	Hou Po	Magnolia Bark
	Lian Qiao	Forsythia
	Nan Mu	Southern Chinese Cedarwood
	Qing Pi	Green Mandarin Tangerine Peel
	Ru Xiang	Frankincense
	Song Zhen	Pine Needle
	Su He Xiang	Styrax
	Xi Xin	Asarum
	Xing Ren	Apricot Kernel
	Yin Chen Hao	Redstem Wormwood
	Yun Shan	Black Spruce Needle
	Zhang Nao	White Camphor
	Zi Su Ye	Perilla Leaf
	Zi Su Zi	Perilla Seed
Nervine	Bai Yu Lan Ye	Magnolia Leaf
	Bai Zi Ren	Biota Seed
	Cang Zhu	Atroctlyodes Rhizome
	Huo Xiang	Patchouli
	Jiang Xiang	Rosewood
	Ju Hua	Chrysanthemum
	Lian Qiao	Forsythia
	Mei Gui Hua	Rose
	Nan Mu	Southern Chinese Cedarwood
	Qi Li Xiang	Orange Jessamine
	Song Zhen	Pine Needle
	Wu Zhu Yu	Evodia Fruit
	Xun Yi Cao	Lavender
Neuroprotective	Du Huo	Angelica pubescentis Root
	Gou Qi Zi	Goji Berry
	Hou Po	Magnolia Bark
	Hu Lu Ba	Fenugreek Seed
	Mu Xiang	Saussurea
Neuroregenerative	Du Huo	Angelica pubescentis Root
Neurotonic	Long Nao	Borneol
	Rou Gui	Cinnamon Bark
Osteopromotive	Bi Cheng Qie	Litsea Fruit

Pharmaceutical Action	Pinyin	Common Name
	Ce Bai Ye	Biota Leaf
	She Chuang Zi	Cnidium Fruit
Platelet Agonist	Ce Bai Ye	Biota Leaf
Prebiotic	Jin Yin Hua	Honeysuckle
Preventative	Ding Xiang	Clove
	Gui Zhi/Gui Ye	Cinnamon Twig and Leaf
	Hu Lu Ba	Fenugreek Seed
	Huo Xiang	Patchouli
	Qi Li Xiang	Orange Jessamine
	Rou Gui	Cinnamon Bark
	Zi Su Ye	Perilla Leaf
Pro-libido	She Chuang Zi	Cnidium Fruit
Psychedelic	Rou Dou Kou	Nutmeg
	Shi Chang Pu	Acorus
	Wu Zhu Yu	Evodia Fruit
Radioprotective	Chuan Xiong	Sichuan Lovage Root
	Ren Shen	White Ginseng
Respiratory	An Shu Ye	Eucalyptus Leaf
	Gui Zhi/Gui Ye	Cinnamon Twig and Leaf
	Hou Po	Magnolia Bark
	Song Zhen	Pine Needle
	Xi Xin	Asarum
	Yun Shan	Black Spruce Needle
Respiratory (Bronchodilating)	Jing Jie	Schizonepeta
Restorative	Du Huo	Angelica pubescentis Root
	Gou Qi Zi	Goji Berry
	Huang Qi	Astragalus Root
	Ren Shen	White Ginseng
Sedative	Bai Zi Ren	Biota Seed
	Bo He	Peppermint
	Chai Hu	Bupleurum Root
	Chuan Xiong	Sichuan Lovage Root
	Hou Po	Magnolia Bark
	Hu Po	Amber
	Man Jing Zi	Vitex
	Mo Li Hua	Jasmine
	Qi Li Xiang	Orange Jessamine
	Ru Xiang	Frankincense
	Shi Chang Pu	Acorus
	Tan Xiang	Sandalwood
	Xiang Fu	Cyperus

Pharmaceutical Action	Pinyin	Common Name
	Zhi Zi	Gardenia Fruit
	Zhi Zi Hua	Gardenia Flower
Smooth Muscle Relaxant	Chen Pi	Aged Tangerine Peel
	Chuan Xiong	Sichuan Lovage Root
	Dang Gui	Angelica sinensis Root
	Mu Xiang	Saussurea
	Zhi Ke	Bitter Orange Fruit
Steroidal	Yi Yi Ren	Coix Seed
	Ze Xie	Alisma
Stimulant	Bai Zhi	Angelica dahurica Root
	Bi Cheng Qie	Litsea Fruit
	Su He Xiang	Styrax
	Zhang Nao	White Camphor
Stomachic	Bai Dou Kou (antireflux)	Round Cardamom
	Bi Cheng Qie	Litsea Fruit
	Ce Bai Ye	Biota Leaf
	Gan Jiang	Dry Ginger
	Huo Xiang	Patchouli
	Rou Dou Kou	Nutmeg
	Xiao Hui Xiang	Fennel Seed
Uterine relaxant	Xiang Fu	Cyperus
Vascular decongestant	Huo Xiang	Patchouli
Vasodilator	Ju Hua	Chrysanthemum
	Su He Xiang	Styrax
	Wu Wei Zi	Schisandra Fruit
Vulnerary	Bai Zi Ren	Biota Seed
	Cang Zhu	Atroctlyodes Rhizome
	Ce Bai Ye	Biota Leaf
	Du Huo	Angelica pubescentis Root
	Hou Po	Magnolia Bark
	Hu Po	Amber
	Jiang Xiang	Rosewood
	Mo Yao	Myrhh
	Ru Xiang	Frankincense

Essential Oils by Chinese Medicine Category

Releasing the Exterior - Wind-Cold or Wind-Heat: Wind-Cold:

- An Shu Ye - Eucalyptus
- Bai Zhi - Angelica dahurica
- Gui Zhi/Gui Ye - Cinnamon Twig and Leaf
- Jing Jie - Schizonepeta
- Xi Xin - Wild Ginger, Asarum
- Zi Su Ye - Perilla Leaf

Wind-Heat:

- Bo He - Peppermint
- Chai Hu - Bupleurum
- Jin Yin Hua - Honeysuckle
- Jing Jie - Schizonepeta
- Ju Hua, Bai Ju Hua - Chrysanthemum
- Lian Qiao - Forsythia Fruit
- Man Jing Zi - Vitex
- Zi Su Ye - Perilla Leaf

Clearing Heat - Purging Fire; Damp Heat; Deficiency Heat; Cooling Blood; Eliminating Toxins.

- Lian Qiao - Forsythia Fruit
- Ye Ju Hua - Wild Chrysanthemum
- Zhi Zi - Gardenia Fruit

Clearing Heat and Eliminating Toxins:

- Jin Yin Hua - Honeysuckle Flower
- Ju Hua, Bai Ju Hua - Chrysanthemum
- Lian Qiao - Forsythia Fruit
- Long Nao - Borneol
- Qing Hao - Sweet Wormwood
- Ye Ju Hua - Wild Chrysanthemum
- Yin Chen Hao - Artemisia scoparia
- Zhi Zi - Gardenia Fruit

Clearing Damp-Heat:

- Nan Mu - Southern Chinese Cedarwood
- Yin Chen Hao - Artemisia scoparia
- Zhi Zi - Gardenia Fruit

Clearing Deficiency Heat:

- Ju Hua/Bai Ju Hua - Chrysanthemum
- Mo Li Hua - Jasmine
- Qing Hao - Artemisia annua
- Zhi Zi Hua - Gardenia Flower

Draining Dampness and Regulating Water

- Cang Zhu - Atractylodes
- Nan Mu - Southern Chinese Cedarwood
- Yi Yi Ren - Coix Seed
- Ze Xie - Water Plantain, Alisma

Dispelling Wind-Damp Bi Obstruction (Relieving Pain, Opening Channels and Collaterals, Strengthening Tendons and Bones)

- Bi Cheng Qie - Litsea
- Cang Zhu - Atractylodes
- Du Huo - Angelica pubescentis
- Gan Jiang - Dry Ginger
- Jing Jie - Schizonepeta
- Man Jing Zi - Vitex
- Rou Dou Kou - Nutmeg
- Rou Gui - Cinnamon Bark
- Song Zhen - Pine Needle
- Yi Yi Ren - Coix Seed
- Yun Shan - Black Spruce Needle

Transforming Phlegm, Stopping Cough and Wheezing

- An Shu Ye - Eucalyptus
- Bai Dou Kou - Round Cardamom
- Bai Yu Lan Ye - Magnolia Leaf
- Ce Bai Ye - Biota Leaf
- Chen Pi - Aged Tangerine Peel
- Fo Shou - Buddha's Hand Fruit
- Gan Jiang - Dry Ginger
- Nan Mu - Southern Chinese Cedarwood
- Qing Hao - Artemisia annua
- Song Zhen - Pine Needle
- Xiao Hui Xiang - Fennel Seed
- Xing Ren - Bitter Almond Kernel
- Yun Shan - Black Spruce Needle
- Zi Su Ye - Perilla Leaf
- Zi Su Zi - Perilla Seed

Aromatic Transforming Dampness

- Bai Dou Kou - Round Cardamom
- Bai Yu Lan Ye - Magnolia Leaf
- Cang Zhu - Atractylodes
- Hou Po - Magnolia Bark
- Huo Xiang - Patchouli

Relieving Food Stagnation, Promoting Digestion and Absorption

- Bai Dou Kou - Round Cardamom
- Bi Cheng Qie - Litsea
- Cang Zhu - Atractylodes
- Chen Pi - Aged Tangerine Peel
- Ding Xiang - Clove
- Fo Shou - Buddha's Hand Fruit
- Gan Jiang - Dry Ginger
- Hou Po - Magnolia Bark
- Huo Xiang - Pachouli
- Jin Yin Hua - Honeysuckle
- Mu Xiang - Saussurea
- Qing Pi - Green Mandarin Tangerine Peel
- Rou Dou Kou - Nutmeg
- Wu Zhu Yu - Evodia
- Xiao Hui Xiang - Fennel
- Zi Su Ye - Perilla Leaf

Regulating Qi

- Chai Hu - Bupleurum
- Chen Pi - Aged Tangerine Peel
- Fo Shou - Buddha's Hand Fruit
- Mo Yao - Myrrh
- Mu Xiang - Saussurea
- Qing Pi - Green Mandarin Tangerine Peel
- Ru Xiang - Frankincense
- Tan Xiang - Sandalwood
- Xiang Fu - Cyperus, Nutgrass
- Xun Yi Cao - Lavender
- Zhi Ke - Bitter Orange Fruit

Regulating Blood, Stopping Bleeding

- Ai Ye - Mugwort, Artemisia argyi
- Ce Bai Ye - Biota Leaf
- Jiang Xiang - Dalbergia

Invigorating Blood, Removing Blood Stasis, Wound Healing

- Chuan Xiong - Ligusticum wallichii
- Ce Bai Ye - Biota Leaf
- Dang Gui - Angelica sinensis
- Du Huo - Angelica pubescentis
- E Zhu - Curcuma zedoaria
- Hu Po - Amber
- Huo Xiang -Patchouli
- Jiang Xiang - Dalbergia
- Mo Yao - Myrrh
- Qi Li Xiang - Orange Jessamine Flower
- Rou Gui - Cinnamon Bark
- Ru Xiang - Frankincense
- Su He Xiang - Styrax

Warming Interior and Expelling Cold

- Bi Cheng Qie - Litsea
- Ding Xiang - Clove
- Gan Jiang - Dry Ginger
- Qing Hua Jiao - Green Sichuan Pepper
- Rou Gui - Cinnamon Bark
- Wu Zhu Yu - Evodia Fruit
- Xi Xin - Wild Ginger, Asarum
- Xiao Hui Xiang - Fennel

Tonifying - Blood, Qi; Yin, Yang / Tonifying, Nourishing Blood:

- Bai Zi Ren - Biota Seed
- Ce Bai Ye - Biota Leaf
- Dang Gui - Angelica sinensis
- Gou Qi Zi - Goji Berry
- Huo Luo Bo Zi - Carrot Seed
- Mei Gui Hua - Rose
- Ren Shen - Ginseng
- Xiang Fu - Cyperus, Nutgrass

Tonifying Qi:

- Huang Qi - Astragalus
- Qi Li Xiang - Orange Jessamine Flower
- Ren Shen - Ginseng
- Ru Xiang - Frankincense

Tonifying, Nourishing Yin:

- Gou Qi Zi - Goji Berry
- Jin Yin Hua - Honeysuckle
- Ju Hua/ Bai Ju Hua - Chrysanthemum
- Mei Gui Hua - Rose
- Mo Li Hua - Jasmine
- Wu Wei Zi - Schisandra Fruit

Tonifying Yang:

- Ai Ye - Mugwort, Artemisia argyi
- Bi Cheng Qie - Litsea
- Ding Xiang - Clove
- Gan Jiang - Dry Ginger
- Hu Lu Ba - Fenugreek
- Rou Gui - Cinnamon Bark
- She Chuang Zi - Cnidium Fruit Seed
- Xiao Hui Xiang - Fennel Seed
- Yun Shan - Black Spruce Needle

Stabilizing and Binding, Astringent

- Qing Pi - Green Tangerine Peel
- Rou Dou Kou - Nutmeg
- Wu Wei Zi - Schisandra Fruit

Calming the Spirit, Nourishing the Heart, Sedating

- Bai Yu Lan Ye - Magnolia Leaf
- Bai Zi Ren - Biota Seed
- Chai Hu - Bupleurum
- Hu Po - Amber
- Huo Luo Bo Zi - Carrot Seed
- Jiang Xiang - Dalbergia
- Jin Yin Hua - Honeysuckle
- Mei Gui Hua - Rose
- Mo Li Hua - Jasmine
- Qi Li Xiang - Orange Jessamine Flower
- Ren Shen - Ginseng
- Song Zhen - Pine Needle
- Tan Xiang - Sandalwood
- Xiang Fu - Cyperus, Nutgrass
- Xun Yi Cao - Lavender
- Yun Shan - Black Spruce Needle
- Zhi Zi Hua - Gardenia Flower

Aromatic Opening Orifices

- Bai Yu Lan Ye - Magnolia Leaf
- Hu Po - Amber
- Long Nao - Borneol
- Shi Chang Pu - Acorus
- Su He Xiang - Styrax
- Tan Xiang - Sandalwood
- Xi Xin - Wild Ginger, Asarum
- Zhang Nao - Camphor

Extinguishing Wind and Stopping Tremors

- Hu Po - Amber
- Long Nao - Borneol

Expelling Parasites

- Bi Cheng Qie - Litsea
- Ding Xiang - Clove
- Hou Po - Magnolia Bark
- Qing Hao - Artemisia annua
- Qing Hua Jiao - Green Sichuan Pepper
- Rou Dou Kou - Nutmeg
- She Chuang Zi - Cnidium Fruit Seed
- Su He Xiang - Styrax
- Wu Zhu Yu - Evodia
- Xiao Hui Xiang - Fennel Seed
- Zhang Nao - Camphor

Index

D

M

N

O

P

U

V

W

Y

Z

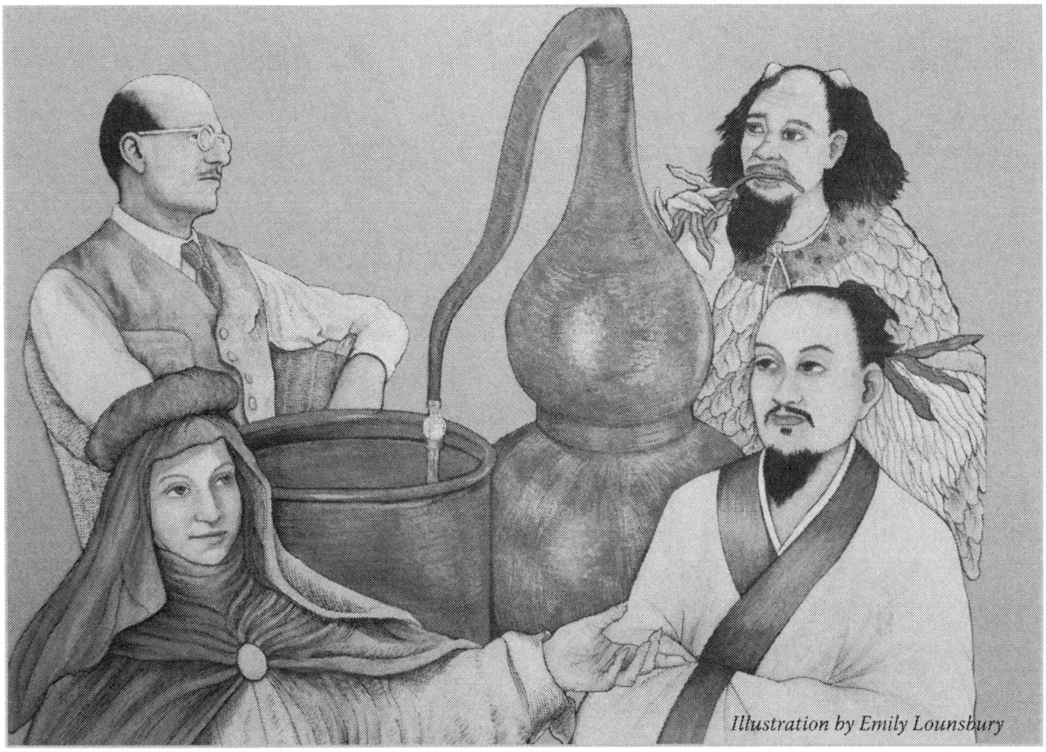

A magical meeting of brilliant minds across time and cultures where a prophetess, a scientist, a God, and an immortal discuss the distillation of essential oils and the merging of alchemy, plant medicine and aromatherapy.

Miriam the Jewess

Also known as Miriam or Maria the Alchemist, and Mary the Prophetess, is believed to be the first alchemist of the Judeo-Christian tradition in history. She is known from the fourth century works of the Gnostic Christian writer Zosimos of Panopolis. According to Zosimos's writings, she lived between the first and third centuries CE in Alexandria, Egypt where she founded a school of alchemy. Mary invented processes and apparatuses that continued to be used for centuries. She made various designs of stills and condensers for working with hot metals and vapours. One device associated with her was a sort of double boiler which she used for boiling mercury or sulphur, then using the condensing vapours to heat copper or lead in a pan above, using high temperature.

Her story became something of a legend in later Arabic and Christian writings. Her work came out of a revelatory recognition of the divine potential in all things. She spoke of mineral substances, the forces of nature and the planets as sacred, living things and referred to alchemy as a blessed art involving the secrets of The Philosophers and of God.

Several cryptic alchemical precepts have been attributed to Mary. She is said to have spoken of the union of opposites: "Join the male and the female, and you will find what is sought." The following was known as the Axiom of Maria: "One becomes two, two becomes three, and out of the third comes the one as the fourth."

Ancient written records of her esoteric teachings and alchemical processes are full of mysterious metaphor. Quotations credited to her are found in hermetic writings such as *The Dialogue of Mary and Aros on the Magistery of Hermes* by an anonymous Christian philosopher. Operations are described in this document which would later become the basis of alchemy, such as leukosis (whitening) and xanthosis (yellowing). The document describes, for the first time, an acid salt and other acids. There are also several recipes for making gold from plants (mandragora, for example). Here is an excerpt, translated in the style of old English:

> *"...there are the two fumes comprehending the two Lights, and project upon that the complement of the Tinctures of the Spirits, and the weights of Truth, and pound it all, and put it to the Fire, and you shall see wonderful things from them. The whole government consists in the temper of the Fire, O how strange it is, how it will be moved from one colour to another, in less than an hour of the day, until it arrive at the mark of redness and whiteness, and cast away the Fire and permit it to cool, and open it and you will find the clear pearly Body to be of the colour of the Poppy of the Wood mixt with whiteness and that is it which is incerating, liquefying and penetrating, and one golden piece thereof, the weight of a small golden coin, falleth upon a thousand thousand and two hundred thousand. That is the hidden secret."*

RENE-MAURICE GATTEFOSSÉ

Rene-Maurice Gattefossé is considered to be the father of aromatherapy, was a little known French chemist and scholar born in Montchat near Lyon, France in 1881. In July 1910 he discovered the healing properties of lavender oil after severely burning his hands in a laboratory explosion. This led him into a lifetime of research into essential oils. Gattefossé is credited with being the person who coined the word aromatherapy in the 1920s using it for the title of his book, *Aromathérapie: Les Huiles Essentielles, Hormones Végétales*, the first modern work on aromatherapy. An English version, Gattefossé's Aromatherapy was published in 1993.

Gattefossé believed that the power of essential oils not only restored the body but could also have a beneficial healing effect on the mind. What he discovered was that essential oils applied to the skin can be absorbed into the blood stream, where they may interact with the body's own chemistry. Ahead of his time, he held the view that the essential oils were more efficient and safer to use when 'complete', rather than when extracted and used as isolated chemicals.

SHEN NONG

Venerated as the father of Chinese herbal medicine along with Fuxi and Huang Di, the Yellow Emperor, Shen Nong is one of the three legendary Emperor Gods at the roots of the development of Chinese medicine. It is thought that he lived from 2737 BCE to 2697 BCE, nearly 5,000 years ago. The name, Shen Nong means "Divine Farmer." He was so named because he taught society to sow the five grains by inventing the cart and plow, taming the ox, yoking the horse, teaching people how to choose arable land, and clear the land by fire. He is therefore credited with establishing a stable agricultural society in China.

Shen Nong investigated herbs by ingesting them himself to learn how they affect the body, mind and spirit. These sometimes included toxic substances. He also discovered antidotes using herbs such as licorice and ginger. So deep was his union with nature that he is most often depicted with small horns growing out of his head and clothing made of leaves. Shen Nong's *Ben Cao Jing* (神農本草經), *The Divine Farmer's Materia Medica* is the oldest known book on agriculture, and medicine utilizing plants, as well as mineral and animal substances. Originally passed along by oral tradition, it was later compiled and organized by the Daoist physician, Tao Hong Jing (452-536 CE) into the version that is still read today. This classic Chinese materia medica records 365 medicinal substances. It was the first to describe them by their five flavors, natures (temperature), functions, and indications. It introduced the method of classifying Chinese medicines by grades: superior grade herbs corresponding to heaven which govern the maintenance of life, middle grade herbs corresponding to humankind which benefit human nature and include medicinal functions, and inferior grade herbs corresponding to earth which cure diseases.

Ge Hong

Ge Hong is a Daoist Immortal. He was an alchemist and priest of the Ling Bao tradition who lived from 283 to 343 BCE during the early Jin Dynasty period. During the later part of his life he retreated from society to Mount Luo Fu in southern China where he devoted his life to study and practice. Ge Hong developed systems of internal and external alchemy as pathways to longevity and transcendence. Two of his illuminating written works, *Bao Pu Zi (The Sage Who Embraces Simplicity)* and *Tai Qing Jing (Treatise on Great Clarity)* are classics of Daoist alchemy, spiritual cultivation and Confucian morality which have had a deep influence on the Daoist traditions that followed. He used external alchemical techniques to cultivate internal alchemical transformation and developed the nine stages of alchemy. He created a cauldron made of seven stones and learned to regulate time and temperature in order to transmute minerals for alchemical elixirs. He worked with substances such as cinnabar, sulfur, arsenic, orpiment, malachite, magnetite and hematite.

He envisioned the body as a sacred landscape, with its own internal cauldron in the lower burner, and taught internal alchemical techniques to cultivate the fire needed to enable the combustion and transmutation of Jing into Shen, in other words the return to spirit from matter. He taught about areas and points on the body which could be potentiated using meditation involving projection, visualization and Qi Gong. He also used herbs in his cultivational practices and wrote works on herbal medicine for the benefit of society including the Zhou Hou Bei Ji Fang (肘後備急方) containing prescriptions of readily available herbs to be used as home remedies for acute illnesses and emergencies .

Made in the USA
Monee, IL
12 November 2026

6b976331-5986-4c34-862e-a8fade6ee6b2R01